The Treatment of Psychiatric Disorders
REVISED FOR THE *DSM-III-R*

by

William H. Reid, M.D., M.P.H.

with contributions by
George U. Balis, M.D.
James S. Wicoff, M.D.
Jerry J. Tomasovic, M.D.

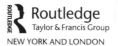

Routledge
Taylor & Francis Group
NEW YORK AND LONDON

First published 1989 by BRUNNER/MAZEL, INC.

Published 2014 by Routledge
711 Third Avenue, New York, NY 10017
27 Church Road, Hove, East Sussex BN3 2FA

First issued in paperback 2015

*Routledge is an imprint of the Taylor & Francis Group,
an informa business*

Copyright © 1989 by William H. Reid

All rights reserved. No part of this book
may be reproduced by any process whatsoever
without the written permission
of the copyright owner.

Newbridge Book Clubs

Library of Congress Cataloging-in-Publication Data

Reid, William H., 1945–
  The treatment of psychiatric disorders : revised for the DSM-III-R
  William H. Reid ; with contributions by George U. Balis, James S.
Wicoff, Jerry J. Tomasovic.
    p. cm.
  Rev. ed. of: Treatment of the DSM-III psychiatric disorders.
c1983.
  Includes bibliographies and indexes.
  ISBN 0-87630-536-2
  1. Mental illness—Treatment. 2. Diagnostic and statistical
manual of mental disorders. I. Reid, William H., 1945– Treatment
of the DSM-III psychiatric disorders. II. Title.
  [DNLM: 1. Mental Disorders—therapy. WM 400 R359t]
RC480.R4 1988
616.89'1—dc19
DNLM/DLC
for Library of Congress   88-19468
                                                                CIP

ISBN 13: 978-1-138-86908-0 (pbk)
ISBN 13: 978-0-87630-536-2 (hbk)

To Merrill T. Eaton, M.D.
to Elise
and to the memory
of Ann Alhadeff

Contents

Acknowledgments — viii
Contributors — ix
Introduction to the Revised Edition — xi
Prologue — xiii

SECTION I: DISORDERS USUALLY FIRST EVIDENT IN INFANCY, CHILDHOOD, OR ADOLESCENCE
by James S. Wicoff — 3

1. Developmental Disorders (Axis II) — 7
2. Disruptive Behavior Disorders — 16
3. Anxiety Disorders of Childhood or Adolescence — 25
4. Eating Disorders — 29
5. Gender Identity Disorders — 33
6. Tic Disorders — 36
7. Elimination Disorders — 38
8. Speech Disorders Not Elsewhere Classified — 41
9. Other Disorders of Infancy, Childhood, or Adolescence — 42
   References for Section I — 45

SECTION II: ORGANIC MENTAL DISORDERS
by George U. Balis — 49

10. Delirium and Dementia — 59

11. Syndromes Similar to Functional Disorders	88
12. Withdrawal and Intoxication	112

SECTION III: PSYCHOACTIVE SUBSTANCE USE DISORDERS
by George U. Balis — 131

13. Psychoactive Substance Use Disorders	133
References for Sections II and III	147

SECTION IV: OTHER ADULT DISORDERS
by William H. Reid — 161

14. Schizophrenia	163
15. Delusional (Paranoid) Disorder	197
16. Psychotic Disorders Not Elsewhere Classified	200
17. Mood Disorders	204
18. Anxiety Disorders (Anxiety and Phobic Neuroses)	245
19. Somatoform Disorders	259
20. Dissociative Disorders (Hysterical Neuroses, Dissociative Type)	266
21. Sexual Disorders	273
22. Sleep Disorders *(by Jerry J. Tomasovic)*	296
23. Factitious Disorders	311
24. Impulse Control Disorders Not Elsewhere Classified	314
25. Adjustment Disorders	321
26. Psychological Factors Affecting Physical Condition	328
27. Personality Disorders	332
28. V Codes for Conditions Not Attributable to a Mental Disorder That Are a Focus of Attention or Treatment	352
References for Section IV	357

Appendix A: Drug-Drug Interactions	383
Appendix B: Generic and Trade Names of Medications	389
Name Index	393
Subject Index	404

List of Tables

Table 1: Causes of Organic Mental Disorders   54
Table 2: Drugs Capable of Causing Delirium   61
Table 3: Equivalent Doses of Neuroleptics   166
Table 4: Sleep Hygiene   297
Table 5: Benzodiazepines Frequently Used in the Treatment of Insomnia   299

Acknowledgments

R. James Willis ably organized our clinical office to accommodate this project, juggling schedules and tasks as needed. Vicki Spencer typed and retyped most of the manuscript, and was available with her word processor seven days a week. Medical student David Genecov assisted in library research. Several colleagues read and corrected early drafts.

All of these are acknowledged with thanks, but none more than my wife, Elise, who tolerated my multiple personalities of physician, medical director, writer, editor and husband—each with attendant moods and foibles—up to 18 hours a day, week in and week out, for far too long.

Contributors

William H. Reid, M.D., M.P.H., Medical Director, Colonial Hills Hospital; Clinical Professor of Psychiatry, University of Texas Health Science Center, San Antonio, Texas.

George U. Balis, M.D., Professor of Psychiatry, University of Maryland School of Medicine, Baltimore, Maryland.

James S. Wicoff, M.D., Clinical Psychiatry Faculty, Department of Psychiatry, University of Texas Health Science Center; Child and Adolescent Unit Medical Chief, Colonial Hills Hospital, San Antonio, Texas.

Jerry J. Tomasovic, M.D., Clinical Associate Professor of Pediatrics, Child Neurology Section, University of Texas Health Science Center, San Antonio, Texas.

Introduction to the Revised Edition

When I was asked to prepare a revision of *Treatment of the DSM-III Psychiatric Disorders*, in which the therapeutic modalities would be updated and keyed to the *DSM-III-R*, I asked the same questions with which the earlier volume was begun: Is there a need for this book? What is the appropriate format?

The broad readership of the first book implies a clear need. A general acceptance of its format (with notable exceptions which have been addressed herein) seems to mean that we were on the right track.

The primary author and other contributors assume that the reader is familiar with psychiatric evaluation and with the diagnostic format of *DSM-III-R*. He or she should be pursuing treatment approaches with clear working diagnoses in mind before picking up this book. The text recommends, describes, and briefly expands upon treatment modalities; however, *we make no attempt to present a complete discussion of specific treatment modalities*. This book is a guide, not a reference text.

Several thousand references, most published after 1983, were consulted. Almost 1,000 are listed within these pages. It is strongly recommended that the clinician consult these and other standard sources for more detailed information.

Virtually all standard treatment modalities, and a number of esoteric ones, have been included. Some experimental or unproved therapies are mentioned; every effort has been made to identify them as such.

It is important for the reader to note that this volume takes the extremely simplistic stance that the disorder to be treated has been accurately diagnosed according to *DSM-III-R* criteria, and that the *DSM-III-R* criteria are clinically adequate. As every clinician knows, initial diagnostic impressions are not cast in stone. A patient's response to a particular treatment may confirm, refute, or add to one's diagnosis.

In addition, it is vital that the clinician (or other reader of this book) be aware that the *DSM-III-R* is not the last or only word in our understanding of mental disorders. Diagnosis and treatment are dynamic and multifaceted, and not nearly so concrete as a lay reader might assume.

There is no real substitute for psychiatric training and experience in the treatment of most psychiatric disorders. Accordingly, although this book may be useful for general physicians or certain nonmedical mental health clinicians, it is not intended to take the place of consultation from or referral to a psychiatrist, nor is it intended for use by superficially trained counselors. The treatment techniques are for the most part intended for clinical environments, and not lay counseling centers or self-help settings.

There is particular danger of misunderstanding diagnostic and treatment concepts in legal settings. It should be made clear from the outset that this book, like the *DSM-III-R*, should not be used in the legal arena without psychiatric consultation.

Finally, there are many ways to approach the writing of a book such as this. One is to have each section or subsection written by a different expert. Although this works well for large, comprehensive texts, the variability and loss of continuity that one finds in edited texts was considered unacceptable for our purposes. I hope that readers and reviewers will agree.

William H. Reid, M.D., M.P.H.
San Antonio, TX

Prologue: The Treatment of Psychiatric Disorders

Before we present the disorders and their treatments, it is appropriate that a number of concepts that override specific treatments, and that appear again and again in the care of psychiatric patients, be discussed.

Hospitalization
Whether or not to hospitalize the patient is often a critical treatment decision. The various purposes of hospitalization include protection or monitoring of the patient, protection of others in the environment, increasing the effectiveness or efficiency of treatment, and providing certain kinds of care not available outside the hospital. Modern medical practice has given rise to some other, less acceptable reasons for hospitalization as well: convenience for the physician, convenience for the family, and increased reimbursement from third-party payers.

This creates something of a paradox. We are taught in medical training, and the public is convinced through the news media, that unnecessary hospitalization produces a tremendous drain upon our financial resources. Health care costs, which appear to be borne by insurers, employers, and governments, are in the last analysis actually carried by the taxpayer and employee. Waste and increased costs of health care are universally decried.

On the other hand, the providing of health care and its accoutrements is big business. Those whose incomes depend upon hospitalized patients, prescribed medications, or expensive procedures encourage the doctor or other clinician to use them. Thus in the private sector, one sometimes finds incentives to hospitalize which are not related to the patient's clinical needs. In the public sector (and in that portion of the private sector that is driven by cost control mechanisms such as capitation), one finds discouragements for hospitalization, many of which are not related to clinical need either.

The decision to hospitalize should be made by the *physician*, and not by administrative, political, marketing, or profit motives. The questions to ask are fairly simple. Is hospitalization the best way to treat my patient? If cost is a factor, pro or con, can cost be appropriately weighed in the clinical balance (e.g., would money saved by treatment on an outpatient basis be justified by the treatment received?)? Am I being honest with the patient and the payer in my explanation of the clinical benefits of hospital care?

The type of hospital or clinical service one uses is perhaps just as important as the decision whether or not to hospitalize. The usefulness of certain kinds of inpatient milieux in various disorders is discussed at various points in this book.

One finds considerable pressure from payers to make hospitalization as brief as possible. Most psychiatric training stresses an acute-care setting followed by outpatient or partial hospital management. For many patients, this is best. It would be a serious mistake, however, to ignore the dangers of premature discharge and the benefits of lengthy hospitalization for some patients. It has long been known that a common source of relapse is incomplete inpatient treatment, coupled with slipshod transition to the outpatient environment.

Partial Hospitalization
Partial hospital settings are very effective for some patients. It is important that the clinician seek partial hospitalization as an active, dynamic treatment setting in which the patient is clearly moving from need for the institution toward ability to function independently. This requires specialized settings, staff, and therapeutic concepts.

Unfortunately, two problems are eroding public (and payer) confidence in the partial hospitalization concept, and threaten loss of funding for these programs. One is that the common partial hospital "program" is really a halfway house for chronically ill patients. Although such settings may provide sheltered living, they must be differentiated from programs whose goal is actual patient growth.

The second problem is the program that has been specifically created to increase funding to a hospital or clinical entity. It is a fact of life that as reimbursement for some forms of treatment, such as inpatient care, becomes scarce, programs such as partial hospitalization may be established more for financial than for therapeutic reasons.

Other Treatment Settings
There are a number of treatment settings that psychiatrists use every day, but may not recognize as such. The importance of paying attention to, and sometimes guiding, the home, school, or work environment has been particularly brought out in Dr. Wicoff's section. One should always remember that the patient spends far more time with his family, his work, or his schooling than he does with any therapist. Understanding their usefulness, and sometimes their pitfalls, is critical to optimal care.

Kinds of Treaters
As mentioned in the introduction, this book is written primarily for the psychiatrist or psychiatric subspecialist. Psychiatrists in training and general physicians or medical students learning about the specialty are included in this group.

Psychiatry realizes, perhaps more than any other specialty, the importance of integrating the biological, psychological, and social facets of the patient's disorder and his life. This leads to the many advantages of multidisciplinary treatment teams, and to the psychiatrist's acceptance of the fact that some aspects of care may best be carried out by nonphysicians. The clinical psychologist or social worker trained in psychotherapy, for example, can provide treatment for many kinds of patients. Some highly specialized nonphysicians offer modalities, such as biofeedback or covert sensitization, which are often not available in the psychiatrist's office.

All of the nonmedical professionals to whom this book refers should, like psychiatrists and other physicians, be aware of the limits of their expertise and ability to help particular patients. The availability of consultants in other fields, and the willingness to use them, is very important. One's familiarity with his or her consultants should include not only knowledge of their training and credentials, but also of clinical reputation, rapport with patients, and professional ethics.

Many other people, some professional and some not, come into the treatment environment. All deserve the clinician's cooperation, in the patient's interest and in the interest of simple courtesy. Issues of privacy and confidentiality should be considered in all communications with therapists, counselors, clergy, friends, and family.

Patients and Clients

The word "patient" is used throughout this book to describe those people who have come to us for help or who are being treated. The word "client" is popular in some psychotherapeutic and counseling environments. One advantage of "client" is that it connotes a partnership between the clinician and the person being treated, providing the latter with a certain respect and responsibility for his life and care. On the other hand, it is this author's belief that the "doctor-patient" relationship has many advantages in most therapeutic and treatment settings. One's status as "patient" should not be used to infantilize or demean him or her; however, the expectations (some of which are legal ones) of "doctor" and "patient" have great value to patient care.

Diagnostic Accuracy in Treatment

Diagnosis is a cornerstone of effective treatment. The practice of psychiatry and psychotherapy is not an informal, "let's-try-this-and-see-if-it-works" endeavor. Our treatment modalities are not so broadly successful that they can be applied to anyone who happens to have particular symptoms.

The other side of the same coin is the recent effort to reduce diagnostic methods to such pseudoscientific levels that diagnoses can be made, literally, by computer. While there can be no doubt that the *reliability* of diagnosis can be improved with the use of highly standardized checklists and the like, the result is only a statistical one, and often lacks *validity*. One can program the computer to add two and two and come up with five time after time. Nevertheless, the result will not be valid.

Diagnosis must blend the best scientific methods with clinical experience, to lead to treatment decisions most likely to help the patient. If one's diagnosis is wrong, then the treatment is likely to be ineffective, partially effective at best, or even harmful. It is not so simple as merely trying a treatment to see if it works, then abandoning it after a few hours or days. Many of the treatments used in psychiatry—biological as well as psychotherapeutic ones—are complex, easy to apply incorrectly, and/or take considerable time to evaluate.

Psychiatric disorders rarely exist in a vacuum. This is true in other medical specialties as well; the pediatrician knows that while treating strep throat, he or she must consider the possibilities of kidney damage, rheumatic heart disease, and medication side effects and interactions. Psychiatric disorders seem often to be even more confusing, and present more often in combination, than many other illnesses.

It is thus extremely important that the reader not become enamored with the apparently "cookbook" style with which this book follows the DSM-III-R diagnoses. There are warnings and suggestions throughout the book regarding this; however, it bears mention here as well. The patient's overt symptoms and signs are often part of an Axis I disorder. All of this is laid over the patient's personality, which may or may not imply an Axis II diagnosis. Axis III diagnoses may be critical to one's understanding of the patient. Finally, the Axis IV and Axis V considerations of the *Diagnostic and Statistical Manual of Mental Disorders* should always be considered as one attempts to plan the best overall treatment for the individual patient.

Continua in Diagnosis and Treatment

The concept of related symptoms and disorders, and that of symptoms being laid over personality styles, organic illness, sociocultural issues, and so forth, sometimes make one think of some disorders as on a "continuum" of diagnoses. For example, at one time it was thought that neurotic illnesses, personality disorders, and psychotic illnesses merely represented differences in degree of the same basic emotional problems.

With some notable exceptions, the concept of diagnostic continua has more problems than advantages for the person who is learning about psychiatric diagnosis and treatment. It is better to understand separately, for example, the characteristics and treatment of schizophrenic patients, schizoid patients, "borderline" patients with brief psychotic episodes, and severely anxious patients whose symptoms reach psychotic proportions. When exceptions to this general rule exist, they will be mentioned in the text.

Pessimism vs. Realism in Treatment

Although, taken as a group, psychiatric disorders have about the same rate of cure or amelioration of discomfort as those found in other medical specialties, they are often viewed more pessimistically. The vast majority of patients with psychiatric disorders *are* treatable, given appropriate diagnosis and resources for treatment. It is important to recall that the relief of pain, mental or physical, with or without a "cure," is often the physician's highest calling.

Treating the "Myth of Mental Illness"

Psychiatry is perhaps the only clinical field in which aberrant behavior or emotions alone can warrant a "diagnosis" and "treatment." Although this author acknowledges the importance of sociocultural factors in determining whether a particular feeling or behavior (or even an hallucination) is or is not normal, mental illness is not a "myth." The longer a clinician works with patients; sees the interaction of biological, psychological and social factors in their pain; and sees the patterns of disturbance which appear over and over; the more he or she becomes convinced that mental disorders deserve consideration beyond labels of maladaptation or "problems in living."

On the other hand, the clinician who has the social (and perhaps legal) authority to diagnose and treat such disorders must take this responsibility very seriously. The international literature is rife with situations in which social or political behavior is confused with illness. The issue of using psychiatry to control behavior is one that deserves more space than is available in this book; however, one should be particularly careful when treating children, adolescents, the elderly, and people whose behavior is deemed "antisocial."

The Treatment of Psychiatric Disorders

REVISED FOR THE *DSM-III-R*

Section I:
Disorders Usually First Evident in Infancy, Childhood, or Adolescence

by

James S. Wicoff, M.D.

Several factors must be taken into account that are somewhat limited in treating children and adolescents and may call for a different perspective from that used in treating adults. First of all, the rapidly changing physical and psychological makeup of the child often influences the choice of treatment for a particular psychopathology. Second, while chemical research has progressed a great deal in general psychiatry and application to adults, research about and application to children still lag quite far behind. This is due, in part, to regulations governing experimentation with medications in children, as well as to the above-mentioned rapidly changing nature of the child's physiology. Psychotropic intervention, therefore, is not as well documented in either clinical trials or long-term follow-up studies. The third factor that is unique to treating children and adolescents is the routine inclusion of family members in the treatment process. Family therapy and/or education is generally crucial to any therapeutic approach used with children and adolescents.

DRUG TREATMENT IN CHILDREN

Although the body of knowledge regarding psychotropic medications has expanded tremendously over the last 30 years, the use of these medications in children has not been nearly as well studied. Many factors contribute to this, including the rarity in children of some disorders such as manic-depressive illness and schizophrenia and parents' resistance to the use of psychotropic medicines. Studies of the medication effects on control groups are difficult to find.

Nevertheless, there is growing use of the full range of psychotropic medications in child and adolescent psychiatry. Clinicians prescribing for this age group should be well aware of the developmental variations, both physical and psychological, seen in children and adolescents and the effects these have on the presentation of their disorders. There should also be careful consideration of the family's influence on the placebo effects of the medication. Children are strongly influenced by the introduction of the medication and family support for their taking it.

Education of both the child and the family about the medication and what it can and cannot accomplish is crucial to obtaining optimal effects of the drug. Questions about short- and long-term side effects and possible predisposition to substance abuse in adolescents should be answered straightforwardly and the drug should not be started until the family is in support of its use. During the first few weeks of treatment the family should be encouraged to call whenever they have questions. The physician should be readily available and able to answer questions regarding side effects, interactions with other medications, and other concerns of either parent or child.

Whenever possible, a single daily dose should be given to avoid having the child leave class to take medication. Initiation of medications is generally best done at doses below therapeutic amounts, to avoid initial side effects and related rejection of the drug. The dose should be increased systematically once or twice a week until positive therapeutic effects are noted, or unacceptable side effects are experienced.

Assessment of efficacy must often be done through communication with the school. This is the one place where the child experiences a consistent and repetitive level of task orientation, peer interaction, and academic stress. Teachers, however, may have previously fixed opinions about the use of medications in children. One should use structured rating methods such as questionnaires which allow for objective monitoring of the child's progress.

The preschool child who is taking medication often develops behavioral toxicity. This usually takes the form of either increased or decreased activity, loss of appetite, or general irritability. Symptoms such as these should lead the clinician to reduce the dosage or eliminate the medicine for several days, then try restarting at a lower dose.

Long-term side effects are often asked about by parents who have seen reports in popular magazines or on television. Although systematic studies of most drugs are at best inconsistent, we can say that side effects such as extrapyramidal signs and tardive-dyskinesia-like syndromes are not seen as often in adolescents as they are in adults, and that the frequency generally decreases with the age of the child. This is also true for impaired liver functioning, jaundice, and bone marrow damage. Stunting of growth by stimulants is also brought up quite often. Follow-up studies to the original paper that postulated growth retardation have indicated that stimulants may reduce weight gain, but that height is not affected (Gross, 1976; McNutt et al., 1976; Quinn & Rapoport, 1975). Side effects with methylphenidate generally do not occur if the dose remains around 0.3 mg/kg/day. When the dose is increased to 1.0 mg/kg/day, over 50% of children have some side effect (worsening of behavior, weight loss, or general irritability).

One should consider discontinuing stimulants for one to two weeks in the fall after the first six weeks of school and in the spring a few weeks before or after spring break. This allows determination of continuing necessity of the drug. The teacher should be informed of the trial period in order to be more observant and tolerant of the child's behavior during this time. Should the behavior be intolerable after only a few days, medication can easily be restarted.

Two medications that are used quite often by pediatricians and should be considered in behavior control are chloral hydrate and diphenhydramine. Chloral hydrate can be prescribed in doses of 25–50 mg/kg/day, divided into two or three doses for sedative and/or hypnotic effects, in emergency situations or treatment of insomnia. Diphenhydramine is usually given in much smaller doses for an antihistaminic, but can be used in dosages from 3–26 mg/kg/day for behavioral control. This is particularly effective in children with hyperactivity who are not responsive to other medication approaches.

Lithium carbonate is being used more and more in childhood disorders that are either diagnosed as bipolar illness or resemble it in terms of severe mood swings. Lithium has not been found to be effective in the Attention Deficit-Hyperactive Disorder child. Prescribing lithium for children should be limited to psychiatrists with experience with both children and the medication, and good laboratory evaluation should be available. Hospitalization for establishment of dose ranges is often needed.

Therapies using megavitamins, "natural" diets, sugar restrictions, or hypoallergenic diets have been suggested for several disorders. To this point, none has proved consistently effective.

Medication usage in children and adolescents is often warranted for the more severe behavioral disorders and, in particular, for hyperactivity. Medicine by itself, however, is never the sole treatment for these children and should be prescribed in conjunction with individual, family, group, or educational therapies.

ADULT DISORDERS IN CHILDREN

Several adult diagnoses found in *DSM-III-R* (American Psychiatric Association, 1987) will occasionally be applied to the child or adolescent. Schizophrenia is rarely found in early childhood, but when it does occur it is severely disruptive to the entire family. Treatment often involves hospitalization, the use of neuroleptics, and long-term therapy. Family therapy is essential to evaluate the psychopathology of the environment, to determine changes that may be necessary in the child's placement, or to ameliorate aberrant communication or disturbance in the parents.

The same can be said of bipolar illness in children. This diagnosis should be considered more often when there is a clear family history of bipolar illness. Lithium carbonate can be valuable in the treatment of these children.

Major Affective Disorder, Dysthymic Disorder, and the Personality Disorders are also diagnosable in children and adolescents, but are rare compared to most others that we diagnose.

Chapter 1

Developmental Disorders (Axis II)

The use of the term "Developmental Disorders" may be misleading to the parent or lay individual. The concept of a developmental disorder may indicate to them that their child will "grow out" of the problem. While this may be true at times, these disorders are generally chronic in nature and persist in some form into adult life. The use of ongoing evaluative procedures and new diagnostic workups every 18 months to 3 years is helpful not only in evaluating one's therapeutic interventions, but also in being able to answer family members' questions with regard to possible prognosis.

1A: MENTAL RETARDATION

There are no changes in the diagnosis of Mental Retardation from what is described in *DSM-III*. *DSM-III-R* indicates that the essential features of this disorder are:

> (1) Significantly subaverage general intellectual functioning accompanied by (2) significant deficits or impairment in adaptive functioning, with (3) onset before the age of 18. The diagnosis is made regardless of whether or not there is a co-existing physical or other mental disorder. (p. 28)

There have been numerous studies demonstrating the high frequency of psychiatric disorders in the mentally retarded. Emphasis has been placed on the much-increased prevalence (47% by some studies) of these disorders in the severely retarded. Childhood psychosis, severe Stereotypy/Habit Disorder, Pica, Behavioral Disorders, and isolated habits all appear to be more common than in normal intelligence children. The psychiatrist, therefore, must be prepared to deal therapeutically with a wide range of emotional and behavioral disturbances, and yet a diminished ability of the individual to deal verbally or behaviorally with stress. Assessment and treatment, however, should start with the same techniques one uses with the normal intellect child and then be modified according to the patient's particular limitations. The following guidelines help define treatment choices:

317.00 Mild Mental Retardation

This category of individuals comprises approximately 85% (American Psychiatric Association, 1987, p. 32) and, therefore, the largest group of mentally retarded individuals. Advances in the understanding and treatment of mental retardation have led to much higher goals for this group which used to be termed "educable." Parents can now be told that these children, with good intervention and programming, can generally live successfully in the community as adults either "independently or in supervised apartments or group homes" (American Psychiatric Association, 1987, p. 32). The key to achieving this goal for the mildly retarded is a team approach with careful testing to properly place the child in a situation that he or she can handle. Early diagnosis helps this a great deal, and careful explanation to the parents of their child's academic and social limitations and potentials will help the parents not only adjust their expectations, but also be realistic advocates for their child in school and social environments. Avoiding excessive exposure to failure through unrealistic parental or environmental expectations can help the individual child or adolescent immensely (Carr, 1980).

When psychiatric disturbances do occur in the mildly retarded, they are generally handled with more emphasis on family therapy and behavior modification, but individual psychotherapy and use of medication are also quite important. Individual therapy is often in the form of play therapy, to circumvent the need for frequent verbal responses by the individual and also as a more developmentally appropriate technique. Any drug therapy should be monitored closely, because of the patient's difficulty at times verbalizing side effects and the tendency of those around the child toward complacency in letting the drug become the sole therapeutic agent. Here again, family education is very important, as the parents will often be the ones to note side effects in their children that others in the environment may not perceive.

Behavioral modification is a cornerstone for the treatment of many psychiatric disturbances in the mildly retarded, such as Conduct Disorders and Stereotypy/Habit Disorders (Yule & Carr, 1980). Parents who are willing and able to learn the tenets of behavioral modification often become quite creative behavioral therapists and are able to handle many of the day-to-day problems that arise with their children without the need for professional help.

318.00 Moderate Mental Retardation

This group of individuals (formerly referred to as "trainable") is more severely limited verbally. Thus, treatment interventions shift toward the increased use of behavioral interventions and environmental support systems. Psychopathology is often more prominent and requires institutionalization more often than in the mildly retarded.

Supportive therapy with parents in dealing with their despair and sense of helplessness is very important. Community agencies can often be beneficial in alleviating the financial and emotional stresses that these families undergo. Respite programs in local hospitals or mutual support groups among parents often give families a needed rest from taking care of their handicapped child. This in turn allows them to give energies to their marriages and/or their nonhandicapped children, helping avoid the buildup of anger and resentment that often occurs when a severely handicapped child is in the home.

318.10 Severe Mental Retardation

This group of individuals, a small minority of the people with Mental Retardation, need a much more extensive network of support in the community and at home. They will need constant supervision even as adults, but can often adapt well to life in the community. Almost half of these individuals will at some time develop a psychiatric disorder and be in need of a mental health specialist. Drug therapy and behavior modification are the most frequently used interventions with these disorders, whether it be childhood psychosis or Attention-Deficit Hyperactivity Disorder. The drugs used are no different than those used to treat the same psychiatric disturbances in the regular population. Proper dosages, however, seem to be quite difficult to maintain. The mentally retarded child often has an initial reduction of symptoms, but then seems to need larger doses of medicine than his or her average-intellect counterpart (Lipton et al., 1977). There appears to be a very narrow range of efficacy for the major tranquilizers. Thioridazine and haloperidol have become the two most commonly used medications. Thioridazine has been particularly helpful in reducing stereotypy and tics. Haloperidol has been useful in treating psychosis, both because of its potency and its ease of administration in colorless drops, or intramuscularly. Minor tranquilizers and antidepressants are generally not indicated in retarded children. Exceptions to this statement would be clearcut evidence of affective illness or use of imipramine for nocturnal enuresis. Stimulant medications are not as effective for the most part in controlling hyperactivity as one sees in their use in normal children. There is also an increased risk of stereotyped behavior when stimulants are used in the severely retarded patient.

In all cases, a behavior modification program is essential as an adjunct to any drug therapy. The use of operant conditioning techniques can often reduce the need for medications. These techniques involve careful analysis of the retarded child's behavior, in both its antecedents and its consequences. The child's particular intellectual level will dictate whether more sophisticated systems such as the use of tokens can be employed. Individual therapy can be used at a very basic play therapy level. Family education becomes crucial in teaching the families to adapt to particular limitations of the individual and also to continue a home treatment program after any kind of institutionalization.

318.20 Profound Mental Retardation
These individuals comprise approximately 1%-2% of those with Mental Retardation and are generally institutionalized. They need a great deal of structure in their environment and if they develop psychiatric disorders, they often need institutionalization in a facility trained to deal with the "dually diagnosed" mentally retarded. Therapeutic interventions center around medications to control violent physical outbursts or self-destructive habits. Behavior modification, here again, is a cornerstone of working with these individuals and someone with higher level training in this area is generally needed to set up a program to deal with the sometimes complex behavioral problems. These may range anywhere from encopresis and enuresis to psychotic outbursts.

319.00 Unspecified Mental Retardation
This category is used for infants and those who are untestable but presumed to be mentally retarded. The above mentioned tenets of therapeutic intervention still apply in this category. Diagnostic evaluations (neurological, genetic, biochemical) will often dictate the direction in which therapeutic intervention proceeds.

Drug Therapy in Mental Retardation

The use of medications in the mentally retarded is often more complex than when treating a child or adolescent of normal intellectual abilities. The lack of verbal feedback regarding the child's experience of side effects or understanding of the purpose of the medication often handicaps the physician in evaluating his or her treatment. In addition, it has been demonstrated that the mentally retarded often have unusual responses to medications, or very small therapeutic windows. Complicating matters even further is the increased incidence of neurological problems, such as epilepsy. Anticonvulsant therapy needs to be monitored quite closely with blood levels for possible toxicity and/or side effects, as well as interactions with psychotropics such as phenothiazines which can change the seizure threshold. The high doses of neuroleptics often needed for reduction of self-destructive behavior in the mentally retarded make these individuals at increased risk for long-term side effects, such as tardive dyskinesia, blood dyscrasias, and liver disorders. Regular blood counts and chemical profiles followed by complete physical checkups by a physician are all very important in the treatment. The prescribing physician should also be quite cautious about lapsing into the complacency of "medication only" intervention. This can lead to higher and higher doses of neuroleptics when behavioral interventions or decreased dosage could possibly reduce or eliminate the need for medications.

Perhaps the most disturbing psychiatric syndrome that develops in the retarded is severe self-destructive behavior such as head-banging, biting of oneself, or other self-mutilation. Newer medication approaches to these symptoms are currently revolving around the use of lithium, propanolol, or carbamazepine. All of these medications are used in dosages that can either be increased to the maximum recommended blood levels, as in the case of Tegretol and lithium, or until side effects or improvement is seen in the case of propanolol. Psychotic symptoms in the individual should point toward a first-line use of major tranquilizers. Thioridazine and haloperidol are chosen medications by many physicians dealing with the retarded, but this is often because of their availability in a palatable liquid form. Other major tranquilizers can be equally effective.

1B: PERVASIVE DEVELOPMENTAL DISORDERS

This diagnostic category in *DSM-III-R* is being used to pull together a number of different early childhood disorders characterized by "qualitative impairment in the development of reciprocal social interaction, in the development of verbal and nonverbal communication skills, and in imaginative activity" (p. 33). Old diagnostic terms such as atypical development, symbiotic psychosis, childhood psychosis, childhood schizophrenia, and autism will all now be subsumed under Pervasive Developmental Disorders. Careful attention should be paid to the introductory pages in the *DSM-III-R* which help one to understand the thinking behind this diagnostic category and the complications involved in differential diagnosis and prediction of future adaptation and general prognosis.

299.00 Autistic Disorder

Please note the revised criteria for diagnosis of this disorder. The old diagnosis of Childhood Onset Pervasive Developmental Disorder is now included under autism and the age of onset criterion has been dropped because of the inability of researchers to validate this as a predictable criterion.

Treatment of autistic disorders over the past 30 years has varied greatly as a result of conflicting theories regarding etiology, diagnosis, and prognosis. Experimentation with physiological interventions such as LSD, ECT, and numerous other medications reflects the confusion that has existed. Currently, the use of fenfluramine (a drug that reduces serotonin levels) is being considered. Thus far, the results seem to be short-term and difficult to replicate, but have been occasionally encouraging. The overall treatment of autism is summarized quite well by Rutter and Hersov in *Child and Adolescent Psychiatry* (1985).

Treatment is centered around the long-term benefits of an intensive, behaviorally oriented treatment program. Emphasis is placed on the use of techniques appropriate to the level and pattern of the children's cognitive handicaps. A child's IQ level is deemed important in terms of possible goals. An IQ below 50 generally indicates an inability, no matter what the program, to attain any kind of useful skill in reading, writing, and arithmetic. Following are the goals, strategies, and principles of treatment summarized by Rutter (1985):

The Fostering of Normal Development. This involves attending to the cognition, language, and socialization areas of development and finding ways to reduce or circumvent the effects of autism in these areas. Language development and socialization skills are concentrated on through behavioral techniques and teaching parents alternative methods of being directly and, sometimes intrusively, involved in their child's development in these areas.

The Promotion of Autistic Children Learning More Generally. Teaching the autistic child involves breaking down learning tasks into very small steps with high rates of success. Autistic children tend to retreat into stereotypys when they face failure.

The Reduction of Rigidity in Stereotypy. This problem is best approached with a very stimulated environment that goes about accomplishing changes through very small steps, each of which by itself does not upset the child as it does not indicate any noticeable change in their environment. Stereotypies can be reduced and/or modified to more acceptable expressions through this technique.

The Elimination of Nonspecific Maladaptive Behaviors. These involve behaviors such as tantrums, aggression, bedwetting, and encopresis. The behavioral approaches used for these problems are also used in the case of autism with some minor modifications.

The Alleviation of Family Distress. This may be the most important component of the treatment in that family understanding of the child's problems and needs helps create a more supportive environment both from the parents and from siblings. Several sessions should be spent with the family going over diagnostic studies and talking about the future.

Drug intervention with the autistic child should be for the specific type of problem manifested. This is difficult, however, when one speaks of symptoms such as attention deficit and stereotypy/habits that require knowledge of not only the autistic symptomatology, but also comparative developmental levels. There is some indication that attention deficit in the autistic child, for instance, does not respond to normal levels of stimulant medication. One must weigh, therefore, the benefits and risks of high doses of medications like methylphenidate when trying to help the autistic child to have a longer attention span in an academic or home setting. In general, stimulants are contraindicated as a treatment of hyperactivity because they tend to increase stereotypy/habit disorders.

Self-mutilation is the symptom that causes the most concern in the autistic child's environment. Use of protective devices (helmets, gloves, etc.), drug intervention, and behavioral modification can generally reduce or eliminate the self-mutilating behavior. Phenothiazines are considered safer than the butyrophenones, although the latter can be more powerful.

299.80 Pervasive Developmental Disorder Not Otherwise Specified

This category of individuals is considered a diagnostic dilemma, but is used for children who have enough qualitative impairments in development that they deserve a Pervasive Developmental Disorder diagnosis. The long-term outcome for these children is much more variable; continual evaluation and the therapeutic interventions outlined above are essential to allowing the highest level of potential for the individual.

1C: SPECIFIC DEVELOPMENTAL DISORDERS

These disorders are much more specific for a certain type of developmental problem such as academic, language, speech, or motor skills than the foregoing.

ACADEMIC SKILLS DISORDERS

315.10 Developmental Arithmetic Disorder
315.80 Developmental Expressive Writing Disorder
315.00 Developmental Reading Disorder

LANGUAGE AND SPEECH DISORDERS

315.39 Developmental Articulation Disorder
315.31 Developmental Expressive Language Disorder
315.31 Developmental Receptive Language Disorder

MOTOR SKILLS DISORDER

315.40 Developmental Coordination Disorder
315.90 Specific Developmental Disorder Not Otherwise Specified (NOS)

Therapeutic intervention for these disorders is generally not handled by the mental health professional. Education specialists or perhaps neurologists are the first people to see these children. The psychiatrist or mental health professional is often brought in when associated psychiatric disturbances are suspected. Psychiatric presentation most commonly takes the form of Conduct Disorders. The child with a

Developmental Disorders (Axis II) 15

specific developmental disorder often develops low self-esteem and becomes a problem at home and at school if not worked with properly to help him overcome his handicap. Often these disorders are not diagnosed until the child has developed behavioral problems that bring him to the attention of a psychologist or a psychiatrist, and special education testing is ordered. This becomes a therapeutic intervention in itself.

Parents who understand their child's limitations are able, with help, to set up a positive academic and social environment for their child. Emphasizing the child's strengths and helping him or her deal with weaknesses leads to a healthier relationship between the child and his or her environment. Medication is occasionally helpful. There is some indication that stimulants can increase learning, but certainly not unless indicated by other symptomatology, such as a short attention span. The primary intervention should always emphasize special education and behavioral modification. When concurrent psychiatric disturbances exist, medication for symptomatology other than the specific developmental disorder often leads to improvement in learning simply because the behavioral disturbance has been helped.

Chapter 2

Disruptive Behavior Disorders

314.01 Attention-Deficit Hyperactivity Disorder (ADHD)
This disorder has received a great deal of publicity in the media. For this reason, it is even more important than usual for the psychiatrist to review the past history for medications and different diagnoses. Terms such as "minimal brain damage" and "minimal brain dysfunction" were quite confusing to parents in the past and still linger in certain literature. The use of stimulants has been quite controversial at times, and has led to sensationalistic reports on television and in the press. The clinician will be asked about the long- and short-term side effects of the medication and should be ready to answer many questions.

First, one must understand that this disorder is not a simple physiological problem and it must be viewed as a multiply handicapping disorder for the child. The symptoms of short attention span and hyperactivity make for very difficult adjustment in school, at home, with peers, and in practically any social situation. The damaging effects, therefore, lead to a tremendous disruption of family life and lowering of self-esteem, and concomitant behavioral problems may develop. Treatment will center around the following major areas:

1. Family therapy
2. Proper educational setting
3. Behavior modification
4. Medication
5. Individual therapy

Family Therapy. The focus of family therapy in the family with an Attention-Deficit Hyperactive Disorder child is both educational and supportive. The educational component is extremely important because parents quite often describe feelings of failure and defeat, and even difficulty feeling warmth and love for their child. In addition, there is often anger at those around them who have made simplistic suggestions, such as that they should simply discipline their child. Helping these parents to understand the physiological nature of the disorder and that treatment can be beneficial is the first step in combating the negative environment that has been created.

The therapist should be aware of the higher incidence of disorders such as alcoholism, antisocial behavior, and hyperactivity in primary relatives. Families are often sensitized because of the existence of hyperactivity in a relative who has "turned out bad." Sometimes there will be resistance to treatment because the father or mother was hyperactive as a child and "made it through okay without any drugs or seeing any shrinks." Sensitive areas such as these, and perhaps resistance to medication for other reasons (TV, magazine articles, etc.), should be explored by the therapist in a nonconfronting, supportive manner. Once the resistance is worked through, one is likely to be able to help both the family and the child, having taken the time to understand how this disorder has affected them. One can then begin to teach the parents how to be advocates for their child and help him or her secure the other treatment interventions that are necessary.

Proper Educational Setting. This is extremely important to the hyperactive child because his or her sense of self-esteem is most often based on being able to compete—socially and academically—in the classroom. Good educational testing is helpful in delineating subtle learning disorders that may be present in addition to the attention deficit and hyperactivity and in planning special education if necessary. Small special education classrooms with teachers who are trained in working with hyperactive children are ideal. These should not, however, be exclusively recommended, as the hyperactive child can often be mainstreamed with other children if he or she is well controlled on medication.

The teacher must understand the critical need for positive reinforcers for these children. The regular classroom or special education teacher needs to be informed regarding the child's short attention span and the need for immediate and specific reinforcers or consequences.

Good communication between teacher and parents is extremely helpful. This is best done through a combination of daily reports to the parents and conferences between teacher and parents every three to six weeks. One relatively simple technique is to take a 3 x 5 index card and put down four or five daily goals (such as turning in homework, getting along with peers, and listening in class) on one side of the card and comments from the teacher on the other side. This can then be sent home each day with the teacher's initials and a rating from excellent to poor in each of the categories.

This kind of daily communication between teacher and parents is especially helpful for corroboration of symptoms, mutual support, and clarification of the child's severe disorganization. Parents and teacher must both adjust their expectations and find a level of "stress" that pushes the child to accept responsibilities, but does not demand more than he or she is truly capable of doing. This is difficult to do and often involves trial and error, but good communication between the two settings helps a great deal. The teacher is often a good, reliable source of feedback regarding the effectiveness of medication. Questionnaires for behavioral rating, such as the Conners Questionnaire, can be quite helpful and are more objective than simply asking the teacher to write out observations and comments. Special education teachers will note that many hyperactive children do quite well with one-on-one intervention. This seems to be because of the immediate focusing and increased individual stimulation. The parents can help with some one-on-one contact at home—for example, in helping organize the child's homework and prepare for the next day.

Parents usually should not be "teachers" at home, however, but rather be organizers and provide the structure that helps the child attend to homework and other tasks. The parents all too often become so involved in *making* the child learn that a battleground is created, with nothing but tears and anger as the result. Sometimes individual tutoring in certain subjects is helpful and removes the intense feelings that can develop between parent and child.

Behavior Modification. Most studies indicate that behavior modification is a key to working with Attention-Deficit Hyperactive Disorder children in any setting. However, one should remember the basic tenets of positiveness and specific, consistent consequences and rewards. The younger the child, the less he or she will understand long-term goals and/or consequences. The four- or five-year-old, for instance, can only benefit from a time-out or other behavioral consequence if it is extremely short and given immediately after the undesired behavior. These children do not respond to warnings because their impulsiveness leads them to act first and think later. A good behavioral approach can lead to longer delays in impulse discharge and help the child deal with day-to-day expectations, both in the classroom and at home. Concrete reminders such as "star charts," "stickers," and other colorful and/or graphic representations of success are quite helpful to the child with a short attention span.

The older child or adolescent with Attention-Deficit Hyperactivity Disorder often tolerates more delay of reward or consequence but, here again, generally not as delayed as his peers. The adolescent becomes a special problem if his hyperactivity continues. These teenagers are very difficult to manage and often develop severe Conduct Disorders. They may well need intensive psychotherapeutic intervention, and perhaps institutionalization for brief periods. The tenets of behavior modification still apply, however, and should be kept in mind in the setting in which the adolescent is placed.

Medication. The use of drug therapy has long been advocated in these children and dates back to 1924, when brain-damaged children were noted to have increased activity levels. Currently, stimulants appear to be effective in approximately 80% of well-diagnosed children. The other 20% may respond to either antidepressants or neuroleptics, depending upon concomitant psychiatric problems. Perhaps the most difficult child to treat is one who is extremely anxious and/or depressed and hyperactive. This child may need higher doses of a stimulant, and sometimes needs not only stimulant medication but also a neuroleptic.

Methylphenidate is still the best stimulant to use in the treatment of hyperactivity. Dosages are generally about 0.3 mg/kg and range from 10–60 mg per day, depending upon the severity of the hyperactivity syndrome. At doses below 10 mg, methylphenidate must be given in split doses approximately four hours apart. This can be given through the day with no major side effects. Some children will have problems with lowered appetite and/or insomnia, but these are usually temporary and disappear within approximately four weeks. If they do not, then the medication should probably be discontinued. Moodiness, tearfulness, and explosive outbursts may also result and generally suggest discontinuation of the medication. Sometimes more talking than usual is noted, but this is often due simply to a better ability to communicate.

One criticism of methylphenidate has been the lack of a sustained-release form. A 20 mg sustained-release tablet that is given once in the morning and lasts from seven to 15 hours, depending upon the metabolism of the child, is now available.

Pemoline is also a long-acting stimulant, but has not been as effective as methylphenidate. It is given in chewable tablets from 18.75 mg–150 mg. The literature suggests that pemoline should be given for two to four weeks before determining whether or not it is effective. Some clinical experience indicates that it is generally effective within one to two weeks or not at all.

Dexedrine has been given to hyperactive children for a number of years, but is much less favored now because of side effects and potential for abuse. It comes in spansule form and can be given in 5 mg or 10 mg dosages.

The use of antidepressants has been advocated more and more for the hyperactive child who either does not respond to stimulants or whose symptoms include significant anxiety. Imipramine is most commonly recommended in doses from 10–150 mg per day, depending upon the age and size of the child. Doses should generally not exceed 5 mg/kg. The use of adult blood levels makes treatment more reliable.

The side effects are similar to those seen in adults, with drowsiness, dry mouth, and dizziness being the most common in children. Sometimes parents will report a distressing "zombie" effect, usually a result of a high sensitivity to the medication and/or excessive dosage. Desipramine often has fewer side effects and may be more acceptable, particularly to adolescents.

Major tranquilizers such as thioridazine or haloperidol are sometimes used with the extremely anxious, hyperactive child. These can be used concomitantly with methylphenidate or by themselves. The psychotic child or adolescent who is also documented to be an Attention-Deficit Hyperactive Disorder child often is given both the stimulant and the major tranquilizer in an attempt to deal with the multiple symptomatology.

Lithium carbonate, the "Feingold" diet, carbamazepine, reduced sugar in the diet, and multivitamins have all proved unreliable in the treatment of hyperactivity (Evans, et al., 1987; Greenhill et al., 1973; National Institutes of Health, 1982; Weiss et al., 1971).

The use of medications and, in particular, stimulants in children has led to a great deal of controversy in recent years. Parents often ask about reports of stunted growth and possible predisposition to increased drug abuse. One can generally reassure them that routine prescriptions are relatively safe with regard to growth pattern, with reported problems only occurring after prolonged period of high dosage.

Even then there appears to be minimal danger of long-term adverse effect.

There is little indication of significant increase in drug use or abuse among children who have been on stimulants (Beck et al., 1975). Increased alcohol consumption, however, has been reported in some of these children when they become adolescents.

"Drug holidays" should be used when the child is mildly to moderately hyperactive. This is done either by giving weekends, holidays, or summertime reductions or eliminations of the medication. Parents should be encouraged, however, to give the medicine as prescribed whenever they feel the child would benefit greatly from being more behaved and able to attend to task. The social consequences of taking the medicine as needed outweigh any currently known benefits from drug holidays.

Another question that often arises is whether or not the child will see the medication as making him behave, rather than taking responsibility for his own behavior. Both the parents and the child should look at the medication as something that gives a child the *choice* of behaving but cannot, in and of itself, make him behave. Children exhibit various forms of resistance to taking the medication; education is important to understanding and compliance. Helping them understand the physiological nature of their difficulties with attention span and hyperactivity can help them accept a need for medical intervention.

One should be quite sensitive to the child's needs for privacy. When resistance begins to occur, one should consider the possibility that the child is being teased by siblings or peers at school. This is an area in which the family can help, often through education of the siblings. Comments from siblings or others such as, "You need to take your hyper pill," should be dealt with very firmly by the parents.

Individual Therapy. Individual therapy in Attention-Deficit Hyperactivity Disorder is generally recommended on the basis of individual need rather than the *DSM-III-R* symptoms. However, helping a child with supportive and sometimes insight-oriented therapy with regard not only to the disorder, but also to the depression he or she is experiencing and the coping mechanisms he or she develops, can lead to a better long-term outcome.

Outcome. The outcome for individuals with Attention-Deficit Hyperactivity Disorder is generally poor for those children who do not spontaneously remit by puberty. There is a high incidence of later antisocial behavior and academic failure. Adults with this disorder often have difficulty relating to society and maintaining relationships. Intervention helps reduce problems, but the prognosis is still guarded. Approximately half of the children will have a spontaneous remission of their symptoms at puberty and seem to have no further problems. Three factors—low IQ, aggressive symptomatology, and low socioeconomic status—seem to predispose children to worse outcomes.

CONDUCT DISORDERS

312.20 Group Type
312.00 Solitary Aggressive Type
312.90 Undifferentiated Type

Treatment of Conduct Disorders over the years has been both confusing and disheartening to the mental health professional. Long-term outcome studies have indicated that delinquent youths not only did not benefit from many of the interventions attempted, but many also appeared to be worse than those delinquents who were left alone (McCord, 1978). These studies led to a reevaluation of treatment approaches and further research into the presumed outcome of severe Conduct Disorders.

Approximately 75% of delinquents do not adopt an antisocial behavioral pattern in adulthood (McCord, 1978). This large group should generally be dealt with through improved education, probation programs, and social and vocational skills programs. Institutionalization does not seem to benefit either this group or the 25% that continue to be antisocial later in life. The evidence suggests institutional care only for those youths who are repeatedly violent in their crimes or who are obviously unable to stay within the law or in community-based programs (Palmer, 1974).

Delinquency research has pointed to the need for a very thorough physical, psychological, and neurological workup. It is important to understand any biochemical problems that may be associated with a child's or an adolescent's behavior. The use of stimulants in those with Attention–Deficit Hyperactivity Disorder often results in much improved behavior in group, institutional, school, or home settings. A higher proportion of Conduct Disorder children and adolescents than normals have abnormal EEGs. Possible episodic dyscontrol syndromes may benefit from medications such as carbamazepine.

Major depression also appears to be increased in Conduct Disorders. This leads to a much higher suicide risk when combined with the impulsiveness of the Conduct Disorder. When the combination is diagnosed, the patient should generally be hospitalized and may respond to treatment with tricyclic antidepressants. Evidence is beginning to mount for a different biological substrate for these young men and women, as contrasted with adults. Studies concentrate on the extremely low or zero level of dopamine beta hydroxylase and the need to raise the abnormally low anxiety level found in many delinquent adolescents (Rogeness et al., 1986). Imipramine is often the most effective medication, although desipramine is also used and has fewer side effects. Dosage can range up to 5 mg/kg in the child under 12, with adult doses appropriate for most pubescent or older adolescents.

Psychotherapeutic approaches are generally not effective for delinquents. Environmental interventions which improve family or home life, social skills, and/or educational achievement have a much higher impact. Work with schools and social systems that deal with the patient should emphasize the need for consistency, firmness, and realism in one's expectations of the child, taking into account their true abilities. The tough, angry, "I'll show you who's boss" parent, community worker, or teacher is not nearly as effective as the warm but consistently firm adult who helps the child set concrete, achievable goals.

One must bear in mind that concomitant psychiatric disorders such as Attention–Deficit Hyperactivity Disorder, psychoses, and learning disorders are common in these children. Combinations are more difficult to treat. Careful history-taking regarding the development of the Conduct Disorder can lead to a different therapeutic intervention than one might use for the single diagnosis.

Assessment of the family and social environment is also very important. Treatment of severe maternal depression or adult alcoholism, and separation from antisocial influences in the family, can be just as valuable as individual treatment of the child. The group type of Conduct Disorder, for instance, may involve children or adolescents who are quite capable of attachment and of responding to some form of individual therapy if removed from the delinquent group. However, putting them into an institution full of delinquent peers only serves to increase their recidivism.

313.81 Oppositional Defiant Disorder

This is a new term which expands on the old *DSM-III* Oppositional Disorder to include the term "defiant" and therefore define it as a more disruptive behavior. Here we find a child who is generally most troublesome within his or her own home or at school, but has not had the flagrant conflicts with the law or obvious disdain for the rights of others. Although it is felt that Conduct Disorder is a very common complication of Oppositional Defiant Disorder, there are no statistics thus far on outcome. These children are often moody, with low self-esteem and frequent temper outbursts. When one does a careful history, the description of a difficult temperament in infancy or childhood is commonly elicited.

Treatment for Oppositional Defiant Disorder must be differentiated from that of Conduct Disorder in a number of ways. Psychotherapy was not particularly effective with these children until the development of sophisticated family therapy. This, plus behavioral intervention in both school and home, helps a number of children to be in much better control. Use of token systems, reinforcement of acceptable behavior and consistent ignoring of aggressive or disruptive behavior, and development of a highly consistent and systematic approach to reward and discipline in all areas of the child's life can be dramatically effective. The skill of the therapist in relating to the child and the adults involved in administering the rewards and consequences is an important factor. The therapist must also be sensitive to signs of emotional disturbance which may require treatment in the adults. Maternal depression is particularly common. Brief individual or group therapy can be quite helpful. Although generally not capable of insight, these children do seem to respond to the warm, supportive adult who "believes in them."

There is an increased incidence of Attention–Deficit Hyperactivity Disorder in these children. Imipramine is recommended should signs of severe depression be present. Psychological testing should be done to screen for more serious emotional disorders and learning disorders.

Chapter 3

Anxiety Disorders of Childhood or Adolescence

309.21 Separation Anxiety Disorder
This is a relatively common disorder in children between the ages of five and 15. Many parents' own conflicts about separation interfere with mental health intervention for their children until symptoms reach a point of interference with either the child's school attendance or the parents' ability to go to work. "School phobia" has been used to describe a number of these children, although it should be seen as a subset of Separation Anxiety Disorder. These children often have the same level of anxiety during the summer vacation time.

Treatment is quite complicated and often involves coordination between the general practitioner or pediatrician, school personnel, and family members. The psychiatrist or mental health professional must be willing to spend time coordinating a behavioral desensitization program for return to school if that is a problem. Medication may also be an issue for the child, and possibly for one or more family members. (Imipramine is most often used, possibly for one or more family members.) There is often severe maternal depression; treatment of the mother may be the primary intervention. A careful history often reveals a panic disorder or past separation anxiety in the mother. The father can be crucial to the separation process. A father who is psychologically or physically absent contributes to the sense of abandonment or tension experienced by both the mother and the child. The therapist must be acutely aware of the family dynamics.

There is a fine line between empathic but firm insistence in implementing the desensitization program and harsh breaking of the dependency existing between child and adult. Often the mother, in particular, becomes a "doctor shopper" until she finds a general practitioner or therapist who will collude with her resistance to separation from her child.

A crisis may develop when the breadwinner in the family is unable to go to work or the child has missed so much school that academic failure is imminent. Hospitalization or day hospital treatment may need to be implemented at this time. Generally, the child responds well after the initial separation. The therapy then takes on a more psychodynamic approach in helping the mother with her depression and preparing the family system for the return of the child. This particularly involves reducing the "power" of the child's symptom and helping the adults in the family (and sometimes the siblings) to be more resistant to it. They must firmly support the child's ability to separate and be independent.

When working with school personnel, one should remember to consult not only to the teacher but also to the principal and to the counselor. These are the people who will control the administrative tolerance of the school system for special programs that might be needed.

Most behavioral programs emphasize getting the child through the school doors initially, and not demanding full classroom attendance the first day. Depending upon the child's particular resistance, the reinstigation of classroom attendance should proceed at 30 minutes to an hour per day, increased daily until full attendance has been achieved. The therapist may need to consult to the school in person in order to indicate support for the personnel implementing the program.

One should listen to the child's description of his or her school fears. Separation anxiety is a phobic reaction based upon a traumatic experience at school. Should this be the case, manipulation of the school environment is well worthwhile. School personnel can often be helpful in identifying areas of trauma.

Psychopharmacologic treatment generally revolves around the use of antidepressants. A number of these children have a good response to imipramine if they fall into the depressive or panic disorder subset of Separation Anxiety Disorder. Doses up to 5 mg/kg can be used. This, plus the placebo effect for both the child and the parent of having a medication for the disorder, often helps the child get through the initial barrier of resistance. Alprazolam has also been suggested, particularly in adolescents, but further research remains to be done.

Engaging the mother or other maternal figure is often a good initial therapeutic maneuver. Empathizing with her difficulty in putting her child through the pain of separation is essential for therapeutic alliance with the mother. This helps the child, while at the same time allowing the parent to experience her own pain of separation.

313.21 Avoidant Disorder of Childhood or Adolescence

The actual incidence of this disorder is unknown because milder forms are never treated; the child is simply considered overly shy and allowed to develop socially at a slower pace. Adults who describe having the disorder in their childhood often use the term "painful" and indicate that there was generally a desire to be more involved with those outside their family but a seeming inability to overcome the anxiety that this generated.

Therapeutic intervention should begin with a careful study of the case history to delineate any precipitating factors that may have led to a worsening of the disorder. Occasionally, this will be in the form of a death in the family, illness, physical harm having come to a loved one, or perhaps an attempt at social contact which resulted in severe embarrassment and teasing.

Family and/or individual therapy is often helpful. The ability of the therapist to bond with the child in a trusting, supportive way can lead to generalization of increased trust to teachers and other adults. Group psychotherapy is occasionally helpful, but one should be cautious not to have the patient be "group isolate," the only shy or retiring child in the group.

Medication is used only if a child has developed other symptoms which indicate panic, depression, or sleep difficulties. These should all be treated symptomatically. The use of benzodiazepines or imipramine in low doses is sometimes helpful.

313.00 Overanxious Disorder

Children with this disorder are constantly anxious to excess and worry about many aspects of their life. The disorder must be present for six months or longer and interfering with the daily relationships and performance of the individual.

These children often need multimodal treatment approaches. Medications, family therapy, individual therapy, and behavior modification have all been recommended. Individual therapy should usually be brief and focus on the origins of the anxiety. Family psychotherapy should involve evaluation for increased anxiety in the entire family and also for treatment needs in the parents. The child's basic temperament should be assessed to determine if he or she is "naturally" anxiety prone and will need a more understanding home and educational environment. Behavioral methods can be used to teach relaxation techniques, desensitization, and autosuggestion, and to help with anticipatory anxiety. Should the child's symptoms reach an extreme state, psychiatric hospitalization may be necessary. Low doses of phenothiazines, benzodiazepines, or imipramine can be helpful.

This disorder is often long-term and may require intermittent psychotherapeutic intervention for a number of years. Changes in one's environment (e.g., new school, move to a new neighborhood or city, divorce) or in one's body (e.g., puberty) may precipitate extreme levels of anxiety. These should be anticipated if possible, and perhaps treated preventatively.

Psychotherapy in the Anxiety States
Reisman (1973) published a very useful outline of principles that even today should underlie a psychotherapeutic approach to the three childhood anxiety states just discussed.

1. Therapy should be based on a careful assessment of the actual psychological mechanisms which underlie each child's problems rather than on the basis of theoretical considerations.
2. The psychotherapy situation should be structured to facilitate communication and the therapist should allow the child ample opportunity to express his feelings and beliefs.
3. The therapist should communicate his understanding of the child and his wish to be of help.
4. The therapist and the child should define the purpose or goal of their meeting.
5. The therapist must make clear what is ineffective or inappropriate in the child's behavior.
6. When dealing with behavior that is dependent on social interaction, the therapist may modify it by focusing directly on the interactions and where they take place (this may mean conjoint family interviews, group therapy, or contact with the school teachers, according to where the problem lies).
7. Treatment should end when the advantages of ending outweigh the advantages of continuing. (This may mean finishing before the child is fully better.) (cited in Rutter & Hersov, 1985, p. 371).

Chapter 4

Eating Disorders

307.10 Anorexia Nervosa

The treatment of Anorexia Nervosa is extremely complicated. It should be undertaken by a psychiatrist who is comfortable and experienced with the numerous and often dangerous physical sequelae that can develop. One must always keep in mind that this disorder has a high rate of mortality (studies indicate anywhere from 5%–18%) and cannot be taken lightly. This is particularly important when talking with the parents, who have often begun colluding with their child, denying the severity of her symptoms.

The first task of the therapist is, therefore, to inform the patient and her (or, in rare cases, his) parents that the disorder is a serious one. At the same time, one must develop a trusting relationship which will lead to cooperation with the entire family. There should never be a time when the clinician goes along with the patient's frequent rationalization that the problem is not really the anorexia, but something else which is disturbing her. It must be clear that the problem is "not eating."

The single-episode anorectic patient is generally the easiest to treat. She usually responds well to individual and family psychotherapy and returns to a normal weight relatively quickly (in a matter of months). This does not mean that her basic psychological health is restored, but simply that the symptom of anorexia has been taken care of and she is ready for further psychotherapy if she will accept it. Medications are sometimes helpful; imipramine is often used when there is a significant depressive component.

Recurrent or unremitting anorexia is more severe. The patient often needs hospitalization. Hospitalization that results from a trusting relationship with the psychiatrist, and from the belief that inpatient care is both necessary and in the best interests of the patient, is most likely to succeed.

Once hospitalization is accomplished, the psychiatrist must work closely with the nursing staff and consulting specialists such as an endocrinologist or internist. The most desirable hospital setting is a special unit on which the staff is experienced with the treatment of anorexia and a behavior modification program has been developed. The patient should be informed of the need for different medical tests, reduced exercise, and caloric intake which is often greater than that of an average adult (3,000–4,000 calories daily). Nutritional advice should be part of the program. Normal eating patterns should be established before discharge. The patient should be told that calories will be reduced once maintenance weight has been achieved; anorectics are often frightened by the amount of food being prescribed in order to gain weight.

Initially, the nursing staff takes full control of the patient's bodily functions, including trips to the bathroom, the appropriate amount of food to be eaten, and the time and duration of eating times. This maximum control is necessary because of the extreme manipulativeness that can occur in anorectic patients. The staff must be careful, however, to be supportive in implementing the program rather than emphasizing their control. Acceptable weight gain usually takes one to two months. During that time there should be a programmed, progressive attainment of patient independence. By the time of discharge, she should be able to choose her own menu, go on passes for meals, and maintain her weight without supervision for at least one week.

It is crucial to keep the family well informed during the entire hospitalization, and to monitor any disruptive family interactions that occur. Parental guilt, particularly in the mother, can lead to premature discharge if there is not a good therapeutic bond with the psychiatrist and the entire treatment team.

Family therapy has been quite promising in anorexia. The family and therapist may meet for the first few times over a dinner or lunch, which allows observation of eating patterns and dynamics. The therapist can observe other family issues as well, which may have caused family tension even before the anorexia developed.

Individual therapy alone has been largely unsuccessful when concentrating solely on the eating disorder. Issues of weight gain are too easily seen as a power struggle between patient and therapist. The therapist must be very skillful to avoid this and concentrate on psychological conflicts that are present in addition to those of the body image and refusal to eat. These often center around relationships within the family, sexual identity, concerns about the future, and concerns about leaving home.

Medication, if prescribed, is aimed at either anxiety reduction or treatment of depression, panic, or obsessive compulsive symptoms. Phenothiazines may be indicated for very severe anxiety, benzodiazepines for milder symptoms of anxiety, and antidepressants such as imipramine for depressive or obsessive compulsive symptoms.

Endocrine manipulation has not been very successful in altering anorectic symptoms (Brook, 1982). Often, however, there is great concern in the prepubescent or adolescent female regarding breast growth and menstruation. She needs to be reassured that both will occur eventually, but may be delayed by the illness. Adult women who request treatment may be given small doses of ethinyl estradiol, gradually increasing to 20 micrograms daily. Once this level is reached, cyclical withdrawal bleeding is induced and an oral contraceptive tablet is substituted (Brook, 1982; Russell, 1983).

307.51 Bulimia Nervosa

This disorder is unpredictable and very difficult to treat. It is more resistant to treatment than Anorexia Nervosa. Hospitalization is usually required to control the habitual overeating and purging. The nursing care plan is similar to that described for Anorexia Nervosa, and results in quick regulation of the disorder when the patient is confined to the ward and has no access to other food. Once regulation is clearly established, the patient is discharged for outpatient follow-up.

Cognitive therapy seems to be the most promising individual treatment at this point, although this disorder has a poor prognosis for actual cure (Fairburn, 1983). The patient should also be encouraged to maintain a healthy weight rather than the unreasonably low one which she usually sets as her goal. Treatment may take years. The mortality rate is unclear at this point. The therapist should be aware that suicide is the most likely cause of death in both Anorexia Nervosa and Bulimia Nervosa.

307.52 Pica

Most children affected by this disorder are seen by pediatricians rather than mental health professionals. The pediatric workup involves screening for lead poisoning or other physical effects caused by whatever the child has ingested. The psychiatrist is often brought in when there is a need for family therapy to increase the family's coping and child supervision skills. Very little work is done with the children themselves unless they are old enough for educational and psychotherapeutic intervention. If the family is capable, a behavioral modification program is often successful. Medication is not recommended.

307.53 Rumination Disorder of Infancy

This disorder is first seen by the pediatrician, who attempts to rule out physiological causes such as pyloric stenosis or infectious disease. Once the absence of these factors has been established, the psychiatrist may be asked to work with the child and/or nursing staff or family.

A careful history should be taken to understand the feeding patterns that have developed and the mother's feelings toward the child. Negative feelings have often developed because of the child's seeming rejection of the mother's offer of food. The vomitus, the smell, and the constant sense of failure the mother is experiencing are complicating factors. The therapist should work closely with the mother. She should be helped to understand the problem and to begin a behavioral program that includes nurturing activity. The child's intake should be scheduled in very small amounts every two to three hours while awake.

Response to treatment should begin in two or three days. If this does not happen, a specialist who deals often with this disorder should be called upon to develop a more sophisticated behavioral program. A more detailed description of behavioral approaches in severe cases is found in a classic paper by Lang and Melamed (1969).

307.50 Eating Disorder Not Otherwise Specified

These disorders are essentially variants of Anorexia Nervosa and Bulimia Nervosa, and the same general tenets should be used in approaching their treatment, although hospitalization may not be necessary. If hospitalization is used, the nursing care plan and therapeutic approach are similar to those just described.

Chapter 5

Gender Identity Disorders

302.60 Gender Identity Disorder of Childhood

This is a new diagnosis in *DSM-III-R;* there is very little written about it thus far. Treatment approaches generally involve family and individual therapy, but are not based solely on the goal of changing the child's sexual orientation. As indicated in *DSM-III-R,* a significant percentage of boys, but not so many girls, with this disorder develop a homosexual orientation during adolescence.

Work with the family may include answering questions concerning future sexual orientation and the family's ability to accept the child and work toward a healthy resolution of the disorder (rather than rejecting the child). Questions regarding proper role modeling and encouragement of normal gender activities should also be addressed in family therapy.

Green (1985) has done extensive work in evaluation and treatment of childhood sexual identity conflicts. His studies indicate that "feminine" boys are at a much higher risk for transsexual, transvestite, or homosexual outcomes as adults. He also indicates that the severe maladjustment of the adult transsexual mandates intervention with the young male with a gender identity disorder. The boy should be made aware of the gestures and feminine mannerisms that lead to his being called a "sissy." A more accepting male peer group should be sought, and the parents should be encouraged to find other boys who do not fit into the assertive, sports-oriented world. Green also suggests working to reduce the alienation between father and son, and helping both find activities that they can share.

Family reinforcement for the boy's femininity is an important topic of treatment. The parents sometimes encourage the child to show off while cross-dressing and even take pictures for the family album. These and other more subtle forces tend to encourage the boy in his feminine pursuits; the parents need to be sensitized to their reinforcing behavior. Cross-dressing should be stopped without question.

Even with the above-mentioned interventions, long-term outcome for these boys is unclear. Therapy does not appear to affect sexual orientation per se, but does seem to reduce the severity of conflicts within the family and the individual.

"Tomboy" girls have a much lower incidence of gender identity disorder, but whether this is due to society's acceptance of girls dressing more like boys or there is in fact a lower number of cases is unclear. When "tomboyism" persists into adolescence, there may be a higher incidence of lesbianism during adulthood. Little data are available on the treatment of this syndrome in girls, but one would expect that a similar approach to that used in boys could be valuable.

Psychological testing or monitoring for more severe developmental disturbances should be included in the treatment program.

302.50 Transsexualism

This disorder is included for the first time in disorders of childhood and adolescence because invariably the transsexual reports an early childhood gender disorder that may not have been publicly apparent until adolescence or later. When the diagnosis is made in adolescence, the psychiatrist should try to engage the patient in a long-term perspective of his or her disorder rather than in any way condoning the adolescent's urgent request for sexual surgery or body-altering hormones.

Psychotherapy should be geared toward helping the patient understand the conflicts that he or she is experiencing and, if the family has not been informed, to help the adolescent consider doing so. Although group therapy has been recommended for adults with this disorder, there is little published regarding adolescent group therapy (Keller, Althof, & Lothstein, 1982). This is primarily because of the adolescent's extreme reluctance to talk about the problem (which contributes to its uncommon diagnosis before adulthood). Helping the teenager establish a stable lifestyle and normal goals for success in relationships, school, and work increase the likelihood of successful adjustment to adult life.

Sex reassignment surgery should not be considered in the adolescent except in cases of ambiguous genitalia. Even in adults, this surgery should be considered a last resort and only done after all other avenues have been explored by specialists in the field (Lothstein, 1982).

302.85 Gender Identity Disorder of Adolescence or Adulthood, Nontranssexual Type

The treatment for this disorder is similar to that for the childhood type. The therapist is encouraged to be involved not only with the individual but also with the family. Cross-dressing, which often occurs, is extremely upsetting to the parents, who have a difficult time understanding that it is not for the purpose of sexual excitement. Subtyping the disorder as asexual, homosexual, or heterosexual is also important in dealing with the individual's adjustment to society and the parents' concerns about future outcome.

302.85 Gender Disorder Not Otherwise Specified

Very little data are available on the treatment of these disorders. Each has unique characteristics and should be approached according to its symptoms and underlying psychodynamics.

Chapter 6

Tic Disorders

307.23 Tourette's Disorder
The treatment of this highly disabling disorder has been primarily symptomatic rather than curative. The likelihood of a lifelong course is terribly depressing to both family and child; many of the same dynamics develop that one sees in other disabling chronic illnesses such as diabetes, juvenile arthritis, and serious injuries. Some hope, however, is held out for possible spontaneous remission.

The primary successful treatment for the symptoms of Tourette's disease is haloperidol in low doses (0.5–1.5 mg t.i.d.) to suppress the tics (Shapiro et al., 1978). Unfortunately, the side effects of haloperidol can be significant, including sedation, depression and, in particular, akathisia. It is often difficult to distinguish between akathisia and the uncomfortable restlessness patients sometimes describe when their tics are suppressed. If dystonic side effects or akathisia are present, treatment with an anti-Parkinsonian drug is indicated.

Other medications have been suggested when haloperidol is either not successful or the side effects are too great. One of these is the dopamine-blocking drug pimozide, given in very low doses of 1.0–4.0 mg per day. The noradrenergic agonist clonidine has also been recommended, in doses of 0.1–1.0 mg daily. Both of these are second-line medications and successful only in a small group of patients with Tourette's Disorder. Clonidine should be used with care, and it should be understood that tolerance and withdrawal symptoms may occur.

In addition to medication to suppress the tics, behavioral programming and supportive psychotherapy are recommended to deal with the impact the disease has on the school, social, and family life of the child (Turpin, 1983).

307.22 Chronic Motor or Vocal Tic Disorder
Treatment for this disorder is essentially the same as that for Tourette's, in that it is considered part of a continuum of all tic disorders that last over one year.

307.21 Transient Tic Disorder
Treatment for this disorder is generally aimed at the reduction of stress in the child's environment. This can be accomplished through psychotherapy or environmental manipulation and, occasionally, with medication. Haloperidol is not usually needed. Minor tranquilizers (anxiolytics) or relaxation techniques can be effective. The disorder should be monitored carefully for development of Tourette's Disorder or Chronic Motor or Vocal Tic Disorder.

307.20 Tic Disorder Not Otherwise Specified
There is no specific treatment recommended here other than those already discussed.

Chapter 7

Elimination Disorders

307.70 Functional Encopresis
The treatment of functional encopresis can be divided into basic behavioral programming for the primary type (a child who has not ever been fully toilet trained) and more complicated treatment for the secondary type (which often involves more severe emotional problems).

In **primary encopresis,** the pattern is usually seen in younger children from families with social or psychological problems. Simple procedures such as "star charts" and regular toilet use every two or three hours with no emphasis on defecation can often correct the problem. The use of a "star chart" is most often beneficial in children under the age of eight. The parent is instructed to buy several hundred stars of the child's color choice which have a gummed backing so the stars can be licked and put on a simple chart with the days of the week. Each day is divided into two parts and the stars are applied by the child at the end of each half day that he has been successful in proper toilet use and freedom from soiling. Prior to beginning this procedure, a two-week baseline is acquired to document the frequency of soiling. The goal for the child is then set at 50% improvement in the first week and increased by 10% or more each week thereafter. The parent is encouraged to give praise—not for production of stool in the toilet, but for freedom from soiling and for generally appropriate use of the bathroom. A concrete reward for a perfect week can be offered. This should be a toy or a trip to a restaurant chosen by the child. Use of the chart can be discontinued after three successive perfect weeks without soiling.

Secondary encopresis, which occurs in different forms, is much more difficult to treat. The soiling is usually a secondary overflow around partial blockage caused by fecal mass. Sometimes, however, there is active soiling with obvious angry intent; feces are found in clothes drawers, behind couches, or on parents' beds. This generally indicates a much more severe psychological problem and a full workup for other psychiatric disorders should ensue. In cases of soiling by secondary overflow, the first step is to clear the bowel with mild enemas. The child is then placed on a regular program of going to the bathroom, along with a stool softener and close work with the family to eliminate any negative interactions that occur around the soiling. Care should be taken to avoid punitive washing out of underwear or aversive techniques. These tend to increase the power struggle between parent and child and allow the parent to express his or her anger inappropriately.

One must inform the family that the soiling is a chronic problem and follow-up should continue for several years before the child is considered cured. Parents can be reassured that the vast majority of cases disappear by the age of 16. (This might seem quite late, but can be helpful to parents who have been frustrated with their child's soiling problem for four to five years already.)

No psychotropic medications are recommended unless additional disorders such as depression or Attention–Deficit Hyperactivity Disorder are concurrent with the encopresis.

307.60 Functional Enuresis

The first step in the treatment of enuresis is always to obtain a two-week baseline observation during which the parents and the child carefully record dry nights or days. These should be duly noted for the younger child with "smiley faces" or "stars" and, for the older child, with similarly reinforcing social or material rewards. The child with a very mild problem often responds to this simple intervention technique and no further treatment is required.

The most effective form of treatment for nocturnal enuresis appears to be the "bell and pad method." This involves an alarm system which is connected to a sensing pad that goes under the child's sheet in the approximate area of the genitals and is sensitive to the first drops of fluid that reach it. An alarm sounds which wakes the child. Careful instructions are given with the bell and pad on how to then get the child out of bed, wake him or her up, and help him or her empty the rest of his bladder into the toilet. Dry sheets are then put on the bed and the procedure is duplicated for the child that wets a second time early in the morning.

When used correctly, the bell and pad method can be extremely successful within three to six weeks. The clinician should do an initial follow-up a few days after starting the procedure in order to answer any questions. Parents should be told that some children do not wake up with the alarm; they may need louder alarms or the parents may have to wake up and then wake the child. Once the child is dry for two continuous weeks, he or she should be challenged for two more weeks with a two-pint fluid load each night before retiring. This apparently decreases the relapse rate from about 35% to 11%. Should the fluid overload result in a complete relapse, the procedure should be abandoned and other forms of treatment tried. One form of bell and pad is available through the Sears catalog. Techniques reviewed by Dische (1973) many years ago remain practical today.

Drug treatment for enuresis primarily centers around the tricyclic medications, particularly imipramine (Rapoport et al., 1980). This is indicated when the bell and pad are either not available or are not tolerated by the family or the child, or when more rapid response is required for environmental or social reasons. Dosages can start as low as 10 mg each night and then be raised to 3.5 mg/kg/night in the child under 12 years of age. Adolescents may be given a starting dose of 25 mg each evening and be raised to 100 mg per night.

Since the relapse rate with medications is relatively high, this should not be used as a long-term solution. Wetting is suppressed in about 85% of the children and completely eliminated in about 30%. No matter what schedule is used in stopping the drug, the relapse rate is almost 100% within three months of stopping treatment. The effect of long-term treatment has not been established. Medications should not be used in children under the age of four and dosages of 3.5 mg/kg/night are the highest recommended before EKG monitoring is needed.

Daytime wetting is more difficult to treat. Behavioral approaches are generally suggested. These include regular visits to the toilet, both at school and at home, and social reinforcement for dryness. Care should be taken to evaluate causes of anxiety in the child's environment. When found, either environmental manipulation or treatment of the child's overanxious responses should be instituted.

Chapter 8

Speech Disorders Not Elsewhere Classified

307.00 Cluttering
307.00 Stuttering
These two speech disorders are not considered emotional in their etiology. Mental health professionals generally become involved because of impairment of social functioning, anxiety and frustration associated with the disorder, and low self-esteem. Helping the child's family to deal with the disorder and to be supportive of their child is important. It is also important to rule out associated disorders, such as Attention–Deficit Hyperactivity Disorder or Dysthymic Disorder. Speech and language evaluations should be done, but as is pointed out in *DSM–III–R*, approximately 80% of people recover from stuttering, typically before the age of 16. This generally occurs no matter what the treatment, age of onset, or severity. Recovery is more common in females than in males.

Chapter 9

Other Disorders of Infancy, Childhood, or Adolescence

313.23 Elective Mutism
This extremely rare disorder is associated with a high degree of family psychopathology. Kolvin and Fundudis (1981) discuss this and other details of a large epidemiological study, which breaks down the neurological, sociological, psychiatric, and intellectual components of both family and individual child. Behavioral problems are quite frequent, and family therapy and behavior modification are often indicated. Straughan, Potter, and Hamilton (1965) and Reid and colleagues (1967) discuss behavior modification techniques for Elective Mutism. These involve very tangible rewards for the child's speaking in social situations. This approach meets with mixed results, depending upon the ability of the family to follow through with the program and the level of reinforcing psychopathology in the family environment. The psychiatrist or other clinician (or treatment team) should be prepared to deal with multiple systems, including school, family, individual, and community resources interacting with the family environment.

313.82 Identity Disorder
This disorder is included in the child and adolescent section because its age of onset is commonly in late adolescence. The severity of the symptoms being experienced by the adolescent should not be minimized by the therapist; careful evaluation is necessary to prevent misdiagnosis of patients as borderline personality or schizophrenic.

Intensive psychotherapy is often needed to help resolve the patient's tremendous ambivalence. Supportive use of anxiolytics and sometimes even major tranquilizers may be needed. Dosages for postpubescent adolescents are similar to those for adults. Adolescents may resort to extreme forms of behavior to deal with their anxiety and search for identity. The therapist is cautioned to watch for splitting by the patient to justify his or her actions. Should an endogenous depression be present, antidepressant treatment is generally routine.

The key to the treatment of Identity Disorder is the reduction of anxiety. The therapist's own sense of urgency must be considered, as these patients often idealize the therapist initially and expect that within a few sessions they will feel much better and everything will be resolved. The disorder generally lasts at least three months, and sometimes much longer. The therapist needs to keep this chronicity in mind during the treatment process.

313.89 Reactive Attachment Disorder of Infancy or Early Childhood

The definition of this syndrome in *DSM–III–R* directly indicates the etiology of grossly pathogenic care of the child or infant. Treatment is initially environmental and involves (1) stabilizing the home or hospital setting and (2) ensuring a primary caregiver who is responsible and who adequately perceives the child's physical and emotional needs. This may include a substitute caregiver or, more commonly, training of the regular caregiver who may simply be deficient in his or her abilities. Psychiatric evaluation of the parents should include intelligence testing, which helps determine the ability of the nurturing parent to understand his or her child's needs. Involvement of social agencies is often required; follow-up in the child's home by trained personnel can often prevent recurrence or related child abuse or neglect.

307.30 Stereotypy/Habit Disorder

This disorder is generally seen in more severely disturbed patients and has a much higher prevalence in institutionalized people with mental retardation. There is also a higher prevalence in autistic adolescents and adults. The severity of the disorder can be extreme and life-threatening. Self-injurious behavior demands immediate and powerful therapeutic intervention. This usually takes the form of major tranquilizers (neuroleptics); haloperidol is the most consistently successful. Dosage is titrated according to reduction of symptoms, and can reach 15–20 mg or more per day (Campbell, Cohen, & Small, 1982; LeVann,

1969). Most research indicates that the diminution of symptoms is due to the sedative properties of the tranquilizer rather than to any more specific biochemical action. Lithium carbonate and the narcotic antagonists naloxone or naltrexone have frequently been studied. Dramatic results have been reported with lithium levels of 0.6 mEq/L. The narcotic antagonists have been proposed because of the possibility that self-injurious behavior raises the patient's level of endogenous beta endorphins. These beta endorphins may naturally reinforce the behavior; if blocked, the patient might perceive more normal pain. Very little has been done in this area other than individual trials, and treatment with narcotic antagonists remains experimental.

Behavior modification is extremely important in Stereotypy/Habit Disorder. This is a very sophisticated problem, however, and should only be approached by psychologists or psychiatrists who have been well trained in operant techniques. Severely aversive conditioning is sometimes necessary for self-injurious behavior. The combination of behavior modification and medication may be the most successful approach.

314.00 Undifferentiated Attention-Deficit Disorder

This is a new category which is being used to classify disorders of attention which are not fully classifiable in Attention-Deficit Hyperactivity Disorder, Mental Retardation, or other disorders in *DSM-III-R*. There is no recommended treatment because of the lack of clarity regarding the validity of the diagnosis.

V CODES COMMONLY USED IN CHILDHOOD AND ADOLESCENT DISORDERS

The V Codes are used fairly often in the initial diagnosis of children and adolescents coming into the mental health professional's office. Family circumstances, school problems, and a more specific parent-child problem cannot always be attributed to an emotional disorder for the child; further investigation is often needed. A situation of child abuse, for instance, may involve more psychopathology in the adult than in the child. The child, however, would still benefit from treatment in most cases and, therefore, warrant a V Code diagnosis. Family and environmental therapies are most common in the treatment of children falling under V Code diagnoses.

References for Section I

American Psychiatric Association: *Diagnostic and Statistical Manual of Mental Disorders, Third Edition, Revised.* Washington, DC: American Psychiatric Association, 1987.
Brook, C. G. D.: Management of disorders of growth and sexual development. *Prescribers' Journal*, 22:143-150, 1982.
Campbell, M., Cohen, I. L., & Small, A. M.: Drugs in aggressive behavior. *Journal of the American Academy of Child Psychiatry*, 21:107-117, 1982.
Carr, J.: *Helping Your Handicapped Child.* Harmondsworth, England: Penguin, 1980.
Dische, S.: Treatment of enuresis with an enuresis alarm. In I. Kolvin, R. MacKeith, & S. R. Meadow (Eds.), *Bladder Control and Enuresis. Clinics in Developmental Medicine*, London: Heinemann/Spastics International Medical Publications, Nos. 48/49, 1973, pp. 211-230.
Evans, R. W., Clay, T. H., & Gualtieri, C. T.: Review Article. Carbamazepine in pediatric psychiatry. *Journal of the American Academy of Child and Adolescent Psychiatry*, 26(1):2-8, 1987.
Fairburn, C. G.: The place of a cognitive behavioural approach in the management of bulimia. In P. Darby, P. E. Garfinkel, D. M. Garner, & D. V. Coscina (Eds.), *Anorexia Nervosa: Recent Developments in Research*, New York: Alan R. Liss, 1983, pp. 393-402.
Green, R.: Atypical psychosexual development. In M. Rutter & L. Hersov (Eds.), *Child and Adolescent Psychiatry: Modern Approaches.* Boston: Blackwell Scientific Publications, 1985, pp. 638-649.
Greenhill, L. L., Rieder, R., Wender, P., et al.: Lithium carbonate in the treatment of hyperactive children. *Archives of General Psychiatry*, 28(5):636, 1973.
Gross, M. D.: Growth of hyperkinetic children taking methylphenidate, dextroamphetamine or imipramine/desipramine. *Pediatrics*, 58:423, 1976.
Keller, A. C., Althof, S. E., & Lothstein, L. M.: Group therapy with gender-identity patients—A four year study. *American Journal of Psychotherapy*, 36(2):223-228, 1982.
Kolvin, I., & Fundudis, T.: Elective mute children: Psychological development and background factors. *Journal of Child Psychology and Psychiatry*, 22:219-232, 1981.
Lang, P. J., & Melamed, B. G.: Case report: Avoidance conditioning therapy of an infant with chronic ruminative vomiting. *Journal of Abnormal Psychology*, 74(1):1-8, 1969.
LeVann, L. J.: Haloperidol in the treatment of behavioral disorders in children and adolescents. *Canadian Psychiatric Association Journal*, 14(2):217, 1969.

Lipton, M. A., Nemeroff, C. B., Bisette, G., & Prange, A. J., Jr.: The role of drugs in the prevention and treatment of mental retardation. In P. Mittler & J. M. de Jong (Eds.), *Research to Practice in Mental Retardation, Vol. III.* Baltimore: University Park Press, 1977, pp. 203–212.

Lothstein, L. M.: Sex reassignment surgery: Historical, bioethical, and theoretical issues. *American Journal of Psychiatry,* 139(4):417–426, 1982.

McCord, J.: A thirty year follow-up of treatment effects. *American Psychologist,* 37:284–289, 1978.

McNutt, B. A., et al.: The effects of long-term stimulant medication on the growth and body composition of hyperactive children. II: Report on 2 years. Paper presented at the Annual Early Clinical Drug Evaluation Unit Meeting, Psychopharmacology Research Branch National Institute of Mental Health, Key Biscayne, Florida, May 20–22, 1976.

National Institutes of Health. Consensus development conference statement: Defined diets and childhood hyperactivity. *Journal of the American Medical Association,* 248:290–291, 1982.

Palmer, T. B.: The Youth Authority's Community Treatment Project. *Federal Probation,* 38:3–14, 1974.

Quinn, P. O., & Rapoport, J. L.: One year follow-up of hyperactive boys treated with imipramine or methylphenidate. *American Journal of Psychiatry,* 132(3):241, 1975.

Rapoport, J. L., Mikkelsen, E. J., Zavardil, A., et al.: Childhood enuresis II. Psychopathology, tricyclic concentration in plasma, and antienuretic effect. *Archives of General Psychiatry,* 37:1146–1152, 1980.

Reid, J. B., Hawkins, N., Keutzer, C., McNeal, S. A., Phelps, R. E., Reid, K. M., & Mees, H. L.: A marathon behaviour modification of a selectively mute child. *Journal of Child Psychology and Psychiatry,* 8:27–30, 1967.

Reisman, J.: *Principles of Psychotherapy with Children.* London: Wiley, 1973.

Rogeness, G. A., Hernandez, J. M., Macedo, C. A., Amrung, S. A., & Hoppe, S. K.: Near-zero plasma dopamine-beta-hydroxylase and conduct disorder in emotionally disturbed boys. *Journal of the American Academy of Child Psychiatry,* 25(4):521–527, 1986.

Russell, G. F. M.: Delayed puberty due to anorexia nervosa of early onset. In P. L. Darby, P. E. Garfinkel, D. M. Garner, & D. V. Coscina (Eds.), *Anorexia Nervosa: Recent Developments in Research,* New York: Alan R. Liss, 1983, pp. 331–342.

Rutter, M., & Hersov, L. (Eds.): *Child and Adolescent Psychiatry: Modern Approaches* (2nd Edition). Boston: Blackwell Scientific Publications, 1985.

Shapiro, A. K., Shapiro, E. S., Bruun, R. D., & Sweet, T. R. D.: *Gilles de la Tourette Syndrome.* New York: Raven Press, 1978.

Straughan, J. H., Potter, W. K., & Hamilton, S. H.: The behavioral treatment of an elective mute. *Journal of Child Psychology and Psychiatry,* 6:125–130, 1965.

Turpin, G.: The behavioral management of the tic disorders: A critical review. *Advances in Behavior Research and Therapy,* 5:203–245, 1983.

Weiss, G., Minde, K., Werry, J., Douglas, V., & Nemeth, E.: Studies on the hyperactive child: VII. Five-year follow-up. *Archives of General Psychiatry,* 24:409–414, 1971.

Yule, W., & Carr, J.: *Behaviour Modification for the Mentally Handicapped.* London: Croom Helm, 1980.

SUGGESTED READING

Ballard, M., & Yule, W.: A case of separation anxiety treated by *in vivo* systematic desensitization. *Behavior Psychotherapy,* 9:105–110, 1981.

Beck, L., Langfold, W., & MacKay, M.: Childhood chemotherapy and later drug abuse and growth curve: A follow-up study of 30 adolescents. *American Journal of Psychiatry,* 132(4):436, 1975.

Bell, D., Weinberg, M., & Hammersmith, S.: *Sexual Preference: Its Development in Men and Women.* Bloomington: Indiana University Press, 1981.
Bellman, M.: Studies on encopresis. *Acta Paediatrica Scandinavica* (Suppl.), 170, 1966.
DeMyer, M. K., Hingtgen, J. N., & Jackson, R. K.: Infantile autism reviewed: A decade of research. *Schizophrenia Bulletin*, 7:388–451, 1981.
Dische, S., Yule, W., Corbett, J., & Hand, D.: Childhood nocturnal enuresis: Factors associated with outcome of treatment with an enuresis alarm. *Developmental Medicine and Child Neurology*, 25:67–81, 1983.
Doleys, D. M.: Enuresis and encopresis. In T. H. Ollendick & M. Hersen (Eds.), *Handbook of Child Psychopathology.* New York: Plenum Press, 1983.
Doleys, D. M., & Arnold, S.: Treatment of childhood encopresis: Full cleanliness training. *Mental Retardation*, 13:14–16, 1975.
Drotar, D., Malone, C. A., Negray, J., & Dennstedt, M.: Psychosocial assessment and care for infants hospitalized for nonorganic failure to thrive. *Journal of Clinical Child Psychology*, 10:63–66, 1981.
Evler, G. L.: Non-medical management of the failure-to-thrive child in a pediatric inpatient setting. In P. J. Accardo (Ed.), *Failure to Thrive in Infancy and Early Childhood.* Baltimore: University Park Press, 1982, pp. 243–263.
Farber, J. M.: Review article. Psychopharmacology of self-injurious behavior in the mentally retarded. *Journal of the American Academy of Child and Adolescent Psychiatry*, 26(3):296–302, 1987.
Freeman, R. D.: The use of drugs to modify behaviour in retarded persons: A practical guide for parents and advocates. *Monograph Supplement to Mental Retardation.* Ontario: Canadian Association for the Mentally Retarded, 1978.
Fundudis, T., Kolvin, I., & Garside, R. (Eds.): *Speech-Retarded and Deaf Children: Their Psychological Development.* London: Academic Press, 1979.
Harris, J. C.: Non-organic failure-to-thrive syndromes: Reactive attachment disorder of infancy and psychosocial dwarfism of early childhood. In P. J. Accardo (Ed.), *Failure to Thrive in Infancy and Early Childhood.* Baltimore: University Park Press, 1982, pp. 229–241.
Kazdin, A. E., Esveldt-Dawson, K., French, N. H., & Unis, A. S.: Effects of parent management training and problem-solving skills training combined in the treatment of antisocial child behavior. *Journal of the American Academy of Child and Adolescent Psychiatry*, 26(3):416–424, 1987.
Kiernan, C. C., & Woodford, F. P.: *Behaviour Modification with the Severely Retarded.* Amsterdam: Associated Scientific Publishers, 1975.
Moore, J. B.: Project Thrive: A supportive treatment approach to the parents of children with non-organic failure to thrive. *Child Welfare*, 61:389–399, 1982.
Rosenthal, A., & Levine, S.: Brief psychotherapy with children: Process of therapy. *American Journal of Psychiatry*, 128:141–146, 1971.
Rutter, M.: The treatment of autistic children. *Journal of Child Psychology and Psychiatry*, 26(2):193–214, 1985.
Rutter, M., Tizard, J., Yule, W., Graham, P., & Whitmore, K.: Isle of Wight Studies 1964–74. *Psychological Medicine*, 6:313–332, 1976.
Rutter, M., Yule, W., Berger, M., & Hersov, L.: An evaluation of a behavioural approach to the treatment of autistic children. Final Report to the Department of Health and Social Security. London, 1977.
Saghir, M., & Robins, E.: *Male and Female Homosexuality.* Baltimore: Williams & Wilkins, 1973.
Shapiro, A. K., & Shapiro, E. S.: Clinical efficacy of haloperidol, pimozide, penfluridol and clonidine in the treatment of Tourette's syndrome. *Advances in Neurology*, 35:383–386, 1982.
Silva, P. A.: The prevalence, stability, and significance of developmental language delay in pre-school children. *Developmental Medicine and Child Neurology*, 22:768–777, 1980.

Sorensen, T. A.: A follow-up study of operated transsexual females. *Acta Psychiatrica Scandinavica,* 64:50–64, 1981.

Tolstrup, K., Brinch, M., & Isager, T.: The Copenhagen anorexia nervosa follow-up study: General outcome. The tenth international congress of the International Association of Child and Adolescent Psychiatry and Allied Professions, Dublin, July, 1982.

Weiss, G., Hechtman, L., Perlman, T., Hopkins, J., & Wener, A.: Hyperactives as young adults. A controlled prospective 10-year follow-up of 75 children. *Archives of General Psychiatry,* 36:675–681, 1979.

Yule, W., Berger, M., & Howlin, P.: Language deficit and behaviour modification. In N. O'Connor (Ed.), *Language, Cognitive Deficits and Retardation.* London: Butterworths, 1975, pp. 209–223.

Section II: Organic Mental Disorders

by

George U. Balis, M.D.

The format for Section II differs somewhat from that of the other sections. Although an effort has been made to follow the *DSM-III-R* outline of psychiatric disorders exactly, such a format would be unwieldy when addressing the treatment of Organic Mental Disorders. We have accordingly grouped the disorders in a clinically useful way—much as *DSM-III-R* provides early in its section on Organic Mental Disorders.

For those readers who wish to locate specific diagnostic codes, the following table of contents is provided:

DSM-III-R CATEGORIES

Dementias Arising in the Senium and Presenium
Primary Degenerative Dementia of the Alzheimer type, Senile Onset
290.xx General/Uncomplicated .... p. 83

290.20 with Delusions .... p. 99
290.21 with Depression .... p. 105
290.30 with Delirium .... p. 72

Primary Degenerative Dementia of the Alzheimer type, Presenile Onset

290.1x General/Uncomplicated .... p. 83
290.11 with Delirium .... p. 72
290.12 with Delusions .... p. 99
290.13 with Depression .... p. 105

Multi-infarct Dementia

290.4x General/Uncomplicated .... p. 86
290.41 with Delirium .... p. 72
290.42 with Delusions .... p. 99
290.43 with Depression .... p. 105

Psychoactive Substance-Induced Organic Mental Disorders
Alcohol

303.00 Intoxication .... p. 123
291.40 Idiosyncratic Intoxication .... p. 123
291.80 Uncomplicated Alcohol Withdrawal .... p. 114
291.00 Withdrawal Delirium .... p. 114
291.30 Hallucinosis .... p. 92
291.10 Amnestic Disorder................................. p. 89
291.20 Dementia Associated with Alcoholism .... p. 86

Sedative, Hypnotic, or Anxiolytic

305.40 Intoxication .... p. 123
292.00 Uncomplicated Withdrawal .... p. 116
292.00 Withdrawal Delirium .... p. 116
292.83 Amnestic Disorder................................. p. 90

Opioid

305.50 Intoxication .... p. 124
292.00 Withdrawal.. p. 118

Cocaine

305.60 Intoxication .... p. 125

292.00 Withdrawal.......................................p. 120
292.81 Delirium..p. 68
292.11 Delusional Disorder ....p. 97

Amphetamine or Similarly Acting Sympathomimetic

305.70 Intoxication ....p. 125
292.81 Delirium..p. 69
292.11 Delusional Disorder ....p. 97
292.00 Withdrawal.......................................p. 119

Phencyclidine (PCP) or Similarly Acting Arylcyclohexylamine

305.90 Intoxication ....p. 126
292.81 Delirium..p. 69
292.11 Delusional Disorder ....p. 97
292.84 Mood Disorder ....p. 104

Hallucinogen

305.30 Hallucinosis ....p. 93
292.11 Delusional Disorder ....p. 97
292.84 Mood Disorder ....p. 104
292.89 Posthallucinogen Perception Disorder ....p. 95

Cannabis

305.20 Intoxication ....p. 125
292.11 Delusional Disorder ....p. 97

Inhalant

305.90 Intoxication ....p. 127

Nicotine

292.00 Withdrawal.......................................p. 120

Caffeine

305.90 Intoxication ....p. 126

Other or Unspecified Psychoactive Substance

305.90 Intoxication	p.	128
292.00 Mixed Drug Withdrawal	p.	120
292.81 Delirium	p.	70
292.82 Dementia	p.	87
292.83 Amnestic Disorder	p.	90
292.11 Delusional Disorder	p.	98
292.12 Hallucinosis	p.	95
292.84 Mood Disorder	p.	104
292.89 Anxiety Disorder	p.	101
292.89 Personality Disorder	p.	110

Organic Mental Disorders Associated with Axis III Physical Disorders or Conditions, or Whose Etiology is Unknown

293.00 Delirium	p.	73
294.10 Dementia	p.	87
294.00 Amnestic Disorder	p.	90
293.81 Organic Delusional Disorder	p.	99
293.82 Organic Hallucinosis	p.	95
293.83 Organic Mood Disorder	p.	106
294.80 Organic Anxiety Disorder	p.	101
310.10 Organic Personality Disorder	p.	110
Explosive Type	p.	110

DEFINITION

Organic Mental Disorders (OMD) are a category of disorders manifesting disturbances of mental functioning and behavior that result from known or presumed damage or dynsfunction of the brain. The term Organic Mental Syndrome (OMS) is used to refer to a characteristic constellation of signs and symptoms that result from damage or dysfunction of the brain without making reference to the underlying specific etiology. The OMD constitutes an etiological diagnosis, while the OMS constitutes a syndromatic diagnosis. It is the etiological diagnosis that upgrades a syndrome into a disorder and allows for specific treatment.

GENERAL PRINCIPLES OF TREATMENT AND PATIENT MANAGEMENT

The therapeutic approach to the patient with an Organic Mental Disorder is based on a truly biopsychosocial model. Although a biomedical understanding of the underlying disease process is of primary importance, an understanding of the psychosocial aspects of the illness is also of major significance in the treatment and management of these patients (Stern, 1982).

The therapeutic approach to these patients can be divided into *treatment* and *patient management*. Those approaches that utilize specific medical procedures (e.g., drug therapy, surgery, psychotherapy) are referred to as treatment. Treatment is further distinguished into *etiologic* and *symptomatic*, on the basis of whether the therapeutic method aims at eliminating the cause of the disease or merely removing or improving its symptoms respectively. All the nonspecific interventions which are part of the therapeutic effort are referred to as management, and are generally supportive in nature.

Treatment

Etiologic treatment, when such treatment is available, is clearly of overriding significance, since it aims at removing the cause of the disorder and allowing the reparative process to correct the underlying pathology. It is imperative, therefore, that every effort be made to identify and treat the underlying disorder by eliminating its cause, and correcting its consequences, whenever possible. When etiologic treatment is unavailable or the cause of the disorder is still unknown, one is limited to the use of symptomatic treatment. Table 1 lists causes of Organic Mental Disorders.

Symptomatic treatment is directed toward two areas: (1) the removal or control of the physical symptoms of the underlying disorder and the normalization of physiological functioning in all systems affected by the disease process; and (2) the removal or control of psychopathology associated with the syndromes, through the use of various psychiatric treatment modalities which include both pharmacologic and psychosocial approaches. Psychiatric treatment is also directed at restoring the patient's psychosocial functioning to the extent that this is possible, and at improving his or her adjustment to residual cognitive deficits.

Patient Management

Medicine is not only an applied scientific discipline, but also an art that involves the skillful application of management principles as an integral part of treatment. Patient management is a very important aspect of the total effort to provide comprehensive care that meets the current and anticipated needs of the patient and his family. Management interventions aim at reducing morbidity, increasing comfort through relief of suffering, enhancing impaired functions, increasing available

TABLE 1
Causes of Organic Mental Disorders

Intracranial Infections	Epidemic encephalitis (arthropod borne, enteroviruses, lethargica); sporadic encephalitis (herpes simplex, mumps, herpes zoster, infectious hepatitis, rabies); post-infectious encephalitis (influenza, measles, rubella, post-vaccination, chicken pox, scarlet fever, atypical pneumonia, infectious mononucleosis); subacute-chronic encephalitis (Dawson's subacute inclusion body, Von Bogaert's subacute sclerosing leukoencephalitis, subacute sclerosing panencephalitis, Creutzfeldt-Jakob disease, progressive multifocal leukoencephalopathy, kuru); neurosyphilis (meningovascular, general paresis); cerebral abscess; meningitis, AIDS (HIV subacute encephalopathy).
Degenerative	Alzheimer's senile/presenile dementia, Pick's disease, Huntington's chorea, Parkinson's disease, progressive supranuclear palsy, simple cortical atrophy, amyotrophic lateral sclerosis, Shy-Drager syndrome.
Vascular	Thrombosis, embolism, intracerebral and subarachnoid hemorrhage, temporal arteritis, migraine, multi-infarct dementia, carotid artery occlusal disease, Binswanger's disease, subacute bacterial endocarditis (embolism).
Cerebral Injury	Head trauma, radiation, hyperthermia, electric current.
Space-occupying Lesions	Neoplasms, subdural hematoma, aneurysms, colloid cyst, parasitic cyst, tuberculoma, lymphoma.
Epilepsy	Postictal syndromes, epileptic personality, epileptic dementia, epileptic psychosis, psychomotor seizures.
Other CNS Disorders	Multiple sclerosis, normal pressure hydrocephalus, Tourette's syndrome, narcolepsy, Schilder's disease.
Substances/Drugs	Alcohol, sedative-hypnotics, hallucinogens, opiates, sympathomimetic stimulants, cannabis, caffeine, nicotine, phencyclidine or arylcyclohexylamines, cocaine, anticholinergics, antihypertensive drugs, antiarrhythmic drugs, digitalis, cimetidine, anticonvulsants, steroids, etc. (see *Table 2*)

TABLE 1 *(continued)*

Poisons/Chemicals	Heavy metals (lead, mercury, arsenic, thalium); industrial poisons (carbon monoxide and disulfide, organic solvents, methylchloride), inhalants (hydrocarbons).
Systemic Infections Affecting CNS	Pneumonia, typhoid, typhus, acute rheumatic fever, malaria, diphtheria, Legionnaires' disease, brucellosis, Rocky Mountain spotted fever, AIDS, Lyme disease.
Other Systemic Disease Affecting CNS	Systemic lupus erythematosus, hypertensive encephalopathy, rheumatoid vasculitis, polyarteritis nodosa, Sydenham's chorea, porphyria, Paget's disease, Wilson's disease.
Metabolic Disorders	Diabetic acidosis or hypoglycemia; hepatic, renal, and pulmonary insufficiency or failure; dialysis encephalopathy (dementia), dialysis disequilibrium syndrome, jejunoileostomy psychosis.
Electrolytes/Water	Hypo- or hyper-calcemia, hypo- or hyper-natremia, hypo- or hyper-kalemia, hypo- or hyper-magnesemia, hypo- or hyper-phosphatemia, dehydration, overhydration, acid–base disturbance.
Blood Gases	hypoxia/anoxia due to cardiac disease, shock, anemia, pulmonary disease.
Endocrinopathies	Hypo- or hyper-thyroidism, hyperparathyroidism, pheochromocytoma, Cushing's syndrome, Addison's disease, hypopituitarism, hyperinsulinism.
Vitamin Deficiencies	Nicotinic acid (pellagra), thiamine (Korsakoff–Wernicke), B12 and folate (pernicious anemia), A and D hypervitaminosis.
Miscellaneous	Sleep deprivation, sarcoidosis, Sjögren's syndrome, carcinoid syndrome, remote effects of cancer, serum sickness, sensory isolation, severe burns, food allergy.

competence and skills, reducing the need for lost functions, and generally optimizing the patient's psychosocial milieu, including his or her physical environment, family, and social setting. The effectiveness of the clinician in patient management depends on:

1. knowledge of the underlying pathogenic mechanisms responsible for the physiological and psychological disturbances of the syndrome and of the way these disturbances impact upon the patient's personality and behavior;
2. understanding of the patient's personality and, in the face of stress, loss of function, and loss of self-esteem;
3. sensitivity to patient needs and empathic caring in meeting these needs;
4. ability to utilize available resources within the hospital, the patient's family, and his or her community in the effort to treat and rehabilitate him or her; and
5. ability to work cooperatively with other health professionals, independently or within a team approach.

Depending on the type of Organic Mental Syndrome (e.g., Delirium, Dementia), different management approaches must be applied within different settings and varying circumstances. Effective approaches vary according to whether the patient is managed in the emergency room, medical–surgical ward, I.C.U., his or her own home, the physician's office, or a nursing home. The appropriate locus of treatment is determined by the type of care the patient needs: for example, acute care settings (general hospital or psychiatric unit) for acutely disturbed, physically ill, delirious, psychotic, or depressed patients; intermediate care or chronic care settings (nursing homes, halfway houses) for patients with protracted or chronic syndromes requiring a lower level of care, or a sheltered or structured environment; or a home care setting for those who can be managed at home and in the physician's office. The patient's need for particular management skills and interventions may vary during the stages of the clinical course of the syndrome (e.g., acute, convalescent, or chronic phase), as well as according to the prognosis of the syndrome (reversible or irreversible, static or progressive).

The management of patients with cognitive impairment secondary to Delirium, Dementia, and Organic Amnestic Syndrome is of particular significance. These patients require continuous management efforts that aim at reducing need for impaired or lost function and maximizing utilization of available function, as well as preventing regression, dependency, and other reactive psychopathology. The management of those patients who suffer from OMS associated with minimal or no cognitive deficit (i.e., Organic Hallucinosis, Organic Personality Syndrome, Organic Delusional Syndrome, Organic Mood Syndrome, and Organic Anxiety Syndrome) is similar to that of patients with the corresponding functional disorders.

The management of patients whose OMS is secondary to substance abuse is particularly important, especially during the period following recovery from the syndrome. Follow-up treatment and rehabilitation for substance abuse represent an indispensable part of the total therapeutic management.

Finally, the family of the patient, his or her home environment, and the social milieu are, in most instances, a major focus in the effort for effective management. Counseling with family members, especially spouse or primary caretakers, may involve a range of concerns, including advice regarding the care and supervision of the patient, reducing stress and resolving conflict within the family, dealing with unrealistic expectations about prognosis of current and future capacity to function, and assisting family members in effective coping strategies, especially in caring for the chronically demented, psychotic, or impulsive and emotionally unstable person.

Chapter 10

Delirium and Dementia

10A: DELIRIUM

Most of the causes of Organic Mental Disorders listed in Table 1 may result in delirium, acting alone or in combination with several other factors (multifactorial etiology). Its most common etiology involves drugs (Table 2). Various metabolic disorders, infectious diseases, endocrinopathies, systemic disorders, and primary CNS disorders (including infections, head trauma, postictal syndromes, neoplasms, and cerebrovascular disorders) are also relatively common (Table 1).

General Therapeutic Principles

The treatment and management of the delirious patient are generally based upon the following therapeutic principles:

1. Identify and treat the causative factor(s) of the underlying primary disorder;
2. Understand the pathogenic mechanisms of the disease process that led to the development of the delirium;
3. Recognize emergency situations for early treatment intervention (e.g., hypoxia, hypoglycemia) in order to prevent the possibility of irreversible brain damage (e.g., dementia) or death.
4. Recognize and treat those psychiatric symptoms that must be removed as soon as possible in order to provide relief or prevent

accidents or complications (e.g., agitation, combativeness, suicidal behavior); and
5. Understand the particular cognitive state of the delirious patient and factors that may influence it, in order to optimize nonspecific supportive measures in patient management (e.g., impaired capacity for information processing as influenced by an unfamiliar or ambiguous environment) (Balis, 1970; Sakles & Balis, 1978).

Etiologic Treatment
Every effort should be made to identify the underlying causative factor(s), with the aim of instituting specific treatment at the earliest possible time. A detailed history from relatives or friends is most helpful, especially in identifying drug ingestion, alcohol abuse, head trauma, chemical exposure, or already diagnosed disease (e.g., diabetes, epilepsy, drug idiosyncrasies, or heart disease). In hospitalized patients, the diagnostic process is aided by focusing on the setting in which the delirium occurred (I.C.U., recovery room, dialysis unit), the nature of preexisting disease (e.g., pulmonary insufficiency, cardiac failure, hepatic cirrhosis), or the nature of treatment of the primary disorder (e.g., digitalization, hypnotic–sedatives, continuous gastric suction, irradiation).

In view of the fact that the etiology of delirium is often multifactorial, especially in the hospitalized patient, the clinician should make an effort to search for several possible causative factors rather than a singular etiology. Although a single factor may cause delirium, several subthreshold factors acting concurrently may be sufficient to produce the critical physiological derangement that leads to the decompensated state. In this regard, every pathophysiological abnormality should be corrected and every possible etiologic factor eliminated, especially nonessential medications or those for which a less toxic drug can be substituted.

Once the causative factor is removed, the condition may be self-limited with rapid and complete recovery. In some instances, the primary cause may have already ceased to operate (e.g., head trauma, burns, seizures, bleeding, radiation) and only the pathogenic sequelae need to be treated (secondary causes). In others, the primary cause is unknown and only the disease processes are identifiable and amenable to treatment (e.g., effects of unknown drugs, fever of unknown origin). Sometimes all efforts fail to provide evidence of "organic" factors that might be related to a clinical delirium.

TABLE 2
Drugs Capable of Causing Delirium

Antidepressants (anticholinergic effect)

Neuroleptics (anticholinergic effect)

Antiparkinsonians (anticholinergic effect)

Anticholinergic/Antispasmodic
    atropine/homatropine
    belladonna alkaloids
    cyclopentolate (Cyclogyl)—eye drops
    scopolamine

Antihistamine (anticholinergic effect)
    brompheniramine (Dimetane)
    chlorpheniramine (Teldrin, Ornade)
    diphenhydramine (Benadryl)
    hydroxyzine (Vistaril, Atarax)
    promethazine (Phenergan)
    over-the-counter sleep and cold medicines

Anticonvulsant
    ethosuximide (Zarontin)
    phenytoin (Dilantin, others)
    primidone (Mysoline)
    sodium valprate (Depakene)

Sympathomimetic
    amphetamines
    ephedrine
    phenylephrine
    phenylpropanolamine
    phenetrazine
    diethylpropion
    methylphenidate (Ritalin)

Sedative–Hypnotic–Anxiolytic
    barbiturates
    glutethimide (Doriden)
    benzodiazepines
    meprobamate

Cardiovascular
    clonidine (Catapres)
    digitalis (Digoxin, Lanox)
    lidocaine (Xylocaine)
    methyldopa (Aldomet)
    propranolol (Inderal)
    procainamide (Pronestyl)
    quinidine (Quinidine, Duraquin)

(continued)

TABLE 2 *(continued)*

Miscellaneous
    amantadine (Symmetrel)
    aminocaproic acid (Amicar)
    aminophylline (Theo-Dur)
    amphotericin B (Fungizone)
    asparaginase (Wispar)
    baclofen (Lioresal)
    bromides
    carbidopa (Sinemet)
    chloroquine (Aralen)
    cimetidine (Tagamet)
    corticosteroids
    cortisones, prednisone, ACTH
    cycloserine (Seromycin)
    disulfiram (Antabuse)
    isoniazid
    ibuprofen (Motrin, Advil)
    indomethacin (Indocin)
    ketamine (Ketalar)
    levodopa (Dopar)
    lithium
    metrizamide (Amipaque)
    metronidazole (Flagyl)
    phenylbutazone (Butazolidin)
    naproxen (Naprosyn)
    quinacrine (Atabrine)
    theophylline
    5-fluorouracil

While searching for an etiologic diagnosis of the delirium, the clinician is called upon to recognize emergency situations presenting with delirium, either because they may be life-threatening or because of the possibility of irreversible brain damage (dementia) should the condition be prolonged. Early recognition and emergency treatment intervention reduce risk or degree of brain injury, general morbidity, and mortality. Common preventable etiologies associated with such risk include drug intoxication, hypoglycemia, diabetic acidosis, hypoxia or anoxia, thiamine deficiency, intracranial hemorrhage, subdural hematoma, subarachnoid or intracerebral hemorrhage due to ruptured aneurysm, withdrawal delirium, acute cerebral edema, and hyperthermia. Delirium as a complication of serious illness often portends life-threatening or ominous outcome.

Symptomatic Treatment
This is directed toward two areas: psychiatric symptoms of the delirium and the physical symptoms of the underlying disorder. Its purpose is to provide relief, improve morbidity, and prevent complications through an appropriately targeted approach to symptom control. Symptomatic treatment may be the only therapeutic approach available in those instances in which etiologic diagnosis is lacking.

The symptomatic treatment of the delirium is primarily medicinal. It should be emphasized, however, that the clinical picture of many delirious patients may not require any drug treatment other than general supportive management, and that appropriate management approaches may minimize or make unnecessary the use of drugs. For instance, when the clinical picture is characterized by a simple confusional state without symptoms of agitation, fear, or combativeness, medicinal treatment is unnecessary and may even be contraindicated since the psychotropic drugs that are commonly used for symptomatic relief may aggravate the delirium through their depressant, anticholinergic, or hypotensive effects (Heizer & Wilbert, 1974). Even in florid deliria in which the patient's emotional and behavioral reaction to the cognitive impairment dominates the clinical picture, pharmacologic control of symptoms should be judicious and tempered by the realization that appropriately supportive management measures may be of equal or even of greater importance.

Medicinal control of delirium generally involves the relief of distressing symptoms (fear, anxiety, panic, irritability, angry outbursts, illusory and hallucinatory symptoms, delusions) and disruptive behaviors (excitement, agitation, restlessness, combativeness, assaultiveness, hyperactivity, insomnia). Psychotropic drugs have no therapeutic effect on the cognitive deficit and, as mentioned earlier, may even worsen it. Physostigmine will restore cognitive functions in deliria induced by anticholinergic agents. Drugs recommended for the symptomatic control of delirious symptoms include antipsychotic (neuroleptic) and anxiolytic drugs (benzodiazepines). The choice of a particular psychotropic medication is based on several considerations including etiology of the delirium, biometabolism and side effects of the drug, and one's previous experience. Thorough familiarity with a drug's pharmacological actions, pharmacokinetics, biometabolism, and side effects enables the physician to tailor the treatment to the patient's particular needs.

High potency neuroleptics (haloperidol, perphenazine, thiothixene, fluphenazine, and trifluoperazine) show minimal sedative and autonomic (anticholinergic and alpha-blocking) effects, but a high incidence of extrapyramidal reactions (dystonia, akathesia, and parkinsonism). They are effective in the control of the delirious psychopathology including agitation, fear, and psychotic symptoms. The neuroleptic of choice in most cases is haloperidol (Ayd, 1978).

The anxiolytic benzodiazepines (chlordiazepoxide, diazepam, oxazepam, lorazepam, etc.) are safe and effective. They are less sedating than the hypnotics, require high doses to produce CNS depression, and have minimal autonomic action or effect on the cardiovascular and respiratory systems. They have a measurable anticonvulsant activity that may be useful in treating withdrawal deliria. They differ in pharmacokinetics and biometabolism, with oxazepam and lorazepam having a short plasma half-life, and chlordiazepoxide and diazepam lasting much longer. Oxazepam and lorazepam may therefore be the benzodiazepines of choice for treating patients expected to show cumulative effects (hepatic or renal insufficiency or prolonged use of the drug) (Lipowski, 1980a, b).

The prescription schedule of any of these drugs should also take into consideration the fluctuating course of delirium. If the timing of occurrence of the symptoms is characteristic (e.g., at night), it is advisable to prescribe the drug only prior to the onset of symptoms (Dubovsky & Weisberg, 1982).

The dosage and route of administration of these drugs depend on the severity of the symptoms, responsiveness to the drug, the patient's age (the elderly require much lower doses), and other factors. Small, preferably oral dosages are appropriate for moderate anxiety and restlessness. Higher doses, given parenterally, are required for the control of severe agitation, panic states, or assaultive behavior. The art of optimal titration of the drug, in order to be able to meet the changing needs of the delirious patient, requires close monitoring of therapeutic response and knowledge of all factors that may modify drug effects. Common problems associated with a failure to titrate the drug optimally include oversedation ("snowing" effect) resulting in stupor or even coma and respiratory depression, and undersedation with ineffective control of the symptoms.

When the choice of drug is haloperidol, the following approach is generally recommended. In mildly to moderately agitated patients, 2–10 mg given orally twice a day generally suffice. Parenteral administration might be necessary for the uncooperative patient, with the dosage adjusted to about three-fourths of the oral amount. In severely agitated, assaultive, or panicked patients, haloperidol should be given parenterally

(IM), with an initial dose of 2–10 mg, which can be repeated several times a day as needed, observing for adverse effects, until control of agitation is achieved (Lipowski, 1980a,b). The so-called "rapid neuroleptization method" has been suggested as a means of handling emergency situations and is described elsewhere. Doses should be lower than those for nonorganic disorders. The total daily dose required to produce a calming effect may range from 10–40 mg (or higher). Once this effect is achieved haloperidol should be given orally, in b.i.d. doses (Moore, 1977), and be gradually tapered and discontinued within days or weeks.

When benzodiazepines are used, the choice depends primarily on differences in their plasma half-lives and hepatic metabolism. In mildly to moderately agitated patients, 25–30 mg of chlordiazepoxide, 5–10 mg of diazepam, 15–30 mg of oxazepam, or 0.5–1.0 mg of lorazepam given orally every four to six hours as needed is generally sufficient. These doses may be doubled in more severely agitated patients. Parenteral (IM) administration of lorazepam may be required for patients showing severe agitation, panic, or combativeness, at dosage levels comparable to those for oral administration. In emergency situations, slow intravenous injection of chlordiazepoxide (25–50 mg) or diazepam (5–10 mg) may become necessary in order to bring the symptoms under immediate control.

Hydroxyzine, an antihistamine, and paraldehyde, a hypnotic, may also be used for control of anxiety and agitation, in a manner similar to that described for the benzodiazepines. Hydroxyzine may be given orally or parenterally, while paraldehyde is preferably administered rectally.

In addition to the symptomatic control of the psychiatric manifestations of delirium, close attention must be paid to correcting any concomitant pathophysiological derangement, even though not directly related to the primary etiology of the delirium. The symptomatic treatment may involve a broad range of disturbances including fever, insomnia, cardiac arrhythmias, seizures, dehydration, nutritional deficits, and urinary retention.

Patient Management

The management of the delirious patient in a hospital setting is the cornerstone of the total therapeutic approach. Its effectiveness is based on an understanding of the cognitive state of the patient and the factors that may influence it, as well as on an appreciation of the patient's psychological needs. Its goals are: (1) to optimize the patient's environment and the staff's bedside approach as a means of providing support to the patient's cognitive deficit; (2) to provide protection from accidents; and (3) to improve and maintain the patient's physical and mental state through nonspecific supportive measures that provide control and comfort. The key for successful management is the quality of nursing care.

The primary physician must be thoroughly familiar with the management of the delirious patient in a hospital setting (Dubovsky & Weisberg, 1982). In managing a delirious patient, one should be guided by the awareness that the patient is confused and disoriented, has impaired memory and cannot retain new information, has difficulty processing information, tends to misinterpret events and distort their meaning, cannot tolerate either excessive or diminished sensory input, and may be experiencing perceptual distortions in the form of illusions or even hallucinations that are often frightening.

The patient with a mild delirium of known etiology and good prognosis (e.g., idiosyncratic reaction to a drug, febrile illness) is best cared for at home, within a stable and familiar environment, and under the continuous care and supervision of family members. Patients with more serious deliria, and especially those of unknown etiology, require immediate hospitalization. The choice of hospital type depends on several considerations, including etiology of the underlying illness, degree and sophistication of medical and diagnostic requirements, and severity of behavioral disturbances. For instance, patients with a delirium due to serious physical illness (e.g., heart failure) should be treated in a general hospital; in cases of alcohol withdrawal delirium, treatment may best be carried out in a detoxification unit; violent, suicidal, or acutely psychotic patients who show no evidence of serious physical illness require psychiatric hospitalization. Psychiatric consultation is required in most cases for assistance in diagnosis and management.

The physical environment should be stable and unambiguous, with elements that enhance familiarity and orientation, and maintain low sensory input, while at the same time preserving variability through stimulus change. The patient is best cared for in a quiet, simply furnished, and preferably single-bed room, softly lighted at all times, with mild stimulation provided by a radio or television set. A calendar, clock, and some personal articles (family pictures) should be at bedside for orientation and familiarity. Continuous supervision, preferably by a relative or friend who is thoroughly instructed about the requirements of this task, should be provided. Effort should be made to minimize the number of the nursing and house staff involved in the care of the patient, in order to increase the patient's familiarity with personnel. Special attention should be given to the overriding need for constant supervision and for instituting measures for protection from accidents, including suicidal and homicidal precautions when indicated. Physical restraints should be avoided whenever possible, and when applied they should be used for only brief periods. Control of agitation and combativeness is best managed by the personal contact of a supervising family member and by the appropriate use of tranquilizing drugs.

The interpersonal aspects of management are primarily determined by the patient's need to be oriented, to comprehend what is happening to him or her, and to be reassured. Accordingly, every interaction with the patient should adhere at all times to an approach that meets these needs. Professional staff should clearly identify themselves, state their role, remind the patient that he or she is in a hospital, and carefully explain what they intend to do. They should provide reassurance and explanation about everything that the patient experiences as alien, ambiguous, threatening, or frightening.

Upon recovery from the delirious state, the patient may have complete amnesia for the episode or may have spotty or incomplete recollection. If the patient is amnestic, he or she should be helped to understand the nature of the experiential gap and be reassured that his or her memory is now intact in spite of the amnesia. If the patient remembers the psychotic experiences (especially delusions and hallucinations), their nature and benign prognosis should be carefully explained.

SPECIFIC DELIRIA

The preceding section described the symptomatic treatment and management of delirium as an Organic Mental Syndrome (OMS), that is, without reference to etiology. DSM-III-R codes for deliria of unknown etiology include Axis I diagnoses when an unspecified psychoactive substance is suspected (292.81) and Axis III diagnoses for all other unknown etiologies (293.00).

The following section deals with specific treatments of deliria of known etiology. The previously described basic principles of symptomatic treatment and management of delirium are also applicable to these disorders. DSM-III-R classifies deliria of known etiology into three categories: (1) Psychoactive Substance-Induced Deliria; (2) Deliria Complicating Dementias Arising in the Senium and Presenium; and (3) Deliria Associated with Axis III Physical Disorders or Conditions.

1. Psychoactive Substance-Induced Deliria

These are most common and are generally associated with substance use disorders, suicidal or accidental drug overdose, and idiosyncratic reactions to prescribed or over-the-counter drugs. The pathogenic mechanism depends on the pharmacologic action(s) of the drug. Predisposing or facilitating factors include age (the elderly being most susceptible), biological substrate of the host (genetically determined enzyme systems), dosage, route of administration, hepatic function, and other (Balis, 1982). Clinically, these deliria can be classified into dose-related, idiosyncratic, and withdrawal types. This distinction allows definition of different approaches to treatment.

Dose-Related Deliria
These are deliria induced by relatively high blood concentrations of a potentially deliriogenic drug, such as certain psychoactive drugs (e.g., cocaine, amphetamines, phencyclidine) and anticholinergic agents. The major etiologic treatment approach is the elimination or inactivation by an antidote of the causative agent.

Idiosyncratic Deliria
These are not dose-related and can occur early in the course of treatment at therapeutic doses. Genetically controlled enzymatic processes in drug metabolism are thought to be responsible for the induction of the delirium (Balis, 1982). Many prescription drugs may cause idiosyncratic deliria in predisposed individuals (e.g., codeine, diazepam, glutethimide, chloroquine). They clear rapidly without any sequelae. Treatment is symptomatic.

Withdrawal Deliria
This is a special class of substance-induced deliria involving a different pathogenetic mechanism, as well as different *DSM-III-R* coding. These deliria occur in individuals who have developed physiological dependence on alcohol (291.00) or sedative–hypnotic–anxiolytic drugs (292.00), usually following prolonged use, during withdrawal from the agent. Their treatment is discussed in the section on Withdrawal and Withdrawal Deliria in Chapter 12.

The *DSM-III-R* lists on Axis I the following specific psychoactive substance-induced deliria, under the code 292.81.

292.81 Cocaine Delirium
Cocaine-induced delirium may develop in both the naive and the chronic cocaine user. The syndrome occurs almost immediately following in-

travenous injection or smoking ("free-basing"), usually within one hour (but not more than 24 hours) of intake of cocaine. In uncomplicated cases, the delirium clears within six hours. Its treatment is similar to that of intoxication with psychostimulant drugs (see Intoxications in Chapter 12). The patient requires placement in a quiet room where safety measures (e.g., physical restraints) may be applied for the protection of the combative individual. Agitation can be controlled by the use of benzodiazepines (e.g., lorazepam 1 mg IM q 2-4 hours prn) or neuroleptics (e.g., haloperidol 5 mg IM or 5-15 mg po q 2-4 hours prn). It should be noted, however, that cocaine abusers may be sensitive to the extrapyramidal side effects of the neuroleptics because of dopamine depletion (Perry, 1987). The patient's vital signs should be monitored very closely for rising temperature, pulse, and blood pressure. Hyperthermia (above 29°C) requires vigorous treatment with both hypothermic blankets and ice packs to prevent grand mal seizures. If convulsions do occur, the patient should be treated with slowly administered intravenous diazepam 5-15 mg q 15 to 45 minutes to prevent progression to status epilepticus. Uncontrollable severe hypertension (systolic blood pressure remaining above 200 mg Hg for an hour or more) should be controlled promptly with propranolol (Perry, 1987).

292.81 Amphetamine or Similarly Acting Sympathomimetic Delirium

Sympathomimetic drugs with a CNS stimulant action include, besides amphetamine, cocaine, methylphenidate (Ritalin) and diethylpropion (Tenuate). All these psychostimulant drugs may induce delirium within 24 hours of intake, and almost immediately following intravenous administration. In addition to confusional symptoms, associated features include tactile and olfactory hallucinations, labile affect, and violent behavior. The patient needs to be closely monitored for rising blood pressure and temperature and occurrence of convulsions. Treatment of psychostimulant delirium is similar to that of Cocaine Delirium and psychostimulant intoxication.

292.81 Phencyclidine (PCP) or Similarly Acting Arylcyclohexylamine Delirium

The delirium may develop within 24 hours after intake or it may emerge days later after recovery from an overdose. It may last for a week with a waxing and waning course. Associated features are those of phencyclidine intoxication including both physiological changes (e.g., ataxia, dysarthria, muscular rigidity, nystagmus, seizures, elevated blood pressure) and behavioral disturbances (e.g., fluctuations in mood, impulsivity, agitation, assaultiveness).

Treatment is similar to that described in the section of Phencyclidine Intoxication. It includes the provision of a calm environment and adequate restraints for combative behavior, and the use of diazepam or haloperidol for controlling agitation. If seizures develop, diazepam should be given intravenously to prevent status epilepticus. If serious hypertension develops, diazoxide and hydrazine have been reported to be effective in lowering blood pressure (Lewis & Senay, 1981).

292.81 Deliria Associated with Other Psychoactive Substance

Numerous drugs with psychoactive action (CNS effects) may induce delirium as a result of drug idiosyncrasy in predisposed individuals (genetically determined) or altered drug metabolism (e.g., elderly, impaired hepatic function, drug interaction), or because of toxic blood concentrations of the drug (e.g., overdose, cumulative effects, impaired renal excretion). Table 2 (pp. 61–62) lists drugs that are known to cause delirium. Many of these drugs possess an anticholinergic action. An anticholinergic mechanism is implicated in the majority of drug-induced deliria.

Anticholinergic Substance Delirium

Drugs with anticholinergic activity include many antispasmodics (atropine, homatropine, belladonna alkaloids, scopolamine, etc.), antiparkinsonians (benztropine, trihexyphenidyl, biperiden, etc.) analgesics (meperidine), tricyclic antidepressants (especially amitriptyline), neuroleptics (low potency, and especially thioridazine), antihistamines (diphenhydramine, promethazine, etc.), hydroxyzine, cimetidine, and others.

Tricyclic drug overdose is a common cause of anticholinergic delirium. According to Preskorn and Simpson (1982), tricyclic plasma levels exceeding 450 ng/ml produced delirium in six of seven patients. Delirium may also occur as an idiosyncratic phenomenon with blood concentrations within the therapeutic range (Godwin, 1983). The elderly are particularly vulnerable to anticholinergic delirium.

Treatment of anticholinergic delirium is similar to that described in the section on Anticholinergic Drug Intoxication. Physostigmine salicylate 1–2 mg IV or IM will clear the delirium within less than 30 minutes. A second dose of 1–2 mg physostigmine may be given 15 minutes later, and may be repeated every two to three hours if needed (Blitt & Petty, 1975; Eisendrath et al., 1987; Godwin, 1983; Heizer &

Wilbert, 1974; Lewis & Senay, 1981; Mogelnicki, Waller, & Finlayson, 1979; Perry, 1987).

In the case of anticholinergic delirium induced by tri- and tetracyclic antidepressants, one needs to monitor the EKG closely and treat, if necessary, the cardiotoxic effects of these drugs.

2. Deliria Complicating Dementias of the Senium and Presenium

The *DSM-III-R* Axis I provides the following codes for delirium complicating dementias:

> 290.30 Primary Degenerative Dementia of the Alzheimer Type, Senile Onset, with Delirium
> 290.11 Primary Degenerative Dementia of the Alzheimer Type, Presenile Onset with Delirium
> 290.41 Multi-infarct Dementia with Delirium

Delirium is one of the complicating syndromes often superimposed upon a dementia. This syndrome is also known as "acute confusional state." The etiology of these deliria is not uniform, and is generally not related directly to the pathogenic mechanism of the dementia itself. Most of them are drug-induced, often having an anticholinergic mechanism (see Table 2). Other etiologies include metabolic disorders (diabetic acidosis, or hypoglycemia, hepatic and renal insufficiency), hypoxia–anoxia resulting from cardiac or pulmonary disease, and other conditions listed in Table 1. One of the etiologies of delirium complicating Multi-infarct Dementia is the disease process itself, which may result in delirium during transient ischemic attacks (TIAs) and during the acute phase of an occlusive episode secondary to thrombosis or cerebral emboli (small stroke). Acute confusional episodes in the demented elderly that are characterized by transient, delirium-like cognitive disturbances judged to be functional and referred to as "pseudodelirium" by analogy with "pseudodementia" are particularly interesting (Lipowski, 1983). They generally occur in the evening or at night in the form of "sundowner" syndrome, as a result of diminished sensory input and social isolation and/or exposure to an unfamiliar environment (e.g., the hospital). The treatment of the "sundowner" syndrome consists of better orientation, room lights, and of small doses of a high potency neuroleptic (e.g., haloperidol 0.5 to 1 mg) given one or two hours before sundown. The dosage may be gradually increased as needed (DuBovsky & Weisberg, 1982).

290.30 Primary Degenerative Dementia of the Alzheimer Type, Senile Onset with Delirium
290.11 Primary Degenerative Dementia of the Alzheimer Type, Presenile Onset with Delirium

As with other deliria, therapy of delirium in the demented patient suffering from Alzheimer's disorder is both etiologic and symptomatic/supportive. It consists of treatment or removal of the putative deliriogenic condition, while providing symptomatic therapy for agitation, psychotic symptoms, or insomnia, as well as supportive management through good nursing (Bayne, 1978; Lipowski, 1980a, 1983; Liston, 1982; Seymour et al., 1980; Wolanin & Phillips, 1981).

For control of agitation, high potency neuroleptics are recommended, and especially haloperidol in doses 0.5–5 mg po or IM twice daily (Lipowski, 1980b, 1983). If the patient develops intolerable extrapyramidal symptoms, agitation may be alternatively controlled with small doses of a short-half-life benzodiazepine, such as lorazepam (Ativan), which can be given in doses 0.5–1 mg po or IM q 4 to 6 hours prn. If insomnia is present, it may be treated with a short-half-life benzodiazepine hypnotic, such as temazepam (Restoril) 15–30 mg hs prn, or triazolam (Halcion). The clinician should keep in mind that the use of sedative/hypnotics and benzodiazepines, especially those with longer half-life (e.g., flurazepam, diazepam) may worsen the confusion in delirium, especially in the elderly, as a result of drug accumulation. For more information, see section on Dementia (p. 76).

290.41 Multi-infarct Dementia with Delirium

The development of delirium in a patient with multiple infarct dementia is a serious complication because of the patient's poor general health (hypertension, arteriosclerotic heart disease) and because of the possibility that the disease process itself may be causing the delirium as a result of transient ischemic attacks (TIAs) or thrombotic episodes in evolution. The latter etiology requires careful diagnostic evaluation before etiological treatment is instituted, in an effort to abort an irreversible cerebrovascular accident.

TIAs referable to the carotid or vertebrobasilar arterial territories may present with acute confusional symptoms constituting a delirium. TIAs last from a few seconds up to 12 hours and may occur repeatedly, leaving no sequelae or progressing to a thrombotic episode in the form of a small or catastrophic stroke. The treatment of TIAs consists of anticoagulants, aspirin, and vasodilators. Anticoagulant therapy (heparin, warfarin) may prevent TIAs and postpone an impending stroke. Anticoagulants may also arrest the advance of a thrombotic stroke-in-evolution. The use of anticoagulant drugs makes an accurate diagnosis imperative, especially in ruling out intracranial hemorrhage. Other measures that have been used in the treatment of TIAs include aspirin, cerebral vasodilators such as papaverine, nicotinic acid, inhalation of 5% carbon dioxide, aminophylline, and acetazolamide. The use of vasodilators is controversial and of questionable value. On the other hand, the prophylactic use of aspirin is generally recommended.

In the case of a thrombotic episode in evolution, anticoagulation with heparin IV or continuous drip therapy is instituted for several days, followed by oral warfarin at doses sufficient to maintain prothrombin time at twice the control value (Hass, 1979; Mohr et al., 1977). Currently used thrombolytic agents (e.g., fibrinolysin and profibrinolysin activator) have not proved helpful in treating thrombosis-in-evolution (Mohr et al., 1977).

The treatment of deliria of other etiologies that occur in patients with multi-infarct dementia is similar to that described in the general section on Delirium.

3. Deliria Associated With Axis III Physical Disorders or Conditions

Most of the disorders listed in Table 1 may cause delirium, coded as 293.00. Metabolic disorders, systemic and CNS infections, head trauma, and postictal states are common etiologies and are listed in Axis III. Deliria of particular interest include Wernicke's encephalopathy and Neuroleptic Malignant Syndrome (NMS).

Wernicke's Syndrome

This acute encephalopathy is produced by nutritional deficiency involving thiamine, usually secondary to chronic alcoholism. Other conditions leading to Wernicke's syndrome include chronic hemodialysis, thyrotoxicosis, pernicious vomiting of pregnancy, and gastric carcinoma. It usually begins abruptly as a "quiet delirium" and is accompanied by characteristic neurologic signs that include external ophthalmoplegia, nystagmus, and cerebellar ataxia, as well as polyneuropathy. The patient most often appears apathetic, listless, confused, and disoriented.

Treatment of the syndrome consists of parenteral thiamine (50 mg IM) followed by oral doses of thiamine and good nutrition with multivitamin supplement. The ophthalmoplegia and signs of delirium show dramatic improvement within hours and clear completely within a few days after administration of thiamine. Nystagmus and ataxia improve more slowly. The patient emerges from the delirium several days later with an organic amnestic syndrome (Korsakoff's) (Victor, Adams, & Collins, 1971).

Neuroleptic Malignant Syndrome (NMS)
This syndrome presents unpredictably among psychiatric patients as an idiosyncratic response to therapeutic doses of neuroleptics. It is more likely to occur with high potency neuroleptics, especially when given parenterally, and in conjunction with lithium and other drugs. Dehydration and exhaustion are thought to be predisposing factors. In the author's opinion NMS appears to be a state-dependent response to neuroleptics often associated with excitement and agitation. It is thought to be the result of a neuroleptic-induced massive blockade of dopamine (DA) receptors, especially in the striatal, mesofrontal, and hypothalamic DA systems.

Clinically, the patient presents with catatonic-like symptoms of mutism, bradykinesia, and plastic (lead-type) rigidity with counterpull resistance (described by Kleist, 1936, as *Gegenhalten*), suggestive of frontal lobe involvement (mesofrontal DA blockade); often with cogwheel rigidity (basal ganglia DA blockade); autonomic dysregulation manifested by marked diaphoresis, tachycardia, fluctuating blood pressure (hypothalamic DA blockade); hypermetabolic state manifested by pyrexia, elevated serum CPK, leukocytosis, elevated liver enzymes, and cardiac arrhythmias (hypothalamic DA blockade); and confusional symptoms of a waxing and waning course, characteristic of delirium.

Symptoms typically resolve within five to 10 days or longer if depot neuroleptics were used (e.g., fluphenazine decanoate). Complications include rhabdomyolysis with myoglobulinemia resulting in acute renal failure, aspiration pneumonia, and cardiovascular collapse. Mortality has been estimated at 20% (Karoff, 1980; Levenson, 1985; Smego & Durack, 1982).

There are notable similarities between *NMS* and *postanesthetic malignant hyperthermia* (MH). The latter is due to a peripheral mechanism related to an idiopathic dysfunction in sarcoplasmic calcium-ion metabolism resulting in a hypermetabolic state of skeletal muscles (Nelson & Flewellen, 1983). *Lethal catatonia* may also mimic NMS.

The patient is best managed in a general hospital. Placement in I.C.U. may often become necessary during the course of the syndrome.

Treatment of NMS is essentially supportive, consisting of early recognition, immediate discontinuation of neuroleptic medications, and careful attention to the detection and aggressive management of complications: for example, control of hyperthermia with antipyretics and cooling blankets, correction of dehydration and electrolyte imbalance, treatment of intercurrent infection such as pneumonia; dialysis for acute renal failure following rhabdomyolysis; ventilator support in case of acute respiratory failure due to aspiration, infection, or pulmonary emboli; treatment of cardiac arrhythmias; and management of other secondary complications. Since the patient is usually immobile, prophylactic low-dose heparin has been suggested to prevent venous thrombosis and embolic episodes.

Various specific treatments have been advocated in case reports but their efficacy remains unclear. These include anticholinergics, dopamine agonists (e.g., bromocriptine and amantadine), dantrolene, lorazepam, and ECT. The data so far seem to support most strongly the use of bromocriptine and dantrolene. Bromocriptine, a dopamine agonist, has been used in dosages ranging from 7.5–60 mg/day, in divided doses every eight hours, intravenously at the beginning (Dhib-Jalbut et al., 1983; Granato et al., 1983; Mueller, Vester, & Fermaglich, 1983; Zubenko & Pope, 1983). Amantadine, another dopamine agonist, has been used in doses of 100 mg b.i.d. with some anecdotal success (Amdurski et al., 1983; McCarron, Boettger, & Peck, 1982).

Dantrolene has been the most frequently tried; it is a direct-acting muscle relaxant affecting calcium release from the sarcoplasmic reticulum, and used successfully in treating malignant hyperthermia. It has been used in NMS in a dose range of 0.8–2.5 mg/kg every six hours (oral regimens ranged from 100–300 mg/daily in divided doses for two to three days) (Coons, Hillman, & Marshall, 1982; Goekoop & Carbaat, 1982; Kahn et al., 1985; May et al., 1983; Zubenko & Pope, 1983). Anticholinergic agents have not been found to be useful (Karoff, 1980; Levenson, 1985). ECT has been reported to be useful but may result in lethal cardiac arrhythmias (Jessee & Anderson, 1983). Lorazepam may be a safe and useful drug (Fricchione et al., 1983). Further experience is necessary before routinely recommending these agents. Reintroduction of neuroleptics in post-NMS cases must be done very cautiously, preferably with a low potency neuroleptic to avoid possible recurrence of the syndrome (Mueller, Vester, & Fermaglich, 1983; Scarlett, Zimmerman, & Berkovic, 1983). Although NMS cases have been reported to resolve without residual symptoms, the writer has noted two cases followed by permanent brain damage manifested as severe frontal lobe syndrome with catatonic-like symptoms, severe perseveration, gait disturbance, and dementia.

10B: DEMENTIA

The term *dementia*, as currently used, does not carry the prognostic connotation of a progressive or irreversible course implied in the past. Depending on the underlying organic etiology, dementia may be reversible or irreversible. Its clinical course may be progressive, static, or remitting. Most of the causes of Organic Mental Disorders listed in Table 1 may produce dementia, either as a primary disorder (e.g., Primary Degenerative [Alzheimer's type] Dementia) or as a secondary disorder, often progressing from an initial phase of delirium (e.g., protracted cerebral hypoxia, hypoglycemia).

The differential diagnosis of reversible dementias is of great prognostic significance. Early diagnosis of these disorders is of utmost importance. Dementia must be differentiated from delirium (no clouding of consciousness in dementia), Amnestic Syndrome (deficit involves only memory), and from the so-called "pseudodementia," a form of depression masquerading as dementia, which must always be ruled out before the diagnosis is made (Caine, 1981).

General Therapeutic Principles

The following general guidelines apply to the treatment and management of all dementias, with special emphasis on those arising in the senium. Treatment may be etiologic (when the cause is known and treatable) and/or symptomatic.

Etiologic Treatment

In searching for a treatable cause, first consideration should be given to ruling out depressive pseudodementia. A trial treatment with antidepressants may be justified in the absence of demonstrable etiology. The next step is to search for possible treatable organic causes (Cummings, Benson, & LoVerme, 1980), especially when an etiologic diagnosis remains uncertain. This is particularly important in older patients, who are more likely to be diagnosed as suffering from Alzheimer's disease or Multi-infarct Dementia, often in the absence of any objective evidence. A diagnostic battery for screening etiologically treatable dementias often includes the following tests (McAllister & Price, 1982; Wells, 1979):

- Serology test for syphilis
- Complete blood count
- Serum B12, folate, T3 or T4
- Urinalysis
- Metabolic screen
- Drug screen
- Computerized axial tomography (CT-scan)

Additional examination and laboratory procedures may be needed (e.g., magnetic resonance imaging [MRI], serum electrolytes, HIV screening [for high-risk persons]).

Symptomatic Treatment

This is the only therapeutic approach available for those patients suffering from irreversible forms of dementia. Since the cognitive deficit of irreversible dementia is not amenable to any treatment, all therapeutic efforts are directed toward improving impaired functions, promoting general health, and treating psychiatric complications when they develop.

Demented patients, especially the elderly, must maintain the best possible physical health in order to prevent the consequences of physiological derangement of their already compromised cerebral functions. Every effort should be made to restore or improve impaired physical functions (e.g., renal, cardiovascular, respiratory, or endocrine), combat symptoms (pain, insomnia, constipation, impaired mobility), improve impaired hearing and vision, and maintain an optimal nutritional state.

The prevention of toxic effects of medication, prescribed or over-the-counter, is of particular importance, especially those resulting from drug interactions. Elderly patients are particularly susceptible to side effects because of decreased physiologic reserves and slower rates of absorption, metabolism, and elimination of many drugs (Salzman, Shader, & Pearlman, 1970). Demented patients are highly vulnerable to the development of secondary psychiatric disorders, including delirium, depression, and psychosis. The following is a brief review of the treatment of some common psychiatric problems in dementia.

Insomnia. This is a ubiquitous complaint of the elderly. Demented patients often cannot fall asleep as a result of becoming disoriented and frightened when the lights are turned out. The first measure to recommend is leaving a light on all night. Patients with sleep-onset insomnia may benefit from L-tryptophan, which can be prescribed as a pill or provided through high tryptophan foods such as milk or tuna fish.

When drug treatment becomes necessary, antihistamines in low doses are well tolerated (e.g., promethazine hydrochloride 25–50 mg or diphenhydramine 25–50 mg at bedtime) (Salzman, 1982). Antihistamines at higher doses may induce anticholinergic delirium. Thioridazine 25 mg is also effective and well tolerated. Chloral hydrate in doses 250–500 mg is recommended as the next least toxic drug. The hypnotic benzodiazepines (e.g., flurazepam, triazolam, temazepam), although the most widely prescribed hypnotics, work only for a few weeks, and the longer half-life ones (e.g., flurazepam) tend to produce unwanted daytime drowsiness, ataxia, and confusion. Insomnia secondary to another disorder (e.g., depression) should be treated etiologically.

Anxiety. Benzodiazepines are the drugs of choice for treating nonpsychotic anxiety states when psychological approaches fail to control the symptoms. In choosing a suitable benzodiazepine for the elderly demented patient, the clinician must take into consideration the kinetics and biotransformation of the various representatives of this class of anxiolytics (see Symptomatic Treatment section on Delirium). The long-acting chlordiazepoxide and diazepam are undesirable because of cumulative effects. The short-acting oxazepam and lorazepam are preferred, prescribed in approximately one-third to one-half of the younger adult dose. Excessive sedation, apathy, ataxia, incoordination, disorientation, confusion, and dysarthria are common toxic effects (Salzman, 1982).

Agitation. Restlessness, wandering around, and agitation are commonly seen in elderly demented patients. These symptoms tend to be more severe in the evening and at night ("sundowner syndrome") and are often part of a psychosis. Neuroleptics have been shown to be effective. In a recent review by Salzman (1987), neuroleptics show a therapeutic response of "good to excellent" in 60%–70% of elderly agitated patients with a wide variety of organic and emotional disorders. No therapeutic differences among neuroleptics can be inferred.

Delirium. This is the most common psychiatric complication, especially in patients with Multi-infarct Dementia. Various drugs, especially anticholinergic, are very common causes of delirium in the elderly. For treatment, see section on Delirium.

Depression. Treatment of depression includes various psychotherapeutic approaches, antidepressant medication, and ECT (Ban, 1987b; Butler, 1975). In milder forms of dementia, supportive psychotherapy is useful in assisting the patient to grieve and accept cognitive losses and their consequences, and to maintain self-esteem. Psychotherapeutic management approaches are directed toward enhancing environmental–social support throughout the course of dementia.

In the presence of severe depression, tri- or tetracyclic antidepressants have been the preferred drugs. The choice of a specific tricyclic depends on clinical considerations as modified by the altered metabolism of the elderly (Hrdina et al., 1980; Robinson, 1979). Several side effects of the tricyclics are especially hazardous for the elderly, because aging increases plasma half-life and steady-state plasma levels, especially with imipramine and amitriptyline. Side effects include sedation, orthostatic hypotension, anticholinergic effects, and cardiotoxicity.

The higher sedating effects of certain tricyclics (amitriptyline, doxepin) may be desirable in some patients for controlling insomnia, with two-thirds or more of the daily dose given before bedtime. The hypotensive effect of tricyclics does not seem to increase with advancing age (Glassman et al., 1979; Roose et al., 1981); nevertheless, orthostatic hypotension is a very common side effect and may precipitate falls, strokes, or heart attacks. Nortriptyline, compared with imipramine, produces less hypotension (Roose et al., 1981).

Anticholinergic activity is especially prominent with amitriptyline, while desipramine, and to a lesser extent nortriptyline, have the least anticholinergic action. Trazodone has little or none. Elderly demented patients are particularly vulnerable to CNS anticholinergic toxicity, with one-third of patients on tricyclics being reported to develop confusion or delirium (Davies et al., 1971). Cardiotoxicity is of particular concern; tricyclics may produce sinus tachycardia, prolonged intraventricular conduction, and probably decreased myocardial contractility, as well as arrhythmias (Bigger et al., 1978). Imipramine appears to have antiarrhythmic properties.

In view of the above, the tricyclics of choice are desipramine, nortriptyline, and doxepin. Of the three, desipramine is the least anticholinergic, and doxepin the least cardiotoxic (Salzman, 1982; Salzman et al., 1970). The so-called second generation antidepressants (e.g., maprotiline, amoxapine, trazodone) are reported to have fewer anticholinergic and cardiovascular side effects and therefore may present some advantage over the older tricyclics in the treatment of the elderly patient, a claim which has not been well documented (Gerner et al.,

1980). The recently introduced fluoxetine Hcl (Prozac) may prove to be a better tolerated alternative.

The following general guidelines apply in prescribing tricyclic drugs for the elderly demented patient:

1. Obtain a pretreatment electrocardiogram and repeat ECG periodically during course of treatment.
2. Measure seated and standing blood pressure before treatment is started and before each increase in dose.
3. Start with very low doses (e.g., 20–40 mg, imipramine equivalent, daily in divided doses) and raise dose gradually, monitoring both therapeutic response and side effects (50–150 mg, imipramine equivalent, per day is the usual therapeutic range).
4. Give two-thirds of the dose before bedtime to promote sleep.
5. The concurrent administration of volume-depleting diuretics increases risk of orthostatic hypotension.
6. Exercise extreme caution in patients with preexisting cardiovascular disease and patients receiving quinidine or procainamide, and be fully familiar with contraindicated drug combinations (clonidine, guanethidine, or bethanidine).
7. Monitor tricyclic plasma levels regularly, in order to prevent cumulative toxic levels (Salzman, 1982).

Monoamine oxidase inhibitors (MAOIs), such as phenelzine (Nardil) and tranylcypromine (Parnate), have been shown to be effective antidepressants, which are safe and well tolerated by the elderly (Jenike, 1985). Their major advantage over the tricyclics is that they lack anticholinergic and cardiotoxic effects.

Electroconvulsive therapy (ECT) may be indicated in depressed demented patients without posterior fossa space-occupying lesions who fail to respond to an adequate course of antidepressants and patients who cannot tolerate the side effects or adverse effects of tricyclics or MAOIs (Salzman, 1975).

Psychosis. Psychotic symptoms are amenable to treatment with neuroleptic drugs, which, although equally effective in controlling psychotic thinking and behavior, differ in side effects and toxicity (Hamilton, 1966). As with the tricyclics, the choice of a specific antipsychotic agent should be based on considerations regarding toxicity and altered metabolism in the elderly (Salzman, 1982, 1987). Common side effects of neuroleptic drugs which may have serious consequences include sedation, orthostatic hypotension, anticholinergic effects, and extrapyramidal symptoms. Impaired thermoregulation and idiosyncratic reactions should also be noted.

Although the sedative effects of neuroleptics may be used therapeutically to induce sleep at night or tranquilize the agitated patient during daytime, they often produce confusion and disorientation in the elderly. Low potency neuroleptics (chlorpromazine, thioridazine, mesoridazine, chlorprothixene) have the strongest sedative effects, while the high potency neuroleptics (haloperidol, fluphenazine, perphenazine, trifluoperazine, thiothixene) are least sedative. Low potency neuroleptics also have the strongest autonomic effects (hypotensive and anticholinergic) but show fewer extrapyramidal side effects. Conversely, high potency neuroleptics have minimal autonomic effects but very frequent extrapyramidal side effects.

Although high potency neuroleptics are generally safer and the drugs of choice for patients in whom autonomic and sedative effects are most hazardous, low potency neuroleptics (e.g., thioridazine) in small doses may be more appropriate for restless and agitated psychotic patients and those who are sensitive to extrapyramidal reactions (Steele, Lucas, & Tune, 1986). Elderly demented patients are particularly susceptible to orthostatic hypotension (Blumenthal & Davie, 1980), as well as to central anticholinergic toxicity (confusion, delirium) and extrapyramidal effects (Raskind & Risse, 1986; Salzman, 1982; Salzman et al., 1970). Neuroleptic treatment should begin with small amounts of the medication, given in divided doses (e.g., haloperidol 0.5-2 mg daily, or thioridazine 25-75 mg daily).

Patient Management
Effective management of the demented patient demands commitment on the part of the physician to accepting the responsibility for continuing care to a chronically ill and, in most instances, progressively deteriorating patient (Plutzky, 1974). The traditional medical model is expanded to include additional roles required for dealing with social and family problems confronting the patient and his or her caretakers.

The physician is often called upon to coordinate the activities of several caregivers including family members, social workers, visiting nurses, in-house aides, and other social service personnel. Knowledge of available community resources and how they can be utilized in the total care of the demented patient is a prerequisite. Knowledge of the patient's medical and psychological needs, family resources and interpersonal dynamics, assets and liabilities, prognosis, and anticipated problems are all crucial for treatment planning.

The physician should maintain continuing interaction with family members, inform them about the patient's condition, advise them about property management, and involve them in the patient's treatment. He or she should also provide emotional support and assist with their feelings of shame, guilt, or anger, especially when they must make decisions about institutional placement of the patient. Relatives often become highly critical of the physician or nursing home staff as a means of coping with feelings of guilt or helplessness. These reactions can be prevented or resolved through ventilation and moral support.

The doctor–patient relationship should remain a significant focus through the course of the illness. This is most important earlier in progressive dementias and in those patients with nonprogressive dementias, such as those which follow an acute brain insult (e.g., head trauma, encephalitis, anoxia, and hypoglycemic syndromes). The physician should structure each visit with the patient to provide psychological support by allaying fears, counteracting the sense of helplessness, allowing ventilation of feelings, enhancing self-esteem, encouraging independence, strengthening healthier coping mechanisms, and correcting distortions of reality when present.

Rehabilitation through retraining is needed for those patients with milder residual deficit and nonprogressive dementias. Every effort should be made to maintain ambulation and prevent regression to wheelchair or bed. Other guidelines in the management of the demented patient include encouragement of efforts toward maximum feasible independence and self-care; engagement in pleasurable, useful, or productive activities that enhance self-esteem; maintenance of preserved skills and abilities, as well as physical fitness; and appropriate supervision to prevent consequences of poor memory (e.g., fire hazards, getting lost, poor nutrition, deterioration of personal hygiene) or impaired social judgment (e.g., poor management of financial matters and personal affairs).

Appropriate manipulation of the patient's physical environment, whether in an institution or at home, is an important means of supporting impaired cognitive function, such as memory and orientation, and impaired sensory perception. Environmental modulation to establish a "prosthetic environment" for the demented patient includes good room lighting; simple, stable, and familiar furnishings; clocks that sound the time and large calendars on the wall; note pads as memory aids; pill boxes; hearing aids; eyeglasses; dentures; handrails; a walker, and so forth.

SPECIFIC DEMENTIAS

The preceding section dealt with the nonspecific, symptomatic treatment of Dementia without reference to etiology. *DSM-III-R* codes for dementia of unknown etiology include Axis I diagnoses when an unspecified psychoactive substance is suspected (292.82) and Axis III diagnoses for all other unknown etiologies (294.10). The following section discusses specific treatments of dementia of known etiology. The previously described basic principles of symptomatic treatment and supportive management of dementia are also applicable to these disorders.

From a clinical standpoint (prognostic and therapeutic) it is useful to classify dementias into these which are irreversible and reversible.

Irreversible dementias are associated with permanent neuronal damage and may be (a) progressive or (b) residual (nonprogressive). *Progressive dementias* have a relentless course toward a vegetative state and death. They include Primary Degenerative Dementia of the Alzheimer type (Senile and Presenile Onset), Multi-infarct Dementia, and other less common disorders such as Huntington's chorea, progressive supranuclear palsy, and Parkinson's disease. *Residual (nonprogressive) dementias* include those secondary dementias resulting from cerebral trauma, protracted cerebral hypoxia or hypoglycemia, and other permanent but nonprogressive injuries to the brain. The latter are of great clinical significance because the underlying cerebral disorder can be prevented, arrested, or fully reversed or eliminated if appropriate etiologic treatment is applied early (Cummings, Benson, & LoVerme, 1980).

Reversible dementias are syndromes with a treatable underlying organic disorder. They are of great significance prognostically and therapeutically. The substance-induced dementias (e.g., bromides, barbiturates, steroids), for example, are eminently treatable. The *DSM-III-R* classifies dementias of known etiology into the following categories: (1) Dementias Arising in the Senium and Presenium (290.XX); (2) Psychoactive Substance-Induced Dementias (291.20, 292.82); and (3) Dementias Associated with Axis III Physical Disorders or Conditions (294.10).

1. Dementias Arising in the Senium and Presenium

290.xx Primary Degenerative Dementia of the Alzheimer Type, Senile Onset

290.1x Primary Degenerative Dementia of the Alzheimer Type, Presenile Onset

These are the most common dementias in the elderly, affecting 7% of the population over 65 years of age and accounting for 25%–30% of all cases of dementia (Cummings, 1987; Cummings & Benson, 1983). The dementia begins insidiously and progresses slowly, first with symptoms of memory loss followed by progressive intellectual impairment and personality changes, and later with symptoms of aphasia and apraxia, finally reaching a vegetative state after 8–10 years or longer (Reisberg et al., 1987). Compared to patients with Multi-infarct Dementia, patients with Alzheimer's dementia seem to enjoy relatively good physical health.

The etiology of this neurodegenerative disorder remains unknown. Some cases appear to have a familial occurrence (Heston et al., 1981). Recent advances in the neurochemistry of Alzheimer's disease have revealed striking neurotransmitter changes and characteristic cellular proteins (Davies & Wolozin, 1987). Acetylcholine deficit is of particular research and clinical interest, as shown by loss of cortical markers of the cholinergic system: for example, decreased choline acetyltransferase (Davies & Maloney, 1976; Perry et al., 1977), loss of the cholinergic neurons in the nucleus basalis of Meynert (Whitehouse et al., 1982), and decrease of M2 muscarinic receptors (Mash, Flynn, & Potter, 1985).

Apparently, the ventral forebrain cholinergic neurons projecting to the cerebral cortex and hippocampus are the most consistently and severely damaged. Using monoclonal antibodies to ventral forebrain tissue from patients who died with Alzheimer's disease, Wolozin et al. (1986) identified a protein, Az-50, which is an interesting marker of Alzheimer's disease.

On the evidence of a cholinergic deficit associated with Alzheimer's dementia, a number of studies have tested the therapeutic efficacy of the available cholinomimetic drugs. So far, efforts to reverse or arrest cognitive deficit with the use of acetylcholine agonists or precursors have failed to provide significant results. Choline and phosphatidyl choline (PhosChol), dietary precursors of acetylcholine, have been found to be ineffective in improving the cognitive deficit (Thal et al., 1981), probably because these substances do not substantially affect cholinergic activity.

Clinical trials with I.V. physostigmine indicate transient enhancement of memory performance of patients with Alzheimer's disease (Christie et al., 1981; Davis et al., 1982). One major disadvantage of this drug, besides its side effects, is its plasma half-life of only about 30 minutes. Oral physostigmine in doses of 2 mg every two hours for several days was found to be beneficial (Mohs et al., 1985).

Available long-acting cholinesterase inhibitors and cholinergic agonists such as isoflurophate and oxotremorine, respectively, have potentially serious toxicity. Oral tetrahydroaminoacridine (THA), a centrally active anticholinesterase, was recently found by Summers et al. (1986)

in preliminary long-term trials to produce significant cognitive improvement. Several controlled studies using THA are currently under way. There is some interest in studying the efficacy of the so-called nootropic drugs, such as piracetam, and ACTH-4-10 (Cole & Braconnier, 1980; Reisberg, Ferris, & Gershon, 1981; Salzman, 1979), as well as intravenous naloxone (Reisberg et al., 1982).

Numerous other drugs have been used in the treatment of Alzheimer's dementia with questionable results, including central nervous system stimulants (e.g., pentylenetetrazol, amphetamines, and amphetamine-like drugs), cerebral vasodilators (e.g., papaverine), anabolic substances, and dihydroergotoxine mesylate (Hydergine). Hydergine, a dehydrogenated ergot alkaloid, in sublingual doses of 1–2 mg three times daily, has received some support as a means of improving cognitive function in the early phase of primary degenerative dementia (Ban, 1978a; Lehman & Ban, 1975; vonLoveren-Huyben et al., 1984; Yesavage et al., 1979).

Treatment of Alzheimer's dementia continues to be symptomatic-supportive, as already described in the general section of dementia. Proper patient management and family counseling are essential, and the only substantive services the physician can currently offer (Reisberg, 1982; Reisberg, Ferris, & Gershon, 1981).

The use of neuroleptics in the treatment of behavior symptoms in senile dementia of the Alzheimer type has recently been reevaluated. Earlier studies had shown that the target symptoms of agitation, hyperactivity, assaultiveness, irritability, and hallucinations are controlled by neuroleptics in 60% of patients (Rada & Kellner, 1976). However, several recent well designed placebo-controlled studies of neuroleptic medications in behaviorally disturbed dementia patients (mostly primary degenerative) have shown efficacy by global ratings in only one-third of the patients (Raskind & Risse, 1986).

Petrie et al. (1982) found only 32% of loxapine-treated patients (mean dose 22 mg/day) and 35% of haloperidol-treated patients (mean dose 4.6 mg/day) were globally rated as moderately or markedly improved. Target symptoms most responsive to the active drugs included suspiciousness, hallucinatory behavior, excitement, hostility, and uncooperativeness. Similarly, in a study by Barnes et al. (1982), thioridazine (mean dose 62.5 mg/day) and loxapine (mean dose 10.5 mg/day) produced marked or moderate global improvement in only one-third of the patients. Anxiety, excitement, and uncooperativeness were the most drug-responsive target symptoms. Steele et al. (1986) found both haloperidol (1, 2, and 5 mg/day) and thioridazine (25, 50, and 75 mg/

day) effective for managing behavioral symptoms in senile dementia of the Alzheimer type.

290.4x Multi-infarct Dementia
This is the second most common of the progressive dementias arising in the senium. It is characterized by a stepwise deteriorating course, focal neurological signs and symptoms, and evidence of significant cerebrovascular disease. Hypertension is a very common concomitant disorder. It is thought to be due to widespread multiple cerebral infarctions, secondary to cerebral arteriosclerosis. Risk factors predisposing to Multi-infarct Dementia include positive family history, hypertension, high serum cholesterol, serum triglyceride and lipoprotein profile associated with atherosclerosis, obesity, and smoking.

There is no known effective method for reversing or arresting the course of this dementia. Various drugs, such as anticoagulants, vasodilators (Hydergine, papaverine), and lipotropic enzymes have been proposed for altering the course of vascular disease (Cole & Braconnier, 1980; Lehman & Ban, 1975; Salzman, 1982). No reported controlled studies clearly prove the value of any of these agents. Recent reports on the potential usefulness of anti-platelet-agglutinating drugs, such as aspirin, in reducing the risk of infarction in patients with transient ischemic attacks may have some relevance in the treatment of Multi-infarct Dementia (Cole & Broconnier, 1980; Gaitz, Varner, & Overall, 1977; Hass, 1979). See also section on Multi-infarct Dementia with Delirium.

2. Psychoactive Substance-Induced Dementias
These are reversible dementias. The *DSM-III-R* lists on Axis I the following psychoactive substance-induced dementias of known etiology:

291.20 Dementia Associated with Alcoholism
Alcohol dementia is presumed to be caused by prolonged, heavy alcohol abuse. Its etiology is still controversial. It needs to be differentiated from subacute Wernicke-Korsakoff, traumatic, and hepatic encephalopathy. It is associated with greater than 10 years history of drinking and is nonprogressing if alcohol-free. There is evidence for cortical atrophy which may subside following prolonged abstinence (Francis & Franklin, 1987). There is no established specific treatment of this dementia. Abstinence from alcohol, use of thiamine, and good nutrition are recommended.

292.82 Other Psychoactive Substance Dementia

Numerous drugs have been reported to cause reversible dementia following long-term use or chronic intoxication. The most commonly implicated drugs include sedative-hypnotic-anxiolytics, other psychoactive drugs (e.g., lithium carbonate, cyclic antidepressants), beta blockers (e.g., propranolol), methyldopa (especially combined with haloperidol), clonidine (especially combined with fluphenazine), phenytoin, anticholinergic compounds, disulfiram, oral hypoglycemics, anti-inflammatory agents, cimetidine, digitalis, quinidine, L-dopa, diuretics, narcotics (Stoudemire & Thompson, 1981). Steroids can also produce dementia-like decline in cognitive functioning mimicking early Alzheimer's disease (Varney, Alexander, & MacIndoe, 1984). These dementias clear following discontinuation or reduction of medications.

3. Dementias Associated With Axis III Physical Disorders or Conditions

Most of the conditions listed in Table 1 may produce dementia coded as 294.10. They may be irreversible or reversible. Neurologic disorders associated with irreversible dementia include intracranial infections (e.g., encephalitis, Creutzfeldt-Jacob disease, neurosyphilis, HIV subacute encephalopathy in AIDS (Hoffman, 1984; Nichols & Ostrow, 1984), degenerative diseases (Pick's disease, Huntington's chorea, Parkinson's disease, progressive supranuclear palsy [Martin & Black, 1987]), vascular disorders (thrombotic and embolic strokes, Binswanger's disease, etc.), cerebral injury, intracranial space-occupying lesions (tumors, subdural hematoma, colloid cyst, etc.), and other CNS disorders (temporal lobe epilepsy, multiple sclerosis, etc.). Of particular interest are dementias caused by heavy metals and industrial poisons (lead, carbon monoxide), systemic lupus erythematosus, hypertensive encephalopathy, porphyria, Wilson's disease, hypoxia–anoxia, vitamin deficiencies (e.g., B1, B12), normal pressure hydrocephalus, carotid artery occlusal, temporal arteritis, cerebral abscess, Lyme disease, and other disorders. Early treatment of these last mentioned disorders may prevent the development of dementia or reverse it.

Eminently reversible dementias include endocrinopathies (hypothyroidism, Addison's disease), metabolic encephalopathies (diabetic acidosis, hepatic and renal failure, dialysis dementia), electrolyte/water imbalance, hypoxia due to cardiac or pulmonary disease, and Sjörgen's syndrome. It is beyond the scope of this book to review the specific treatments of these disorders.

Chapter 11

Syndromes Similar to Functional Disorders

11A: ORGANIC AMNESTIC SYNDROME
The Organic Amnestic Syndrome is characterized by a selective cognitive impairment in short- and long-term memory. The syndrome occurs in a state of clear awareness (differentiating it from Delirium) and without any significant loss of the remaining intellectual abilities (differentiating it from Dementia).

The syndrome results from bilateral lesions of specific diencephalic or medial temporal lobe structures (e.g., hippocampal formation, mammillary bodies, fornix, and structures in the floor and walls of the third ventricle). The lesions may be reversible or irreversible, depending on the etiology of the causative disorder.

Conditions associated with Amnestic Syndrome of either transient or persistent course include thiamine deficiency (e.g., Wernicke-Korsakoff syndrome), head trauma, carbon monoxide poisoning, subarachnoid hemorrhage, herpes simplex encephalitis, brain tumor, bilateral posterior cerebral arterial occlusion, and cerebral hypoxia. Conditions associated with transient amnestic syndrome include temporal lobe epilepsy, migraine attacks, chronic drug intoxication (e.g., barbiturates, bromides, isoniazid), and electroconvulsive therapy.

Treatment
Treatment is etiologic (when cause is known and treatable) and symptomatic. There is no symptomatic treatment to correct the cognitive

deficit in memory. Physostigmine may improve the Amnestic Syndrome after herpes simplex encephalitis (Peters & Levin, 1977). Memory therapy (teaching the patient to use visual mnemonics) may be helpful to patients with preserved ability to retrieve visual images (Patten, 1972). Specialized rehabilitation programs in "cognitive retraining" are especially valuable, particularly for those with head trauma (Kwentus et al. 1985; Lezak, 1978).

Patient Management
Management approaches are similar to those described for demented patients. However, it should be noted that, compared with demented patients, amnestic patients suffer from a more circumscribed cognitive deficit, maintain relatively intact verbal capacities, and are less vulnerable to developing major psychiatric complications. Although institutionalized custodial care may be necessary for patients with more severe forms, most of these patients can be cared for at home or in a supervised, structured environment. Efforts at rehabilitation of patients with milder syndromes should always be part of the management plan.

SPECIFIC ORGANIC AMNESTIC DISORDERS
The *DSM-III-R* classifies organic amnestic disorders into substance-induced codes on Axis I, and others coded on Axis III.

1. Psychoactive Substance-Induced Amnestic Disorders
The most commonly implicated substances are alcohol and sedative-hypnotic drugs.

291.10 Alcohol Amnestic Disorder
This thiamine deficiency syndrome, also known as Wernicke-Korsakoff syndrome, is the most common amnestic syndrome. It is secondary to the nutritional deficit associated with chronic alcoholism. Brain lesions associated with thiamine deficiency include bilateral sclerosis of the mammillary bodies (Benson, 1978) and degenerative changes in the dorsal nucleus of the thalamus (Victor et al., 1971). In the majority of cases the onset is acute, presenting as a sequela of Wernicke's encephalopathy; a smaller number of patients experience an insidious onset without a preceding acute encephalopathic episode (Adams, 1983).

The reversibility of the Wernicke-Korsakoff syndrome depends on the promptness of instituting specific treatment with thiamine. Thiamine should initially be given parenterally in doses of 50 mg daily for about one week, and then be switched to oral administration, provided that the patient is able to resume a normal diet. This treatment should be continued for several months, with a supplement of B-complex vitamins. A five-year follow-up study by Victor, Adams, & Collins (1971) revealed that 20% recovered completely, 28% were significantly improved, and 25% were slightly improved; the remainder remained unimproved. There is no effective treatment of the residual memory deficit.

Clonidine, an alpha-norepinephrine agonist, has been reported to improve memory and recall at doses of 0.3 mg b.i.d. (McEntee & Mair, 1980; Mair & McEntee, 1986). On the other hand, propranolol, a beta adrenergic blocker, has been used for the control of rage reactions (Yudofsky et al., 1984).

292.83 Sedative, Hypnotic, Anxiolytic Amnestic Disorder

The syndrome develops following prolonged heavy use of this category of drugs. The benzodiazepines are of particular interest because they are extensively used as anxiolytics and night sedatives. Benzodiazepines show significant differences in amnesia-inducing potency, with the short- and intermediate-acting compounds (lorazepam, triazolam) having greater amnestic effects than longer-acting benzodiazepines (e.g., clorazepate) (Brown et al., 1982; Healey et al., 1980; McKay & Dundee, 1980; Scharf et al., 1984). This is particularly relevant to the use of these drugs in the geriatric population. Discontinuation of the drug generally leads to complete recovery (see Intoxication in Chapter 12). Treatment of drug abuse and rehabilitation are indispensable aspects of management (see Psychoactive Substance Use Disorders, Chapter 13).

292.83 Other Psychoactive Substance-Induced Amnestic Disorders

Several other drugs have been reported to produce amnestic disorders, including bromides, isoniazid, and anticholinergic agents. Anticholinergic drugs, including tricyclic antidepressants, antihistamines, and antiparkinsonian drugs, are extensively used and, therefore, more likely to be implicated in amnestic syndromes, especially in the elderly.

2. Amnestic Disorders Associated with Axis III Physical Disorders or Conditions

The following is a brief review of the most significant disorders (coded 294.00) associated with amnestic phenomena.

Transient Global Amnesia (TGA). The syndrome occurs in middle-aged or elderly individuals and consists of sudden loss of recent memory lasting from minutes to hours. It is thought to be due to episodic transient vascular insufficiency of the mesial temporal lobe (Sluping et al., 1980), possibly resulting from stenosis or occlusion of the posterior cerebral artery (Mathew & Meyer, 1974).

Thiamine Deficiency States. Besides alcoholism, thiamine deficiency may be seen in a number of conditions including malabsorption, eating disorders, patients undergoing hemodialysis and patients with disseminated malignancies (McEvoy, 1981).

Neurological Disorders. These include head trauma with damage to diencephalic or temporal regions, brain tumors encroaching on the same cerebral regions, bilateral hippocampal infarctions due to thrombosis or embolism of posterior cerebral arteries, herpes simplex encephalitis, cerebral anoxic states, carbon monoxide poisoning and heavy metal poisoning (lead) (Benson, 1978; Benson, Marsden, & Meadows, 1974; Lipowski, 1980).

The treatment of the above disorders is beyond the scope of this book.

Temporal Lobe Epilepsy. This is characterized by brief amnestic episodes that rarely persist for hours and during which the EEG shows ictal dysrhythmia attributed to seizure foci localized in the limbic system. Treatment aims at control of seizures with anticonvulsant drugs. In selected cases, temporal lobectomy may be indicated for intractable seizures.

11B: ORGANIC HALLUCINOSIS

Organic Hallucinosis is a syndrome characterized by recurrent or persistent hallucinations attributable to specific organic factors judged to be etiologically related to the disturbance. The hallucinations are the only essential feature, occurring in a state of clear awareness (differentiating hallucinosis from delirium) and in the absence of a formal thought disturbance.

Specific conditions producing Organic Hallucinosis include substance abuse (e.g., alcohol, hallucinogens, cocaine), drug toxicity (e.g., levodopa, bromocriptine), temporal lobe epilepsy, space-occupying lesions of the brain, migraine, temporal arteritis, loss of hearing or vision, and other situations involving sensory deprivation. The course and prognosis of organic hallucinosis vary greatly, depending on the underlying pathology.

Treatment

The major focus is on identification of the underlying specific disorder in order to be able to institute appropriate etiologic treatment. The most common etiology is substance abuse, especially alcohol and hallucinogens, but other sources must be sought.

Methods of symptomatic control of hallucinations vary according to the underlying source. For instance, ictal hallucinations and hallucinogen flashbacks may be controlled with antiepileptic drugs or diazepam. A patient suffering from alcoholic hallucinosis or accompanying delusions may require neuroleptics.

Patient Management

Management approaches must be directed toward both the underlying illness and the reactive psychopathology which may be present. Patients with substance abuse, for example, require special efforts to engage them in a comprehensive rehabilitation program (see Psychoactive Substance Use Disorders, Chapter 13). Epileptics, have special psychological, social, and vocational needs that should be dealt with as part of their total treatment plan. Patients suffering irreversible loss of vision or hearing require social stimulation to counteract sensory deprivation.

Reactive psychopathology may require psychiatric management. Anxious, agitated, or frightened patients must be calmed and reassured. Suicidal tendencies or extreme fear or agitation may make hospitalization necessary.

ORGANIC HALLUCINOSIS—SPECIFIC DISORDERS

Psychoactive Substance-Induced Hallucinoses

The most commonly implicated substances are alcohol and hallucinogens.

291.30 Alcohol Hallucinosis

Alcoholic Hallucinosis consists of vivid auditory hallucinations developing shortly (usually within 48 hours) after cessation or reduction of heavy ingestion of alcohol in an individual who apparently has alcohol dependence. The course usually consists of an acute phase typically lasting less than one week, but in some cases (25%) it may be followed by a chronic phase that may last several months, and may be clinically indistinguishable from schizophrenia.

Treatment of the acute phase is similar to that of alcohol withdrawal (see Treatment section on Withdrawal and Withdrawal Deliria, Chapter 12). The "detoxification" procedure includes benzodiazepines, rest, vitamins, and nutritional supplements. The chronic phase is treated with neuroleptic drugs and supportive psychotherapy in a manner similar to that of Schizophreniform Disorder.

305.30 Hallucinogen Hallucinosis

This refers to the typical "trip" induced by hallucinogen intoxication (LSD, MDT, mescaline, psilocybin, etc.). Large doses of cannabis or tetrahydrocannabinol (THC) may also result in hallucinosis. These patients are typically seen in emergency rooms, frequently brought in by friends or the police. The duration of the syndrome varies according to the type of hallucinogen, lasting about six hours for LSD, and from under an hour to a day or two for other hallucinogens. If the syndrome persists longer than 24 hours, it is classified as a Hallucinogen Delusional Disorder or a Hallucinogen Mood Disorder, depending on whether the symptoms are delusional or affective in nature (see corresponding sections below).

The treatment and management of Hallucinogen Hallucinosis are the same as for the "bad tripper" (Berger & Tinklenberg, 1979; Greenblatt & Shader, 1975; Solursh & Clement, 1968; Taylor, Maurer, & Tinklenberg, 1975). The physician should be familiar with the street patterns of drug abuse, the current code names of various illicit drugs, and their clinical manifestations.

The first step is to place the patient in a quiet room, under supervision, for protection from external stimulation and potential consequences of his or her behavior. The second step is to attempt to identify the nature of the drug taken, the amount involved, and the time that has elapsed since it was ingested. It is also helpful to inquire about previous exposures to hallucinogens and the patient's reaction to them. Unfortunately, information obtained from the patient or friends is very often unreliable. Illicit drugs are frequently adulterated ("cut") with other toxic drugs, such as atropine and strychnine, which may present serious treatment complications, especially if the patient is treated with anticholinergic drugs.

The symptom that usually brings the patient to the emergency room is the fear that he or she is going to "lose control" or that he or she will "never come down." This frightening feeling is further aggravated by bizarre illusions and hallucinations, depersonalization, distortions of the body image, and delusions (Balis, 1974). There are two types of treatment approaches in managing the "bad tripper": the "talk-down" method and medications. Generally, "talk-down" is the recommended one, because medications may aggravate intoxication of obscure etiology.

Talk-down. The basic goal is to provide continuing reassurance and defining of reality through the establishment of verbal contact with the patient. The therapist tries to reassure the patient about the transient nature of the experience and the forthcoming "coming down"; provides empathic support; and repetitively defines the reality of the patient's experience, reducing distortions, while the patient is encouraged to describe what is happening to him or her. Communications should consist of repeated, simple, concrete statements. As the patient is improving, he or she should be told to anticipate an "in-and-out" phase during which there is a waxing and waning of awareness. This method requires considerable time and effort that may not be available in an emergency room (Berger & Tinklenberg, 1979; Greenblatt & Shader, 1975; Taylor, Maurer, & Tinklenberg, 1975).

Medications. Medications are recommended when the patient is inaccessible to or fails to respond to verbal contact, or when there is not sufficient time to spare for "talking him down." Neuroleptics are relatively contraindicated, although effective, primarily because they are likely to precipitate an anticholinergic delirium if the illicit drug was adulterated with atropine or another anticholinergic substance (Gershon, Neubauer, & Sundland, 1965).

Benzodiazepines are the drugs of choice (e.g., diazepam 20–30 mg orally, repeated every three to six hours as necessary for controlling anxiety and agitation) (Berger & Tinklenberg, 1979; Taylor, Maurer, & Tinklenberg, 1975). Short-acting barbiturates are also effective, but should be avoided because of risk of respiratory depression.

Upon recovery from the acute episode, the patient should be discharged to the custody and care of a responsible person, with advice to stay home for 24 hours. He or she should also be offered the opportunity for referral to a drug treatment program. Overnight hospitalization may be advisable for the patient who fails to respond to the above treatment approaches and continues to show perceptual and cognitive disturbances. Continuation of these symptoms beyond 24 hours requires a revision of the initial diagnosis (e.g., to Organic Delusional Syndrome).

Chronic hallucinatory psychosis in heavy hallucinogen abusers appears to be refractory to neuroleptic treatment. It has been reported, however, to respond to anticonvulsant drugs (Ifabumuyi & Jeffries, 1976). Treatment with benzodiazepines may also be justified if anticonvulsants prove ineffective after adequate trial.

292.12 Other Psychoactive Substance-Induced Hallucinosis

Most of the drugs listed in Table 2 (pp. 61–62) may produce organic hallucinosis. Those most commonly implicated include amantadine, baclofen, bromocriptine, ephedrine, L-dopa, steroids, propranolol, pentazocine, and levodopa (Lipowski, 1980a). The syndrome is generally benign and transient, rapidly subsiding after discontinuation of the drug. Mild sedation with a benzodiazepine may become necessary for the anxious and agitated patient (see Delirium, Chapter 10).

292.89 Posthallucinogen Perception Disorder

DSM-III-R has elevated hallucinogen-induced "flashbacks" to a new syndrome. The essential feature is the experiencing of one or more of the same perceptual symptoms that were experienced while intoxicated with the hallucinogen. The symptoms are often triggered by emergence into a dark environment, use of cannabis, or use of a phenothiazine. The person maintains insight into the pathologic nature of the symptoms. The symptoms remit within months in half the patients. Others continue to experience the symptoms for years.

The flashback phenomenon is thought to be due to a kindling effect of specific internal or external stimuli on temporo-limbic structures whose seizure threshold was lowered by repeated effects of hallucinogens. Benzodiazepines in low doses have been reported to be effective in controlling hallucinogen flashbacks (Berger & Tinklenberg, 1979), as have anticonvulsant drugs, such as phenytoin (Ifabumuyi & Jeffries, 1976).

293.82 Organic Hallucinosis Associated with Axis III Physical Disorders or Conditions

Temporal lobe epilepsy, migraine, temporal arteritis, space-occupying lesions of the brain, and posterior cerebral artery occlusion may be associated with hallucinosis (Lipowski, 1980a). Of particular diagnostic interest are those patients who experience only hallucinatory auras without a history of psychomotor seizures. Treatment of ictal hallucinosis should be directed toward the primary lesion and the control of seizural episodes with anticonvulsants. The reader is referred elsewhere for the treatment of other conditions.

Visual hallucinations may arise from lesions of the visual pathway (White, 1980) and in patients with bandaging of the eyes following corneal grafting or other procedures. Patients with partial sensory deprivation (loss of vision or hearing) may experience "release-type" hallucinations. Release hallucinations have also been reported in patients with posterior cerebral artery occlusions (Burest & Behemns, 1977). Treatment should be aimed at correcting the primary disorder (e.g., surgery for cataract, hearing aid). If the disorder is not amenable to treatment, an effort should be made to enrich the patient's environment through appropriate social stimulation.

11C: ORGANIC DELUSIONAL SYNDROME

The Organic Delusional Syndrome is characterized by delusions that are judged to be due to a specific organic factor. Diagnosis of the syndrome involves presumption rather than definitive diagnosis. Course and prognosis depend on the underlying pathology.

Treatment

As with other Organic Mental Disorders, the primary focus is on the diagnosis of a specific causative factor. The most common etiologies are phencyclidine (PCP), amphetamine, and cocaine abuse. Other common disorders that should be considered early include epilepsy, pernicious anemia, hypo- or hyperthyroidism, systemic lupus erythematosus, neurosyphilis, and brain tumors.

Symptomatic treatment should control delusions and agitation, as well as the physical symptoms of the underlying pathology (e.g., control of seizures). In general, effective control of the delusions and other psychotic symptoms may be achieved with neuroleptic drugs (see Chapters 14 and 15 on Schizophrenia and Delusional (Paranoid) Disorder). In some disorders, symptomatic treatment of psychosis may involve specific drugs, such as anticonvulsants in epilepsy and propranolol in porphyria (Atsmon & Blum, 1978). Supportive psychotherapy and other psychosocial approaches follow the same general guidelines as those for the functional psychoses.

Patient Management

The management of patients with Organic Delusional Syndrome is similar to that of patients with schizophrenic, schizophreniform, and paranoid disorders.

SPECIFIC ORGANIC DELUSIONAL DISORDERS

DSM-III-R classifies these disorders into (1) Psychoactive Substance-Induced Delusional Disorders (Axis I), (2) Dementias Arising in the Senium and Presenium with Delusions (Axis I), and (3) Organic Delusional Disorders Associated with Axis III Physical Disorders or Conditions.

1. Psychoactive Substance-Induced Delusional Disorders

292.11 Amphetamine or Similarly Acting Sympathomimetic Delusional Disorder

The treatment of the acute phase is supportive, unless the patient is agitated, in which case neuroleptics may be used. Persistent delusions and flashbacks are treated with neuroleptics. Some patients may later experience recurrent flashbacks of delusional ideas, often triggered by small doses of amphetamines.

292.11 Cocaine Delusional Disorder

Rapidly developing persecutory delusions are the predominant feature occurring shortly after use. Tactile hallucinations are characteristic. Delusions last for a week or more, and in some cases for over a year. Treatment of the disorder is similar to that of Amphetamine Delusional Disorder. Symptomatic treatment is based on the use of neuroleptics.

292.11 Hallucinogen Delusional Disorder

Symptomatic treatment of Hallucinogen Delusional Disorder involves the use of neuroleptics and follows the guidelines applicable to schizophrenic and paranoid disorders (see also Hallucinogen Hallucinosis).

292.11 Cannabis Delusional Disorder

Treatment is similar to that of the "bad tripper" (see Hallucinogen Hallucinosis), and may involve the use of neuroleptics in persistent cases or when agitation is present.

292.11 Phencyclidine (PCP) or Similarly Acting Arylcyclohexylamine Delusional Disorder

The symptoms are essentially the same as those in Cocaine Delusional Disorder and closely resemble chronic schizophrenia. Patients with PCP psychosis often require physical restraints during the intoxication because of the risk of violent or suicidal behavior (Perry, 1987).

98 The Treatment of Psychiatric Disorders

The treatment of PCP psychosis involves overcoming psychiatric manifestations and clearing PCP from the body. There is evidence that PCP is stored in lipids of the brain and other organs where it may be retained up to a year after the last known contact (Aniline, Allen, & Pitts, 1981). Urinary acidifiers such as ammonium chloride, cranberry juice, and vitamin C are effective in clearing PCP from the blood. However, acidification for several weeks until no PCP is detectable in the urine or blood does not rid the lipids of stored PCP. Periodic forced urine acidification may be required in an effort to clear the lipid stores of PCP, especially in those patients who experience flashbacks. These emergent symptoms occur with febrile illnesses, exercise, and emotional distress, and are thought to result from reintoxication from mobilized PCP in lipid stores. Urine acidification (pH below 5) can be accomplished by the administration of ammonium chloride in doses of 500 mg three or four times daily until PCP disappears from the urine and blood (Berger & Tinklenberg, 1979; Lewis & Senay, 1981).

During the acute phase, diazepam 10–30 mg orally or lorazepam 1–2 mg intramuscularly may be required to control agitation and violent behavior. Smaller divided daily doses are indicated in the persistent forms. Neuroleptics are effective in controlling psychotic symptoms (delusions, hallucinations); however, the low potency neuroleptics (e.g., chlorpromazine, thioridazine) should be avoided because of the risk of potentiating the anticholinergic effects of PCP. Haloperidol is preferred for the control of both psychotic and assaultive behavior. The rapid neuroleptization method discussed elsewhere in this book may be applied during the acute phase (Berger & Tinklenberg, 1979; Lewis & Senay, 1981). (See also PCP Delirium and Intoxication).

292.11 Other Psychoactive Substance-Induced Delusional Disorder

Numerous prescribed drugs may induce an Organic Delusional Syndrome as a result of excessive dosage or idiosyncratic intoxication. The most common include steroids (Ling, Perry, & Tsuang, 1981), asparaginase, bromocriptine, bromides, chloroquine, cimetidine, corticosteroids, cycloserine, digitalis glycosides, disopyramide, disulfiram, indomethacin, isoniazid, levodopa, methyldopa, pentazocine, phenelzine, propranolol, and sulindac (*The Medical Letter*, 1981). With the exception of bromide psychosis, the psychotic reaction is transient, requiring only brief symptomatic treatment (e.g., haloperidol), following discontinuation of the implicated drug or reduction of the dosage.

2. **Dementias Arising in the Senium and Presenium with Delusions**
290.20 **Primary Degenerative Dementia of the Alzheimer Type, Senile Onset with Delusions**
290.12 **Primary Degenerative Dementia of the Alzheimer Type, Presenile Onset with Delusions**
290.42 **Multi-infarct Dementia with Delusions**

Delusional symptoms may complicate dementias. Their treatment was discussed in the section on Dementia.

3. **Organic Delusional Disorders Associated with Axis III Physical Disorders or Conditions**

Non-substance-induced Organic Delusional Syndromes (293.81) include temporal lobe epilepsy, pernicious anemia, brain tumors, hypo- or hyperthyroidism, hypoparathyroidism, Cushing's syndrome, systemic lupus erythematosus, porphyria, head trauma, Huntington's chorea, and CNS infections (encephalitis, neurosyphilis) (Lipowski, 1975, 1980a). Neuroleptic medications are often effective for symptomatic control (Cummings, 1985).

Epileptic psychosis is an interictal complication of temporal lobe epilepsy, developing in a small percentage of patients many years after the onset of seizures (Balis, 1978; Bear et al., 1985; Blumer, 1975, 1977; McKenna, Kane, & Parish, 1985). Psychotic and seizural episodes may show an inverse relationship in a seesaw phenomenon. During the psychotic episode the EEG may show "forced normalization." Neuroleptic drugs are of limited use, with some notable exceptions.

Reduction of anticonvulsant drug dosage as a means of allowing seizures may be advisable in those patients whose psychosis is inversely related to seizure frequency. Induction of a grand mal seizure by ECT has been suggested. In other patients, raising the dose of the anticonvulsant drugs is recommended, especially in those whose delusional symptoms are paroxysmal. Adding carbamazepine and/or neuroleptics to the treatment regimen may prove helpful. Temporal lobectomy of seizure foci may be considered in some intractable cases.

11D: ORGANIC ANXIETY SYNDROME

The *DSM-III-R* has included a new organic syndrome, the Organic Anxiety Syndrome, whose essential feature is prominent, recurrent panic attacks or generalized anxiety caused by a specific organic factor (MacKenzie & Popkin, 1983). The diagnosis is not made if there is significant cognitive impairment, as in Delirium and Dementia. The course of the syndrome depends on the underlying etiology.

Treatment

As with other Organic Mental Disorders, the primary focus is on the diagnosis and treatment of the disorder presumed to be responsible for the syndrome. Common ones include endocrinopathies (hyperthyroidism, hypoparathyroidism, pheochromocytoma, hypoglycemia), intoxication with psychostimulant drugs (caffeine, amphetamine), temporal lobe epilepsy, and tumors in the vicinity of the third ventricle. In view of the absence of published controlled treatment trials using this new diagnosis, one must rely on case report literature to ascertain response to specific treatment (removal or reversal of underlying organic disorder), as well as to symptomatic control of panic attacks or generalized anxiety through anxiolytic drugs.

Etiologic treatment results in full remission of the syndrome in most cases, including hyperthyroidism (Kathol, Turner, & Delahunt, 1986), temporal lobe meningioma (Ghadirian, Gauthier, & Bertrand, 1986), temporal lobe epilepsy (Balis, 1978; Brodsky et al., 1983; Strub & Black, 1981; Weil, 1959), and hypocalcemia secondary to hypoparathyroidism.

Guidelines for symptomatic treatment are not yet established. There is evidence suggesting that anxiety of certain organic etiology may be refractory to standard anxiolytic drugs (benzodiazepines), especially in syndromes associated with epilepsy, the latter generally responding well to anticonvulsant medication (Brodsky et al., 1983). Failure to respond to anxiolytics should raise the suspicion of organicity. Besides benzodiazepines, other drugs that may prove useful in the symptomatic treatment of anxiety include beta blockers (propranolol) and antidepressants for panic attacks.

Patient Management

No established guidelines exist for the management of these patients. They are generally treated as outpatients, unless there is need for hospitalization to pursue specific diagnostic and treatment interventions. The management of patients abusing psychostimulants, especially amphetamines, is described in the respective section.

SPECIFIC ORGANIC ANXIETY DISORDERS

The following is a brief review of most commonly encountered organic anxiety disorders. They are listed in *DSM-III-R* under two separate codes: (1) 292.89—Other or Unspecified Psychoactive Substance-Induced Anxiety Disorder; and (2) 294.80—Organic Anxiety Disorder Associated with Axis III Physical Disorders or Conditions.

1. Psychoactive Substance-Induced Organic Anxiety Disorders
292.89 Other or Unspecified Psychoactive Substance-Induced Anxiety Disorder

Psychostimulant drugs are the most commonly implicated and include intoxication from caffeine, cocaine, and amphetamine or similarly acting sympathomimetics. The therapeutic approach is based on the treatment of the substance abuse and of underlying psychopathology, if present. The reader is referred to the Substance Abuse and Intoxications section. Organic anxiety disorder may also be associated with withdrawal from sedative-hypnotic-anxiolytic drugs. Treatment is described in the sections on Withdrawal and Substance Use disorders.

2. Organic Anxiety Disorder Associated with Axis III Physical Disorders or Conditions

The following is a brief review of several commonly-implicated disorders.

Endocrinopathies.

Hyperthyroidism. The clinician should always be alert to rule out hyperthyroidism as possible cause of anxiety. Kathol, Turner, and Delahunt (1986) found that 80% of 29 consecutive hyperthyroid patients in a general endocrine clinic met the *DSM-III* criteria for Generalized Anxiety Disorder. More than 90% displayed complete resolution of anxiety symptoms with antithyroid therapy alone. The authors stress the point that this Organic Anxiety Disorder can be treated successfully without anxiolytic drugs. They also noted that thyrotoxic symptoms can be controlled in days to weeks with standard antithyroid therapy, and that remission of anxiety is directly dependent on the ability to control the level of thyroxinemia.

Hypoparathyroidism. Hypocalcemia secondary to hypoparathyroidism is often associated with generalized anxiety and panic attacks (Denko & Kaelbling, 1962). Benzodiazepines have been reported to provide little relief of anxiety symptoms in hypocalcemia. Medical treatment of the hypoparathyroidism results in remission of the anxiety.

Hypoglycemia. Reactive hypoglycemia commonly presents with panic attacks or generalized anxiety related to catecholamine release. The alimentary type, resulting from unusually rapid absorption of glucose, is treated with dietary management. The diabetic type, due to delay in insulin secretion, is treated with a combination of dietary management and oral hypoglycemic agents (Anderson, 1979).

Pheochromocytoma. This relatively rare disorder is diagnosed by its clinical manifestations, measurement of catecholamines in the urine, and angiography. Treatment is based on long-term blockade with alpha adrenergic blocking agents (phenoxybenzamine), and surgery.

Hypercortisolism. Cushing's syndrome is caused by both endogenous (e.g., adrenocortical hyperplasia) and exogenous (e.g., iatrogenic) hypercortisolism. Treatment is directed at the underlying etiology (removal of a demonstrable tumor, discontinuing corticosteroid therapy, etc., as appropriate).

Neurologic Disorders.

Temporal lobe epilepsy. Paroxysmal anxiety symptoms such as fear (Gloor et al., 1982) or panic attacks (Sterman & Coyle, 1984; Strub & Black, 1981; Weil, 1959) are uncommon ictal symptoms of temporal lobe epilepsy. Brodsky et al. (1983) report 10 refractory anxiety patients, of whom nine showed focal paroxysmal EEG abnormalities in the temporal region. All patients improved clinically on anticonvulsant medications. The authors postulated that patients with anxiety attacks who are unusually refractory to anxiolytics and who frequently experience paradoxical reactions to major psychotropic drugs may suffer from epileptiform disorder.

Brain tumors. Tumors in the vicinity of the third ventricle and the temporal lobes may present with anxiety (Balis, 1978; Strub & Black, 1981). Ghadirian, Gauthier, & Bertrand (1986) report on a patient with right temporal lobe meningioma whose anxiety attacks disappeared following removal of the tumor.

Miscellaneous Causes. Other etiologic factors include pulmonary embolus, chronic obstructive pulmonary disease, brucellosis, aspirin intolerance, demyelinating disease, and heavy metal intoxication.

11E: ORGANIC MOOD SYNDROME

Organic Mood Syndrome is also a presumptive rather than a definitive diagnosis. Etiologic factors include medications (e.g., reserpine, corticosteroids), endocrine diseases (e.g., Cushing's syndrome), pernicious anemia, hypothyroidism, infectious diseases (e.g., influenza), brain tumors, Parkinson's disease, carcinoma of the pancreas, temporal lobe epilepsy, and other conditions. These may also produce other Organic Mental Syndromes. Course and prognosis depend on the underlying pathology.

Treatment

Treatment is both etiologic and symptomatic, as is the case with all Organic Mental Syndromes. Etiologic treatment of the underlying pathology does not promptly reverse the affective syndrome. It may persist for weeks or months after recovery from the primary disease. Dexamethasone suppression test in patients with organic mood disorders may show cortisol nonsuppression (Evans & Nemeroff, 1984).

Symptomatic treatment is directed toward the affective syndrome (depression, mania), as well as the physical symptoms of the primary disorder. Treatment of the affective syndrome follows the general guidelines applicable to the functional affective disorders. Psychopharmacological treatment often involves the use of tri- or tetracyclic antidepressants. Monoamine oxidase inhibitors (MAOIs) should be tried in cases refractory to tricyclics. ECT may be advisable in cases refractory to drugs, when suicidal risk is imminent, or when antidepressant drug toxicity is hazardous or intolerable, as in the case of serious cardiac disease.

In some disorders, such as temporal lobe epilepsy, control of the depressive episode may involve drugs of greater specificity (e.g., anticonvulsants). Supportive psychotherapy and other psychosocial approaches follow the same guidelines applicable to functional depressive disorders.

Lithium carbonate has been reported to be effective in various organic manic disorders, including those associated with corticosteroids and other drugs (Falk, Mahnke, & Poskanzer, 1979), Cushing's syndrome, and metabolic disturbances (Krauthammer & Klerman, 1978). Neuroleptics (e.g., haloperidol) may also be effective and should be tried in patients not responsive to lithium.

Carbamazepine has been recently reported to be very effective in bipolar patients. A trial of carbamazepine is justified when the patient fails to respond to lithium or when lithium toxicity is intolerable. It should be the drug of choice for ictal manic episodes in patients with temporal lobe epilepsy (Troupin, 1978). Valproic acid may possess antimanic effects as well (McElroy, Keck, & Pope, 1987).

Patient Management
The management of patients with Organic Mood Syndrome is similar to that of patients with functional affective disorders. Suicide risk or behavioral deterioration in the depressed patient, or socially disruptive behavior in the manic, may necessitate hospitalization.

SPECIFIC ORGANIC MOOD DISORDERS
Organic Mood Disorders may be divided into (1) Psychoactive Substance-Induced (Axis I); (2) Dementias Arising in the Senium and Presenium with Depression (Axis I); and (3) those of other etiology (Axis III).

1. Psychoactive Substance-Induced Mood Disorders
292.84 Hallucinogen Mood Disorder
292.84 Phencyclidine (PCP) or Similarly Acting Arylcyclohexylamine Mood Disorder
The essential feature of both of these disorders is an Organic Mood Syndrome that develops shortly after the use of these drugs (usually within one or two weeks) and persists more than 24 hours after cessation of use. Most common is depression, in which suicide may be a complication. Elation is rare. The course is variable, and may range from a brief experience to a long-lasting episode which is indistinguishable from a Functional Mood Disorder.

Major depressive episodes may call for treatment with antidepressant drugs (tricyclics or MAOIs) or ECT, while manic episodes may require treatment with neuroleptics and lithium. Supportive psychotherapy should be part of the therapeutic regimen. Little is known about the efficacy of such treatments in these disorders. For more information see section on Functional Mood Disorders.

292.84 Other Psychoactive Substance-Induced Mood Disorder
The most commonly implicated are antihypertensive drugs, and steroids. Other drugs include metrizamide, a myelographic substance which may induce both depression (Gelmers, 1979) and mania (Kwentus, Silverman, & Sprague, 1984), indomethacin, and psychostimulants in the withdrawal phase.

Antihypertensive Drugs. Reserpine, methyldopa (Gillespie et al., 1967), guanethidine (Prichard et al., 1968), clonidine, bethanidine, thiazide diuretics (Okada, 1985), and alpha-blockers (propranolol) have been reported to cause depression (Whitlock & Evans, 1978). Reserpine is the most commonly implicated, precipitating a major depressive episode in 5% of patients treated (Simpson & Waal-Manning, 1971; Wells, 1985). Treatment involves discontinuation of the drug and the use of antidepressants or ECT if the depression does not remit. Manic episodes associated with captopril have been treated successfully with haloperidol (McMahon, 1985; Zubenko & Nixon, 1984).

Steroids. Corticosteroids, ACTH, have been reported to cause affective syndromes, both depressive and manic. In manic episodes, reduction of dosage may lead to improvement (Ling, Perry, & Tsuang, 1981).

If the drug cannot be reduced or discontinued, mania can be controlled with neuroleptics or lithium. Lithium may also provide short-term prophylaxis against corticosteroid-induced affective syndrome at serum levels of 0.8–1.2 mEg/L (Falk, Mahnke, & Poskanzer, 1979), and may be considered prophylactically in patients with a prior history of corticosteroid-induced mental disorders who require steroid treatment. Treatment with tricyclics may produce delirium in such patients; small doses and plasma monitoring are advisable (Sergent et al., 1975; Ling, Perry, & Tsuang, 1981). ECT is effective in treating secondary depression (Glaser, 1953).

2. Dementias Arising in the Senium and Presenium with Depression

290.21 Primary Degenerative Dementia of the Alzheimer Type, Senile Onset with Depression

290.13 Primary Degenerative Dementia of the Alzheimer Type, Presenile Onset with Depression

290.43 Multi-infarct Dementia with Depression

Major depression is a common complication of dementias. The syndrome is responsive to tricyclic antidepressants. The latter may produce, however, intolerable side effects related to anticholinergic action and orthostatic hypotension.

There has recently been an upsurge of interest in the use of monoamine oxidase inhibitors (MAOIs) in treating depression in the elderly demented patient. They are effective, well-tolerated antidepressants. One significant advantage over the tricyclics is the MAOI's lack of anticholinergic effects (Jenike, 1985). Their main side effects are orthostatic hypotension and insomnia. They can be used safely in elderly patients when the necessary dietary restrictions are observed (Jenike, 1984).

Electroconvulsive therapy is the treatment of choice for patients who cannot tolerate antidepressant drugs or who are refractory to them. For more information the reader is referred to the section on Dementia.

3. Organic Mood Disorders Associated with Axis III Physical Disorders or Conditions

Other conditions associated with Organic Mood Syndrome (293.83) include endocrine diseases (Gold, Pottash, & Extein, 1981), temporal lobe epilepsy, systemic lupus erythematosus, brain tumors, cerebrovascular lesions, pernicious anemia, Parkinson's disease, Huntington's chorea and other neurologic disorders, carcinoid syndrome, carcinoma of the pancreas, AIDS (Nichols & Ostrow, 1984; Rundall et al., 1986), post-viral syndromes (influenza, infectious mononucleosis, infectious hepatitis, viral pneumonia), lead intoxication (Schottenfeed & Cullen, 1984), and metabolic disorders (Lipowski, 1980a, b). The following is a brief review of the most important disorders.

Endocrinopathies. There are many reports of psychiatric disorders associated with endocrine changes (Haskett & Rose, 1981; Leigh & Kramer, 1984). Hypothyroidism and hyperthyroidism have been found to be most frequently associated with such disorders (Hall et al., 1981).

Hypothyroidism-induced depression (Hall, 1983) is treated with thyroid replacement (T4) alone, and in refractory cases with the addition of tricyclics or ECT (Dackis et al., 1983; Goggans et al., 1986). Several researchers have recently reported depression associated with the so-called "subclinical hypothyroidism," which is characterized by minor degrees of thyroid hypofunction, documented only by elevated thyroid-stimulating hormone (TSH) levels or exaggerated TSH responses to thyrotropin-releasing hormones (TRH). This syndrome may be present especially in anergic patients who fail to respond to antidepressants (Gold & Pearsal, 1983; Krahn, 1987; Targum et al., 1984). The depression seems to respond to thyroid replacement (Cooper et al., 1984; Krahn 1987). Rarely, hyperthyroidism may present with depression (Diaz-Cabal, Pearlman, & Kawecki, 1986).

Hypercortisolism (Cushing's syndrome) is very often associated with psychiatric disorder (Reus & Berlant, 1986), with depression being the most common syndrome (Leigh & Kramer, 1984). Mania and psychosis are also common. Treatment is primarily etiologic. Symptomatic treatment of the psychotic syndromes is similar to that described under corticosteroid-induced mood disorders.

Post-Stroke Depression. Recent studies by Robinson and associates (1983) have shown that major depression and dysthymia are common in stroke victims. Major depression occurs characteristically in left-sided anterior (frontal) lesions (Robinson et al., 1984). Post-stroke depression appears to respond well to tricyclic antidepressants (Feibel & Springer, 1982; Lipsey et al., 1984; Robinson, Lipsey, & Price, 1985), as well as to ECT (Murray et al., 1986).

Other Neurologic Disorders. Other neurologic disorders associated with depression include the subcortical dementias (Parkinson's disease, Huntington's chorea), progressive supranuclear palsy, Shy-Drager syndrome, and normal pressure hydrocephalus. Tricyclic antidepressants and ECT have been of some value in symptomatic treatment (Hales & Hershey, 1984; Martin & Black, 1987). Depression may be a prodromal syndrome of lead encephalopathy, which can be successfully treated with chelation (Schottenfeld & Cullen, 1984).

Manic Syndromes have been reported in right focal thalamic infarctions (Cummings & Mendez, 1984), as well as tumors, trauma, and focal epilepsy (Cohen & Niska, 1980; Forrest, 1982; Jamieson & Wells, 1979; Whitlock, 1982) with a nondominant hemisphere localization (Jampala & Abrams, 1983). Lithium has been reported to be effective for the manic symptoms of these disorders (Cummings & Mendez, 1984; Cohn, Wright, & DeVaul, 1977; Oyewumi & Lapierre, 1981; Rosenbaum & Barry, 1975). Neuroleptics (e.g., haloperidol) are useful for control of acute symptoms.

11F: ORGANIC PERSONALITY SYNDROME

This syndrome is characterized by persistent disturbances in personality and behavior that are judged to be due to a specific organic factor which antedates their onset. The cardinal feature is disinhibition, with impaired control of emotions and impulses. *DSM-III-R* recognizes one major type, the *explosive*, which is also known as "episodic dyscontrol syndrome," characterized by recurrent outbursts of rage or aggression, usually with minimal provocation. Other types include the *pseudopsychopathic* (characterized by emotional lability, impulsivity, and socially inappropriate behavior), and the *pseudo-depressive* (characterized by apathy and indifference). Both are often called "frontal lobe syndromes."

The most common causes of Organic Personality Syndrome are head trauma, cerebrovascular disorders, and intracranial space-occupying lesions. Others include temporal lobe epilepsy, multiple sclerosis, chronic intoxications (e.g., cannabis, LSD, steroids), endocrine disorders, chronic poisoning (e.g., mercury, manganese), neurosyphilis, post-encephalitic parkinsonism, and Huntington's chorea. Chronic hypercalcemia (e.g., from hyperparathyroidism) may induce persistent personality changes that can be reversed with the correction of the hypercalcemia (Peterson, 1968). Cerebral neoplasms, subarachnoid hemorrhage, (especially with anterior communicating artery aneurysm [Storey, 1970]), neurosyphilis, and Wilson's disease are other treatable disorders.

Treatment
Etiologically treatable conditions include endocrine diseases, substance-induced disorders, space-occupying lesions of the brain, epilepsy, and neurosyphilis.

Symptomatic treatment should control the emotional lability and impulse dyscontrol, as well as the physical symptoms of the underlying disorder.

Explosive outbursts of anger and episodes of violent behavior that occur with minimal provocation are the most serious symptoms. Pharmacologic control of these may be possible, with the use of lithium, propranolol, anticonvulsants, (especially carbamazepine), or neuroleptics (Balis, 1979; Elliott, 1977, 1984; Kuhn, 1976; Puente, 1976; Tunks & Dermer, 1977).

Lithium has been reported to have a nonspecific therapeutic effect on aggressive and violent behavior (Marini & Sheard, 1977; Sheard, 1975; Sheard et al., 1976; Tupin, 1978). Propranolol may control violent episodes in patients with closed-head injury or temporal lobe epilepsy (Ratey, Morril, & Oxenkrug, 1983; Schreier, 1979; Williams et al., 1982; Yudofsky, Williams, & Gounan, 1981, 1984).

Anticonvulsants, especially carbamazepine (alone or in combination with propranolol), have been shown to improve irritability and episodic rage in patients with temporo-limbic epilepsy (Kuhn, 1976; Monroe, 1975; Troupin, 1978; Tunks & Dermer, 1977). Neuroleptic drugs, although often used, are usually ineffective.

Psychosocial therapeutic approaches, including individual psychotherapy, group and family therapy, and behavior modification techniques, have been reported to be of value for some of these patients (Eames & Wood, 1985; Mehr & Holi, 1984). They may encourage compliance and help with the transition to a normal life.

Patient Management

The management of the patient with Organic Personality Syndrome is primarily directed toward enhancing behavioral controls and minimizing undesirable conduct. This may be accomplished through direct counseling and family intervention.

Patient counseling should help the patient avoid situations that trigger violent outbursts; abstain from alcohol, which may induce dyscontrol episodes; learn ways to prevent social embarrassment; and make decisions about job changes or early retirement, if necessary. Vocational rehabilitation may be indicated.

Family counseling is an essential part of management. Family members need to be advised about the changes in the patient's personality, especially with regard to behavioral dyscontrol and impaired social judgment (e.g., embarrassing behaviors, shoplifting, sexual indiscretions). The physician should provide emotional support for their caring for the needs of the patient, as well as for their own needs (Lezak, 1978). He or she should advise about proper management of the patient and assist in developing coping strategies and/or avoiding situations that tend to elicit psychopathology.

It is most important that the family understand the interaction of environmental contingencies (e.g., supports and demands of social situations) with the patient's lifelong coping style, in the face of organic disinhibition (Leigh, 1979). For instance, excessive obsessiveness and "viscosity" in the epileptic personality may represent compensatory mechanisms for maintaining control in the face of uncontrollable seizures; "catastrophic reactions" (crying, rage, or cognitive disorganization) may be manifested when the brain-injured person is faced with tasks beyond his or her capabilities.

The patient should be allowed to perform at his or her own level, in his or her own tedious and ruminative style, in a familiar setting that provides routine and predictability. Novel or shifting environments and excessive change of stimulus strain the patient's resources. The ensuing stress often leads to reactive psychopathology and "catastrophic" episodes. Patients who are violent, sexually abusive, or otherwise unmanageable may have to be removed from the home.

SPECIFIC ORGANIC PERSONALITY DISORDERS

DSM-III-R lists two syndromatic categories (substance-induced and other) without any reference to specific disorders.

1. Psychoactive Substance-Induced Personality Disorders
292.89 Other Psychoactive Substance-Induced Personality Disorder

Chronic abuse of cannabis, LSD, and other hallucinogens has been associated with persistent personality changes (Balis, 1974). Therapeutic approaches for patients with substance abuse should include a comprehensive program, with efforts toward social and vocational rehabilitation and resocialization (see Psychoactive Substance Use Disorders, Chapter 13).

2. Organic Personality Disorder Associated with Axis III Physical Disorders or Conditions (310.10)

Treatable organic disorders should be identified in order to be able to institute specific therapies. Symptomatic treatment depends on target symptoms. In the *pseudopsychopathic type*, treatment should be primarily behavioral and supportive, including family counseling.

The *explosive type* is the most common organic personality. Its etiology includes head trauma, complex partial seizures, cerebral tumors, and encephalitis (Elliott, 1984). Alcohol and benzodiazepines are common precipitants, due to their disinhibiting effect. Treatment includes both pharmacological and behavior intervention. Drugs used for explosive rage or aggression include carbamazepine, phenytoin (Tunks & Dermer, 1977), and propranolol (Elliott, 1977, 1984; Ratey, Morril, & Oxenkrug, 1983; Schreier, 1979; Williams et al., 1982).

Elliott (1984) has used propranolol in doses up to 320 mg/day to control aggressive episodes. Some have found in open trials of propranolol that effective treatment requires higher doses (up to 20 mg/kg per day) (Williams et al., 1982; Yudofsky et al., 1981; Yudofsky et al., 1984). Metoprolol, a beta-1 adrenoreceptor blocker, has been reported by Mattes (1985) to suppress aggressive episodes in two patients who failed to respond to propranolol and carbamazepine.

In temporal lobe epilepsy, anticonvulsant drugs (e.g., carbamazepine) may improve hypersexuality and irritability (Troupin, 1978). Propranolol (alone or in combination with carbamazepine) may be effective in controlling rage outbursts of the explosive epileptic (Elliott, 1977;

Kuhn, 1976; Tunks & Dermer, 1977). Psychotherapy and family counseling are of value for some patients (Blumer, 1977).

Behavioral interventions should be part of a comprehensive approach to treating the explosive type personality. Thorough behavioral assessment is a necessary prerequisite to an effective behavior treatment program (Eames & Wood, 1985; Mehr & Holi, 1984).

Chapter 12

Withdrawal and Intoxication

12A: WITHDRAWAL AND WITHDRAWAL DELIRIA
Withdrawal (uncomplicated) includes all manifestations of the "abstinence sickness" except delirium. Common symptoms include anxiety, restlessness, irritability, insomnia, and impaired attention. The nature of the substance determines additional symptoms which are characteristic of that particular substance or of its class. The course of withdrawal is generally self-limited, unless it becomes complicated by Delirium. Withdrawal delirium is a complication of certain substance-specific withdrawal syndromes associated with dependence on alcohol or hypnotic–sedative–anxiolytic drugs. Withdrawal from alcohol or hypnotic–sedative–anxiolytic drugs may also be complicated by grand mal seizures.

General Therapeutic Principles
The ultimate goal is to eliminate physiological dependence ("detoxify" the patient) without allowing the development of the withdrawal syndrome. This procedure is based upon gradually withdrawing an individual from the drug by means of decreasing doses, either of the drug on which the individual is dependent or one that is cross-tolerant to it (Czechowicz, 1978). Loss of substance dependence does not necessarily cure the underlying Psychoactive Substance Use Disorder. The most important factor of substance abuse is the mechanism of psychological dependence, in which complex psychological and sociological determinants are responsible for the development and perpetuation of the

disorder. Detoxification is not a rehabilitative procedure but rather a prerequisite for rehabilitation.

The following general principles are based on detoxification guidelines and procedures established by the National Institute on Drug Abuse (NIDA) (Czechowicz, 1978).

A thorough evaluation of the patient should serve as the cornerstone for developing an appropriate treatment plan. This involves:

1. identification of the drugs used and assessment of the level of tolerance to and the degree of physical dependence on each
2. medical history, with a thorough review of systems
3. psychiatric history and mental status examination
4. physical examination
5. appropriate laboratory tests

The decision regarding the appropriate site of detoxification (inpatient, outpatient, residential) involves a number of considerations including type of substance dependence, available resources, and the individual's lifestyle. In general, opiate detoxification can be done in an outpatient setting. Alcohol should generally be withdrawn in a hospital setting; however, patients with mild-to-moderate withdrawal reactions can be managed at home or in a specialized residential setting. Barbiturate-type, meprobamate, and/or polydrug dependence usually requires a hospital setting in order to prevent life-threatening complications. Amphetamine and cocaine withdrawal may necessitate hospitalization in the presence of significant suicidal risk.

A *detoxification treatment plan* should follow certain general guidelines (Czechowicz, 1978):

(a) Whenever possible, a long-acting drug should be substituted for a short-acting drug of addiction.
(b) The initial amount of the drug required to suppress withdrawal symptoms is determined empirically, by assessing symptom response to repeated drug dosages (e.g., alcohol withdrawal) or through a challenge test (e.g., barbiturate withdrawal).
(c) The detoxification procedure should be safe and geared to provide a comfortable withdrawal through individualized titration and progressive withdrawal of the drug.

(d) The patient should be closely monitored for signs and symptoms of withdrawal or intoxication as a means of titrating dosage and pace of withdrawal schedule.

(e) Before completion of the detoxification procedure, provision should be made for an aftercare plan with appropriate referral for further treatment and rehabilitation.

SPECIFIC WITHDRAWAL DISORDERS

291.80 Uncomplicated Alcohol Withdrawal
291.00 Alcohol Withdrawal Delirium

The severity of the Uncomplicated Alcohol Withdrawal depends on the amount, frequency, and duration of prior alcohol consumption. It is usually benign and self-limited, unless it progresses to a Withdrawal Delirium. Alcohol-dependent patients are preferably withdrawn in specialized detoxification units by the use of benzodiazepines (chlordiazepoxide, lorazepam, etc.). Dosages are titrated at levels suppressing withdrawal symptoms and then gradually tapered. Some alcohol detoxification protocols are based on a prn use of benzodiazepines. The need for or efficacy of concurrent phenytoin has not been supported by controlled studies.

Alcohol Withdrawal Delirium (delirium tremens) is a serious withdrawal complication occurring in about 5% of cases and occasionally leading to death from intercurrent illness (Victor & Adams, 1953). Patients with Withdrawal Delirium must be hospitalized. After medical evaluation (especially for subdural hematoma, pancreatitis, infections, hepatic disease, and malnutrition), treatment should follow the protocol below, or a similar one:

(a) The patient should be sedated with a benzodiazepine (e.g., chlordiazepoxide, diazepam, or lorazepam) (Greenblatt & Shader, 1975; Sellers & Kalant, 1976). Neuroleptics, paraldehyde, and magnesium sulfate have also been successfully used. Barbiturates, although effective, should be avoided. Chlordiazepoxide 25–50 mg or diazepam 5–10 mg may be given orally, or lorazepam 1–2 mg intramuscularly, and repeated every two to four hours as necessary until symptoms are suppressed, and then reduced to half that dose three or four times per day orally. Benzodiazepines and paraldehyde provide an anticonvulsant effect, thus reducing the risk of withdrawal seizures. Neuroleptics, on the other hand, tend to increase the risk of developing convulsions.

Magnesium sulfate has been used by some inpatients with low serum magnesium (below 2 mEq/L). It is given intravenously in a 5% solution in doses up to 2.0 gm, repeated three to four times daily for three days and then reduced to 1.0 gm daily for an additional two to three days (Mendelson, 1970; Stending-Lindberg, 1974).

(b) The patient should be given daily thiamine (initial dose of 100–200 mg I.M., with subsequent doses given orally) and a multivitamine supplement, to combat malnutrition and prevent acute thiamine deficiency that may lead to Wernicke's encephalopathy or cardiac failure (Cade, 1970).

(c) Parenteral fluid administration should be carefully individualized and titrated according to the hydration status of the patient. Fluid retention and overhydration develop during rising blood alcohol levels, while dehydration follows a period of stable high blood alcohol levels. Therefore, many patients may actually be overhydrated, in which case parenteral fluids are contraindicated (Ogata, Mendelsohn, & Mello, 1968).

Dehydration is presumed in cases of vomiting, diarrhea, elevated hematocrit and other objective signs of dehydration. No more than 50% of an initial fluid deficit should be replaced during the first 24 hours, and no more than 6 liters of dextrose-containing fluid should be given in a 24-hour period (Czechowicz, 1978). Fluids should be given orally if the patient is not severely ill and can tolerate oral intake. Any electrolyte deficiency should be corrected.

(d) Hypoglycemia may be present in some patients during the withdrawal period. Patients should be given sufficient carbohydrates in oral fluids (e.g., orange juice). Parenteral fluids, if needed, should contain 5% dextrose (Freinkel & Arky, 1966).

(e) Alcohol withdrawal seizures (grand mal) are generally self-limited and have a relatively benign course. There is no evidence that prophylactic use of phenytoin will prevent withdrawal seizures. Benzodiazepines are effective in lessening the likelihood of seizures and will suffice for the patient who has no history of epilepsy. Prophylactic anticonvulsant therapy is indicated in patients known to have an underlying seizure disorder. In the event that withdrawal seizures occur repeatedly, diazepam 5–10 mg slow IV is recommended.

(f) Concurrent disorders (e.g., gastritis, pancreatitis, anemia) may also require proper evaluation and treatment.

General management of the delirious patient is discussed in the section on Delirium in Chapter 10.

292.00 Uncomplicated Sedative, Hypnotic, or Anxiolytic Withdrawal

292.00 Sedative, Hypnotic, or Anxiolytic Withdrawal Delirium

Barbiturates, similarly acting sedative-hypnotic drugs (ethchlorvynol, glutethimide, methyprylon, chloral hydrate, paraldehyde, methaqualone) and anxiolytic drugs (meprobamate, and benzodiazepines) produce a withdrawal syndrome almost identical to that of alcohol. Threshold doses and time periods necessary for development of physical dependence vary according to the type of drug used. Daily doses of 900 mg or more of pentabarbital for one-to-two months will lead, upon sudden withdrawal, to convulsions in 75% of subjects and to delirium in 65% (Fraser et al., 1964).

Barbiturate withdrawal will begin 12-24 hours after the last dose was taken. Grand mal seizures most often occur between the third and seventh day and may lead to status epilepticus. The withdrawal delirium most often occurs between the fourth and sixth day. Hyperpyrexia, cardiovascular collapse, and death may occur in untreated cases. Convulsions associated with benzodiazepine withdrawal (especially diazepam) may appear several weeks after the discontinuation of the drug.

Detoxification of patients with barbiturate or similarly-acting substance dependence should generally be carried out in a hospital setting. These patients need very close medical supervision because of the life-threatening nature of the abstinence syndrome. Detoxification is accomplished by one of the following procedures: phenobarbital substitution, pentobarbital substitution, or slow withdrawal of the addicting agent (Czechowicz, 1978).

Phenobarbital Substitution. The stabilization dose of phenobarbital to be given daily is tentatively calculated on the basis of the patient's history and by monitoring the patient's response to the drug. The initial daily requirement is calculated by substituting one sedative dose (30 mg) of phenobarbital for each hypnotic dose of any reported sedative-hypnotic. The equivalent of 30 mg of phenobarbital is about 100 mg of short-acting barbiturates (amobarbital, pentobarbital, secobarbital), 500 mg of chloral hydrate, 350 mg of ethclorvynol, 250 mg of glutethimide, 400-600 of meprobamate, 250-300 mg methaqualone, or 300 mg of methyprylon (Smith & Wesson, 1970). The initial total daily dose of phenobarbital should never exceed 600 mg, regardless of the dosage claimed by the patient. The established daily requirement is given in divided doses, three or four times daily. If toxic symptoms occur (sedation, slurred speech, nystagmus, ataxia), the daily dose should be reduced. The patient should be maintained on the stabilization dosage for two days before graded withdrawal is initiated. Once this is achieved, the total daily dose of phenobarbital is reduced by 30 mg per day. During this period, the patient should be closely monitored for signs of withdrawal or for phenobarbital toxicity, so that the dosage can be titrated accordingly.

Pentobarbital Substitution. In cases involving dependence on a short-acting barbiturate, the pentobarbital challenge test helps to establish the degree of barbiturate tolerance (and thus dependence) and determine the initial pentobarbital requirement. A standard dose of 200 mg is given orally at two-hour intervals until signs of barbiturate toxicity are elicited (e.g., nystagmus, unsteady gait, slurred speech). No further treatment is necessary if 400 mg or less results in intoxication. If no signs of intoxication are present, the next step involves the estimation of the daily barbiturate requirement by continuing the challenge test until signs of mild intoxication are produced.

The total amount of pentobarbital given becomes the stabilization dosage level. After a two-day period of stabilization the pentobarbital is gradually withdrawn by 10% of the total drug dosage per day, not to exceed 100 mg per day. Rate and amount of reduction may need to be adjusted if withdrawal or toxic signs occur. Once the stabilization dosage is established with pentobarbital, an equivalent dosage of phenobarbital may be used during detoxification, in preference for a long-acting barbiturate.

In the case of barbiturate withdrawal delirium, the patient should be sedated to the point of mild intoxication and be stabilized (suppression of all withdrawal symptoms) for two days before detoxification is started. In extreme agitation, the initial dose of the sedative is given intravenously (e.g., diazepam 10 mg, or amobarbital 500 mg) (Wulff, 1959).

Slow Withdrawal of the Addicting Agent. This method is applied in patients dependent on benzodiazepines, long-acting sedative hypnotics, or mixed sedative hypnotics. Detoxification may be carried out in an outpatient setting. Initially, the patient is given the addicting drug at the dosage level of his or her daily intake and then he or she is gradually withdrawn at a daily decreasing rate of about 20% of the total dosage per day (Hollister, Montzenbecker, & Degans, 1966; Khantzian & McKenna, 1979).

292.00 Opioid Withdrawal

The time of onset and duration of the syndrome vary depending on the action of the drug used (e.g., shortest course with hydromorphone, longest with methadone). Heroin and morphine withdrawal syndromes begin 8–12 hours following the last dose and gradually subside over a period of 7–10 days. Evidence of dependence may be demonstrated by the naloxone test: Intramuscular injection of 0.4 mg of naloxone (Narcan) will precipitate withdrawal symptoms in an opioid-dependent individual.

Detoxification from opioids can be carried out in an inpatient, residential, or outpatient setting. The following procedure describes management in a hospital setting.

Pretreatment evaluation includes a complete medical and drug abuse history, physical examination, routine laboratory tests, and urine screening for drugs of abuse. Following verification of opiod dependence, the patient is detoxified by methadone substitution. The standard approach is to give an initial dose of 10–20 mg of oral methadone. If withdrawal symptoms are not suppressed, an additional 5–10 mg of methadone may be given. The total dose for the day should not exceed 40 mg.

Once the stabilizing dosage is estimated, the patient is maintained on that level for two or three days, with methadone given in b.i.d. divided doses. Detoxification then begins with a reduction each day by 15%–20% of the total methadone daily dose (usually about 5 mg per day). The withdrawal is completed in 7–10 days. Methadone detoxification is often an outpatient treatment, provided drug access is controlled. Patients with concurrent drug dependencies or concomitant medical or psychiatric problems may require an inpatient setting.

Inpatient detoxification of individuals already on methadone maintenance requires prior confirmation of maintenance dosage and enrollment in a methadone maintenance program. In these patients the detoxification period should last longer, extending several weeks, at a rate of reduction of 3–5 mg per day. Some clinicians, however, recommend that withdrawal from methadone maintenance be conducted on an outpatient basis by a process of gradual detoxification over a period of four to six months, with a dose decrement of approximately 3% per week.

Clonidine Detoxification. Recent reports have documented the effectiveness of the antihypertensive clonidine, about 5 µ/kg, for suppressing the symptoms of opioid withdrawal, by acting on brain regions such as the locus ceruleus that are stimulated by opiates and alpha-noradrenergic agonists (Cami et al., 1985; Gold, Redmond, & Kleber, 1978, Gold et al., 1980). Compared to morphine, clonidine appears to be more effective in suppressing autonomic signs of abstinence but less effective in reducing subject-reported symptoms and discomfort (Jasinski, Johnson, & Kocher, 1985).

Clonidine was also reported by Charney et al. (1981) to be effective in methadone withdrawal, with 80% of patients being withdrawn from methadone by the end of a two-week period, with a peak mean dose of 16 μ/kgm/day. Major side effects from clonidine include hypotension and sedation.

In subsequent studies, Charney et al. (1982) found that *clonidine* and *naltrexone* given in combination provide safe, effective, and rapid withdrawal from methadone therapy. Six days of clonidine treatment, with a peak mean dose of 2.9 mg/day on the second treatment day, attenuated the withdrawal-inducing effect of naltrexone. The latter was gradually increased from an initial 1 mg dose on the second treatment day to a 50 mg maintenance dose on the fifth treatment day.

It appears that clonidine is a reasonably safe and effective drug for detoxifying selected opiate addicts, especially patients being directly detoxified from illicit opioids, or patients who have been stabilized on relatively low doses of methadone. It is best suited for detoxifying patients selected for induction into naltrexone therapy (Gold & Dackis, 1984; Washton & Resnick, 1981). Recent studies have reported the successful use of methadyl acetate (LAAM) as a means of outpatient withdrawal from heroin (Judson, Goldstein, & Inturrisi, 1983; Sorensen, Hargreaves, & Weinberg, 1982).

292.00 Amphetamine or Similarly Acting Sympathomimetic Withdrawal

The syndrome may progress during the first two weeks to a major depression involving significant suicidal risk, which may persist for months. In view of the suicidal risk involved, detoxification from amphetamine dependence should be carried out in a controlled environment and under close observation, preferably in a psychiatric hospital setting. The addicting drug should be promptly discontinued and the patient be placed on suicide precautions, if needed.

If the patient is severely agitated or psychotic (see Intoxication, Delirium, and Organic Delusional Syndrome) upon admission, he or she may be treated initially with moderate doses of a neuroleptic, which should be tapered and discontinued upon control of the target symptoms. If the syndrome develops into a depressive episode, treatment with antidepressants may be necessary, following the guidelines applicable to depressive disorders. In the presence of a concurrent delusional syndrome, tricyclic treatment should be combined with the administration of neuroleptics. Psychotherapeutic management and psychosocial counseling should be provided, as well as referral to a treatment program prior to discharge (Berger & Tinklenberg, 1979; Ellinwood, 1979).

292.00 Cocaine Withdrawal
Treatment and management of cocaine withdrawal are similar to that of Amphetamine Withdrawal (see preceding section). The use of tricyclic antidepressants in follow-up treatment of cocaine abuse is discussed in Chapter 13 on Psychoactive Substance Use Disorders.

292.00 Nicotine Withdrawal
Management of Nicotine Withdrawal is discussed in Chapter 13 on Psychoactive Substance Use Disorders.

292.00 Mixed Drug Withdrawal
In mixed substance dependencies, detoxification should proceed with the gradual withdrawal of one drug at a time, while stabilizing the patient on the other drug(s) on which he or she may be dependent.

In the instance of combined heroin and barbiturate dependence, it is preferable to withdraw the barbiturate first, while stabilizing the patient on methadone. Following withdrawal from the barbiturate, one may proceed with detoxification from the opioid (Czechowicz, 1978).

In the instance of alcohol–barbiturate dependence, the detoxification procedure is similar to other sedative–hypnotic–anxiolytic dependence, since the substances are cross-tolerant and have an additive effect. One must calculate the phenobarbital equivalent of alcohol (15 mg phenobarbital for 1 ounce of 80–100 proof alcohol) and add it to the phenobarbital equivalent of the sedative hypnotic (Czechowicz, 1978).

In the instance of opiate and alcohol dependence, it is preferable to begin with the alcohol detoxification, while stabilizing the patient on methadone, and then proceed with methadone withdrawal (Czechowicz, 1978).

12B: INTOXICATION
Intoxication is a residual syndrome associated with substance-specific mental disturbances that result in maladaptive behavior. Substance-specific physiological disturbances may lead to serious medical com-

plications including cardiopulmonary impairment, coma, or death. The severity of the syndrome is generally dose-related, although in some instances it may be idiosyncratic in nature (e.g., pathological alcohol intoxication).

General Therapeutic Principles
The following review will focus on the treatment and management of acute episodes of intoxication that involve overdosage with drugs of abuse. The treatment of Psychoactive Substance Use Disorders will be discussed in the next chapter. The general principles below are applicable to acute, severe intoxications seen in hospital emergency rooms (Czechowicz, 1978).

1. Upon admission of the intoxicated patient, determine immediately the adequacy of cardiopulmonary functions and level of consciousness. Begin cardiopulmonary resuscitation and other life support at once, if needed.
2. Establish a working diagnosis on the basis of available information and clinical evidence. Of immediate concern are the identification of the substance used, its route of entry into the body, and its amount. In addition to the history and physical examination, institute urine and blood screening for drugs and other laboratory tests as appropriate to evaluate the nature and seriousness of the intoxication.
3. Apply measures to eliminate the toxic substance from the body, if needed. In cases of ingested substances in which the overdose occurred within the preceding six hours, immediate measures may include induced emesis, gastric lavage, activated charcoal, and cathartics. Induced vomiting is contraindicated in the presence of impaired consciousness or convulsions. Emesis may be induced with ipecac syrup 30–45 ml; this dose may be repeated in 15 minutes if necessary.

    Gastric lavage requires prior endotracheal intubation if the patient has evidence of CNS depression; it is contraindicated if the patient is convulsing. After lavage is completed, introduce activated charcoal into the stomach to absorb any remaining drug. The use of cathartics (e.g., 30 cc of sorbitol or 30 mg of sodium sulfate) is not a well-established procedure (Davis & Benvenuto, 1975).

    If toxic drug levels persist, it may become necessary to apply other measures for the elimination of the substance, for instance by increasing urinary excretion or by the use of aqueous or lipid dialysis (peritoneal lavage or hemodialysis). Urinary excretion may be hastened by administering sufficient fluids to promote urine output, by forced diuresis with IV 20% mannitol at the rate of 50cc per hour or by the alkalinization of the urine with sodium bicarbonate (e.g., in phenobarbital poisoning).

4. Apply measures that reduce the toxic effects of the substance, as needed. Prompt treatment of impaired vital functions (support of respiration and blood pressure) takes precedence over any other intervention. Assure a clear airway and administer oxygen, if necessary. Provide mechanical ventilation by ambu bag or positive pressure respirator if respiration is not present, and then proceed with endotracheal intubation. Rarely, tracheotomy may be necessary.

   Start IV fluids to maintain blood pressure; vasopressors may be used if fluid therapy fails to restore blood pressure. Upon stabilization of vital functions, obtain an EKG to detect cardiac arrhythmias and provide treatment if necessary.

   In every stuporous or comatose patient, the glucose-naloxone test should be administered routinely as a means of ruling out hypoglycemic or opioid-induced coma: Administer intravenously 50cc of 50% glucose and 0.4 mg naloxone (Narcan). Both agents are safe and readily reverse the respective hypoglycemic or opioid-induced coma. Physostigmine (1–2 mg IV) may serve as an antidote to anticholinergic coma; if successful, it will require frequent repeating. Symptomatic treatment may also control seizures, hyperthermia, cardiac arrhythmias, and so forth.

5. Adequacy of treatment should be regularly assessed by monitoring vital signs, arterial blood gases, drug blood levels, and level of consciousness. Continuous EKG monitoring may be necessary in intoxication with cardiotoxic drugs (e.g., tricyclics).

6. In less serious intoxications, the concomitant behavioral disturbances (agitation, combativeness, suicidal attempts) may become the major focus of management. One may first place the patient in a quiet room and secure his or her safety (as well as that of the attending staff) by providing constant supervision and, if necessary, physical restraint. Sedation may be required for the excited or violent patient, but must be used cautiously. In the case of the "bad tripper" (e.g., Hallucinogen Hallucinosis,

Cannabis Delusional Disorder), the "talk-down" method is the most important aspect of management (see respective sections in Chapter 11).

More complete discussion of management of medical emergencies is beyond the scope of this book.

SPECIFIC INTOXICATION DISORDERS

303.00   Alcohol Intoxication
Most cases of Alcohol Intoxication do not require any special treatment. The most common problem requiring management is combative or assaultive behavior and, occasionally, suicidal behavior. The patient should be handled with a nonprovocative, reassuring approach. Physical restraint may become necessary in combative individuals. The use of sedative drugs should be avoided because of their potentiating effects with alcohol. Benzodiazepines may be used cautiously as a chemical restraint.

In more severe intoxications, the CNS depressant effects of alcohol may impair vital functions (see General Therapeutic Principles). If there is evidence of recent drug use, gastric lavage and other symptomatic treatment may become necessary. In the case of alcohol-disulfiram interaction, treatment consists of the IV administration of an antihistamine and symptomatic control of hypotension.

291.40   Alcohol Idiosyncratic Intoxication
This consists of marked behavioral change—usually aggressiveness—resulting from recent ingestion of a subintoxicating amount of alcohol. Brain damage and temporal lobe epilepsy are thought to be predisposing factors. Treatment is primarily directed toward the management of the aggressive or assaultive behavior.

305.40   Sedative, Hypnotic, or Anxiolytic Intoxication
In mild-to-moderate Sedative, Hypnotic, or Anxiolytic Intoxication, if the patient is conscious and ambulatory, the management is primarily directed to monitoring the vital signs and controlling agitation or aggressiveness. The patient should be placed in a quiet room under close supervision; the use of physical restraints may occasionally become necessary in the presence of combativeness. In more serious intoxica-

tions, treatment largely consists of supportive care and maintenance of vital functions (see General Therapeutic Principles).

In overdose by *short-acting barbiturates*, forced diuresis is of no value. On the other hand, forced diuresis can be very effective in *meprobamate* overdosage. Urine alkalinization with sodium bicarbonate can be helpful in *phenobarbital* overdosage, by increasing the urinary excretion of the drug.

In overdose of *nonbarbiturate sedative-hypnotics*, forced diuresis and dialysis may be useful for certain drugs when response to other measures is unsatisfactory (Czechowicz, 1978). Aqueous dialysis is of little value in *glutethimide* poisoning, because of the drug's protein binding and storage in body fat (Davis & Benvenuto, 1975). Glutethimide overdose may cause a coma-wakefulness cycle due to excretion into and reabsorption from the G.I. tract; monitoring should not be stopped prematurely. Gastric lavage, if performed, should be done with a 1:1 mixture of castor oil and water. If hemodialysis is attempted, it should involve a lipid dialysate (Lewis & Senay, 1981). In *methaqualone* overdose, an intact gag reflex may present difficulties during endotracheal intubation; dialysis may be helpful.

305.50 Opioid Intoxication

In more serious opioid poisoning, medical complications include depressed respiration, depressed consciousness, hypotension, and pulmonary edema. Instead of myosis, pupils may be dilated in severe hypoxia or in mixed addictions. Meperidine may cause dilated pupils and is more frequently associated with convulsions. Heroin may remain active for six hours, methadone for 36–48 hours, and 1-alpha-acetylmethadol (LAAM) for 48–72 hours (Berger & Tinklenberg, 1979; Czechowicz, 1978; Lewis & Senay, 1981).

Management of the acute opioid intoxication involves prompt treatment of respiratory impairment and maintenance of vital functions (see General Therapeutic Principles). Naloxone (Narcan) 0.4 mg IV is effective in reversing both respiratory depression and coma. If the initial dose is ineffective, an additional dose may be given in about five minutes, and again in 10 minutes. Failure to respond should raise consideration of other causes for the intoxication. Narcotic antagonists are effective for about two to three hours; repeat doses may be necessary at regular intervals to continue to reverse respiratory depression.

If withdrawal symptoms are precipitated, they should not be treated with methadone. The patient should remain hospitalized under continuous supervision for 24–48 hours. If pulmonary edema occurs, the treatment of choice is oxygen administration, with positive pressure ventilation and intubation, if necessary (Czechowicz, 1978).

305.60 Cocaine Intoxication
305.70 Amphetamine or Similarly Acting Sympathomimetic Intoxication

Medical complications in acute overdose consist of severe hypertension, hyperpyrexia, seizures, syncope, cardiac arrhythmias or respiratory paralysis. Cocaine and amphetamine-like drugs produce very similar intoxication syndromes. An initial characteristic "rush" of well-being is followed after one hour or longer by a period of "crashing." A suicidal depression may ensure as a complication of withdrawal (see Amphetamine Withdrawal).

The management of a mild-to-moderate psychostimulant intoxication syndrome requires a quiet room where safety measures may be applied for the protection of the patient and the attending staff. If reassurance is not sufficient, sedation with benzodiazepines (e.g., diazepam 10–30 mg orally or lorazepam 1–2 mg IM) may control agitation. Physical restraints may become necessary to control combativeness. Vital signs should be monitored closely for rising blood pressure, pulse, and temperature.

In acute overdose, treatment with neuroleptics is recommended when blood pressure, pulse rate, or temperature are rising, or if acute paranoid behavior develops, provided no anticholinergic drugs were involved in the intoxication. Chlorpromazine, although an effective antidote, has strong anticholinergic effects. The drug of choice is haloperidol, 3–5 mg po or IM, with subsequent doses adjusted to the symptoms (Davis, Sekerke, & Janowsky, 1973). Uncontrollable severe hypertension should be treated with intravenous phentolamine, while hyperpyrexia should be treated with standard medical techniques. Increased fluids and acidification of urine with ammonium chloride can significantly enhance the excretion (Berger & Tinklenberg, 1979).

If psychosis and elevated vital signs persist, the patient requires hospitalization. Suicidal depression may develop during Amphetamine Withdrawal, as may persistent psychosis associated with Amphetamine Delusional Disorder (Berger & Tinklenberg, 1979; Ellinwood, 1979). Amphetamine Delirium has already been discussed.

305.20 Cannabis Intoxication

In moderate doses cannabis acts as a sedative drug, while at high doses it acts as a hallucinogen. Hashish, hash oil, and tetrahydrocannabinol

(THC) are much more potent than cannabis and are more likely to induce Cannabis Hallucinosis. The latter, however, is very rare.

Cannabis Intoxication is relatively mild and short-lived and does not generally require treatment (Balis, 1974). Acute panic associated with Cannabis Intoxication is generally managed by the "talk-down" approach, already described in Hallucinogen Hallucinosis. The treatment of Cannabis Delusional Disorder has also been discussed.

305.90 Phencyclidine (PCP) or Similarly Acting Arylcyclohexylamine Intoxication

Severe PCP intoxication is characterized by the following: motor inhibition and catatonic-like states, stupor, or coma with eyes remaining open; seizures; opisthotonos; hyperreflexia; severe hypertension; and respiratory depression. Bloody vomiting should suggest possible contamination by a synthetic intermediate which decomposes to hydrogen cyanide. The absence of mydriasis and the presence of ataxia, hypertension, and nystagmus differentiate PCP intoxication from hallucinogen intoxication (Lewis & Senay, 1981). Delirium, Organic Mood Disorder, and Organic Delusional Disorder may develop.

In lower-dose intoxication, the key to management is sensory reduction and protection from self-harm. The patient should be kept in a quiet room, closely supervised from a short distance. Physical restraint may be necessary if violent behavior occurs. For sedation, diazepam or haloperidol are the drugs of choice. In moderate to severe intoxication, close observation with monitoring of blood pressure, respiration, and level of consciousness is required. If serious hypertension develops, diazoxide and hydralazine have been reported to be effective (Lewis & Senay, 1981). If status epilepticus develops, diazepam in 2-3 mg increments slow IV is indicated.

Acidification of the urine with ammonium chloride or vitamin C markedly enhances PCP excretion (Aniline, Allen, & Pitts, 1981). Continuous or intermittent gastric suction has been recommended as a means of enhancing PCP excretion (Lewis & Senay, 1981). Prolonged psychotic reactions following PCP intoxication are discussed in the section on Organic Delusional Syndromes in Chapter 11.

305.90 Caffeine Intoxication

Toxic symptoms subside rapidly after reduction of intake or abstinence. Mild withdrawal symptoms may occur in chronic heavy users. No pharmacologic treatment is necessary. Massive overdose may result in seizures that can be controlled with IV diazepam. The substitution of a decaffeinated beverage may prove helpful to some (Greden, 1980).

305.90 Inhalant Intoxication

This diagnosis includes intoxication by inhaling the aliphatic and aromatic hydrocarbons found in gasoline, glue, paint, paint thinners, and spray paints, and to a lesser extent, halogenated hydrocarbons found in cleaners, spray can propellants and other volatile substances. Inhalant users are generally adolescents and young adults, and sometimes young children, with a background invariably marked by considerable family dysfunction (Westermeyer, 1987). Polysubstance abuse is common among this population (e.g., alcohol, marijuana).

The essential features of Inhalant Intoxication are similar to those of alcohol and Sedative, Hypnotic, or Anxiolytic Intoxication and include maladaptive behavioral changes (e.g., impulsiveness, assaultiveness, poor judgment) and physical signs of incoordination, nystagmus, slurred speech, unsteady gait, and so forth. The onset is quick and the course is short, lasting one to one-and-a-half hours. During Inhalant Intoxication, users are accident-prone and may engage in criminal acts or self-destructive behavior. The intoxication may lead to serious complications including CNS depression, cardiac arrhythmias, and sudden death.

Because of the short duration of the intoxication, inhalant users are rarely seen in the emergency room. Treatment is primarily directed toward the management of aggressive or assaultive behavior through behavioral interventions, or physical restraints if necessary. In more serious intoxications involving CNS depression, cardiac arrhythmias, or seizures, treatment consists largely of supportive care (see General Therapeutic Principles).

Family assessment is critical in the case of child and adolescent abusers, for obtaining collateral information and for ruling out child abuse or neglect (Westermeyer, 1987). Patients should be assessed for damage to the CNS, peripheral nervous system, kidneys, liver, lungs, heart, and bone marrow. Tests for lead intoxication (in tetraethyl lead gasoline) should be ordered, and if lead poisoning is present, chelating agents should be used.

Although not well documented, withdrawal seizures and withdrawal delirium may occur in heavy chronic users (Westermeyer, 1987). These patients should be treated with phenobarbital or diazepam (see section on Barbiturate Detoxification). For long-term treatment the reader is referred to Chapter 13 on Psychoactive Substance Use Disorders.

305.90 Other Psychoactive Substance Intoxication

It is beyond the scope of this book to review intoxication from other substances, except for those that are relevant to psychiatric practice. This classification includes inhalant intoxication with anesthetic gases (e.g., nitrous oxide, ether), and short-acting vasodilators such as amyl or butyl nitrite. Anticholinergic drugs represent a class of special interest.

Anticholinergic Drug Intoxication. This type of intoxication is of particular interest because of the widespread use of substances with anticholinergic activity (e.g., tricyclic antidepressants, neuroleptics, antihistamines, antiparkinson drugs). Intoxication may be characterized by dilated and unreactive pupils, flushed face, warm and dry skin, dry mouth, paralytic ileus, urinary retention, tachycardia, hypertension or hypotension, increased respiratory rate, seizures, hyperpyrexia, and delirium, hallucinations, delusions, severe agitation and assaultiveness, stupor or coma.

In addition to the above, the comatose patient may show hyperreflexia, positive Babinski sign, and clonic movements (Berger & Tinklenberg, 1979; Goldfrank & Meliek, 1979; Granacher, Baldessarini, & Messner, 1976). Cardiotoxic effects with tricyclics include supraventricular tachycardia, ventricular tachyarrhythmias, cardiac conduction defects and A/V block, and direct suppression of the myocardium (Goldfrank & Meliek, 1979; Granacher, Baldessarini, & Messner, 1976).

Patient management includes the usual measures for overdosage (emesis, gastric lavage, maintenance of cardiopulmonary functions, monitoring of vital signs), continuous EKG monitoring, and symptomatic treatment of anticholinergic effects. Physostigmine salicylate 2 mg IV is capable of reversing the coma, and controlling delirium, hyperthermia, and supraventricular tachycardia secondary to anticholinergic toxicity (Heizer & Wilbert, 1974). A second dose of 1–2 mg physostigmine may be given 15 minutes later, and it may be repeated every two to three hours, if needed, since it is rapidly metabolized. Close monitoring of anticholinergic symptoms is required. Cholinergic toxicity induced by overmedication with physostigmine can be reversed by atropine 0.1 to 1.0 mg IV or propantheline bromide (Probanthine) 15–30 mg IM or IV (Lewis & Senay, 1981).

Agitation in milder cases may be controlled with diazepam, provided vital functions are stable and the patient is fully conscious. Seizures can be controlled with intravenous diazepam. In tricyclic intoxication, cardiac arrhythmias (other than supraventricular tachycardia) are treated with intravenous fluids and alkalinization with sodium bicarbonate or sodium lactate; if there is no improvement, propranolol and lidocaine can be useful. Prolonged EKG monitoring is extremely important for diagnosing cardiac arrhythmias, and as a means of assessing severity or tricyclic intoxication. The latter correlates with the degree of widening of QRS complex and prolongation of QT interval (Goldfrank & Meliek, 1979; Granacher, Baldessarini, & Messner, 1976).

Section III
Psychoactive Substance Use Disorders

by

George U. Balis, M.D.

Chapter 13

Psychoactive Substance Use Disorders

This diagnostic class defines disorders with maladaptive behavioral changes associated with pathological use of psychoactive substances. They are distinguished into Psychoactive Substance Dependence and Psychoactive Substance Abuse.

Psychoactive Substance Dependence has been redefined by new criteria in *DSM-III-R*. The essential feature is a cluster of cognitive, behavioral, and physiologic symptoms that constitute a *dependence syndrome*, indicating that the person has impaired control of psychoactive substance use and continues its use in spite of adverse consequences. The diagnosis of the dependence syndrome requires at least three of nine characteristic symptoms of dependence, some of which have persisted for at least one month, or have occurred episodically over a longer period.

Psychoactive Substance Abuse is a residual category in which maladaptive patterns of psychoactive substance use have never met the criteria for dependence.

Personality disturbance and other psychopathology (e.g., depression, anxiety) are often present as associated features in substance use disorders. Complications resulting from Substance Abuse or Substance Dependence include substance-specific Organic Mental Syndromes, deterioration of physical health due to malnutrition and poor hygiene, and medical complications due to the effects of the substance (e.g., cirrhosis, peripheral neuropathy, acute pancreatitis associated with Alcohol Dependence) or due to the administration of the substance by contaminated needles (e.g., hepatitis, AIDS, vasculitis, septicemia in Opioid Dependence).

General Therapeutic Principles
The field is replete with treatment approaches, based on diverse theories and ideologies, with claims of therapeutic successes that generally lack objective substantiation. The following principles constitute general guidelines for a treatment and management plan.

1. There is no singular treatment modality that can claim high effectiveness for chemical dependence.
2. A combination of modalities is most likely to achieve a measure of therapeutic success.
3. The treatment modalities must be tailored to the individual, taking into consideration his or her specific problems, response to previous treatment attempts, and the resources available.
4. Different treatment and management approaches are administered by a great variety of professionals, nonprofessional practitioners, and lay groups. The physician plays a central role in the initial evaluation and medical diagnosis, management of physical/psychiatric complications, detoxification, and appropriate referral. In follow-up care, the general physician may apply some of the specific methods available, or may collaborate with other practitioners and various agencies involved in the treatment and rehabilitation of the patient.
5. A prerequisite for any treatment plan is the detoxification of the patient (see Treatment section on Withdrawal and Withdrawal Deliria).
6. The presence of associated psychopathology requires specialized psychiatric treatment, especially with regard to affective disorders and personality disorders (e.g., antisocial, borderline).
7. The socially dislocated individual (e.g., unemployed, homeless, legally entangled, or culturally alienated) requires social and vocational rehabilitation, with the goal of reintegrating him or her into the family, community, or work setting.

Treatment modalities currently include:

1. *Pharmacologic methods,* such as disulfiram for alcoholism, tricyclics for cocaine dependence, narcotic maintenance and narcotic antagonists for opioid dependence, and various psychotropic drugs for the short-term management of targeted symptoms of anxiety and depression following detoxification.
2. *Psychosocial methods,* including individual psychotherapy, group therapy, family therapy, conjoint therapy with spouse, contingency contracting behavior modification, aversive conditioning, and relaxation techniques.
3. *Sociotherapies,* such as various therapeutic communities (e.g., Synanon) and other residential programs.
4. *Self-support groups,* such as Alcoholics Anonymous, Al-Anon, Alateen, Narcotics Anonymous.
5. Various therapeutic, educational, occupational, inspirational, or humane programs, supported or sponsored by government agencies, industry, religious organizations (e.g., Salvation Army), and other community and volunteer agencies.

Common factors that appear to contribute to therapeutic success include:

1. Patience, perseverance, and commitment on the part of the therapist while working with a very difficult and frustrating patient who is suffering from a chronic and relapsing disorder. This should be laced with hopeful expectation, kindled by a caring and nurturing but firm attitude, tempered by a realistic appraisal of the patient's potential and limitations, and monitored for transference and countertransference problems.
2. Maintenance of abstinence during treatment and the setting of abstinence as the ultimate treatment goal.
3. A degree of coercion that ranges from subtle measures of substance control to commitment to a treatment facility. It may take the form of "contracts" that the patient is persuaded or forced to make with the therapist, spouse, or employer, in the face of crisis situations. Structured environments, disulfiram administered under supervision, or limit setting in therapy are other examples of therapeutic coercion.
4. Breaking through the defense of massive denial. A major effort during the initial phase of treatment is to help the patient to recognize and accept the problem.

5. Bolstering of the patient's wavering motivation to stay in treatment and remain abstinent.
6. Development of alternative coping styles to handle intense dysphoric affects, especially rage, guilt, anxiety, and depression; and boosting and maintenance of self-esteem.

SPECIFIC PSYCHOACTIVE SUBSTANCE USE DISORDERS

303.90 Alcohol Dependence
305.00 Alcohol Abuse

Detoxification is the first step of treatment of alcoholism. Detoxification and treatment of psychiatric complications of alcoholism (Organic Mental Syndromes) were discussed elsewhere (see Organic Mental Disorders in Chapter 11).

A comprehensive treatment approach is best. Several treatment modalities should be integrated into a treatment plan tailored to the individual and the resources available. The treatment plan may include psychotherapy, group therapy, family therapy, conjoint therapy, support groups, disulfiram, and short-term use of tranquilizers or antidepressants for targeted psychopathology (Gerard & Saenger, 1966). Alcoholics Anonymous is part of most successful programs. Al-Anon provides assistance to spouses of alcoholics through group support, while Alateen serves the needs of children of alcoholic parents. Referral of family members to these organizations should be part of the multiple treatment approach.

Halfway houses may be important treatment resources for patients with placement problems following detoxification and discharge. Vocational rehabilitation and social support agencies may be required for selected cases (Selzer, 1980). In most communities, there are comprehensive alcoholism treatment and rehabilitation programs, many of which are inpatient or residential.

The primary physician plays a crucial role in diagnosis and treatment. Dealing with the patient's denial must be early and decisive. Instruments such as the Michigan Alcoholism Screening Test (MAST) may serve as the first step in loosening the patient's defensive armor (Selzer et al., 1975). With acceptance of the problem and the establishment of a therapeutic alliance, the physician can proceed with negotiating a therapeutic contract (Brady et al., 1982). Long-term abstinence should be the goal. If this is not possible, a trial period of abstinence is an acceptable compromise. The contract should include means of deterrence and ways of monitoring compliance.

Disulfiram is effective in selected cases, especially when relapse is frequent. Baseline laboratory studies should be obtained and the patient fully instructed about the consequences of drinking within four days of ingestion of the drug. Disulfiram is then given, preferably at bedtime, in a loading dose of 500 mg daily for five to seven days, then continued on a daily maintenance dose of 250–500 mg.

A spouse or some other person should be involved in administering the disulfiram at least every three or four days to ensure compliance or the patient may visit the therapist or clinic every three or four days for observed ingestion. After the first month, a new contract is negotiated, with the patient assuming responsibility for control of his drinking (Goodwin, 1982). Disulfiram should not be allowed to take the place of AA or other support and therapeutic activities.

The psychotherapeutic approach is primarily supportive with many patients; the therapist plays an active and nurturing role while maintaining clear boundaries of separateness and setting firm limits that discourage acting out and enforce the abstinence rule (Wurmser, 1979). Family therapy can be crucial in the treatment of the alcoholic in view of the dysfunctional family systems associated with alcohol abuse (see Kaufman, 1985). Behavioral therapy techniques include relaxation, assertiveness training, self-control skills, aversive conditioning contingency contracting, broad spectrum behavioral treatments, and biofeedback (Emrick, 1974).

Benzodiazepines and small doses of low potency neuroleptics are recommended by some, but only for short-term use following detoxification, for control of anxiety (Rothstein, Cobble, & Sampson, 1976). Most clinicians and programs recommend a drug-free treatment regimen, especially during the first two-to-three weeks following withdrawal (Pattison, 1986).

In patients with a "double diagnosis," a concomitant primary psychiatric disorder (e.g., affective disorder) may play a causative role in the development of alcoholism or, conversely, alcoholism may be a major destabilizing factor. Psychiatric conditions most commonly associated with alcoholism include mood disorders (bipolar disorder, major depression, dysthymia), borderline personality, and antisocial personality. Psychiatric treatment, especially of mood disorders, should be provided concurrently with treatment of alcoholism.

304.0x Opioid Dependence
305.5x Opioid Abuse

Treatment programs for the opioid addict (mainly heroin) include methadone maintenance, maintenance with opioid antagonists, therapeutic communities, and various abstinence-oriented recovery programs. Most of these provide a combination of adjunctive approaches, such as group therapy, improvement of social skills, vocational training, job placement, and family counseling.

Methadone maintenance is the most common and most successful treatment for opioid dependence (Mirin & Meyer, 1978). It is offered in special clinics under close supervision and monitoring. Unlike heroin, methadone is long-acting (24 hours), and is orally effective. In usual doses (40–50 mg), it blocks opioid craving, while in much higher doses (100–120 mg) it blocks the euphoriant effects of opioids. The most significant effect for maintenance is the blocking of opioid craving (Goldstein & Judson, 1973).

In spite of some criticism, methadone maintenance is an effective and safe method that allows the opioid addict to change his lifestyle, stabilize his functioning, and reintegrate into the community. Treatment goals are reduction of illicit drug use, reduction of criminal activity, increased employability, increased self-esteem, and improvement in family and community functioning (Berger & Tinklenberg, 1979; Green, Meyer, & Shader, 1975; Kissin, Lowinson, & Millman, 1978).

According to FDA regulations, those eligible for methadone maintenance are individuals whose dependence on heroin has lasted longer than two years. It is indicated for addicts who have an extensive history of drug use and antisocial behavior and who have repeatedly failed to maintain abstinence. A typical methadone maintenance clinic provides daily administration of oral methadone, monitored with urinalysis, plus drug counseling and ancillary services, including in some instances individual psychotherapy and group therapy.

Several authors have noted that the methadone maintenance approach tends to reinforce the addict's identity as a member of the drug subculture and to perpetuate detrimental attitudes towards drug use. (Dole & Nyswander, 1976; Lennard, Epstein, & Rosenthal, 1972). Many patients continue to use other licit and illicit drugs (Ausabel, 1983), the most common being alcohol (O'Donnell, 1969).

Levo-alpha-acetyl-methadol (LAAM) is a long-acting congener of methadone, currently under investigation. It can be administered three times per week, thus affording greater treatment flexibility (Ling & Blaine, 1979).

Maintenance with opioid antagonists—cyclazocine, naloxone, naltrexone, and buprenorphine—is currently undergoing field trials as a new treatment approach. Its goal is to decondition the behaviors of opioid use and relapse (Whitlock & Evans, 1978), by blocking both the euphoria and the relief of conditioned abstinence symptoms of the former opioid abuser, including injection rituals (Resnick et al., 1979).

According to Greenstein and colleagues (1983), patients most likely to benefit from naltrexone therapy are socially stable (employed, married), self-motivated, and stabilized on low-dose methadone before detoxification from methadone and induction with naltrexone. Naltrexone is useful as an adjunct to other therapies.

Naltrexone induction therapy consists of the following steps:

1. Detoxification from heroin or methadone and establishment of a drug-free period of at least seven days post-heroin withdrawal, or 10 days post-methadone withdrawal.
2. Administration of naloxone challenge in the already abstinent patient (e.g., 0.8 mg subcutaneously or IV of naloxone should elicit no withdrawal).
3. An initial dose of 25 mg or 50 mg of naltrexone is administered, once the patient has been shown to be ready for naltrexone induction.
4. Maintenance naltrexone at 350 mg per week, given on a daily (50 mg/day), twice a week (150 mg on Mondays and 200 mg on Thursdays), or three times a week (100 mg on Mondays and Wednesdays and 150 mg Fridays) regimen.
5. Weekly screening of urine for drugs during the initial several months of treatment, as well as periodic physical examinations.

Therapeutic communities (e.g., Synanon, Odyssey House, Daytop, Phoenix House) are drug-free, full-time residential programs that attempt to rehabilitate and resocialize the drug addict through the use of a rigidly defined, experiential lifestyle that emphasizes group interaction, peer pressure, and self-government. Treatment in the typical therapeutic community lasts one to two years and generally focuses on extensive lifestyle change by means of forceful confrontation. Some have criticized this model as being excessively authoritarian (Ausabel, 1983). Others have noted that there is little methodologically vigorous evidence to substantiate the effectiveness of therapeutic communities (Romand, Forrest, & Kleber, 1975).

This model is thought to be most effective for the highly motivated individual who can complete the required program (Mirin & Meyer, 1978; Sells, 1979). In this regard, the model may not be very practical for many addicts. However, it may be a good choice for the addict with legal entanglements that have led to court referral (Klein & Miller, 1986). The current status and evolution of the therapeutic community was recently reviewed by DeLeon (1985).

Abstinence-oriented recovery models in various addiction treatment centers are based on the alcoholic recovery model (Alcoholic Anonymous) and the derivative self-help groups of Narcotics Anonymous (NA) and Chemical Dependency Anonymous (Bill, 1968).

A confrontational approach that aims to break the addict's denial of the seriousness and severity of his illness is essential to this model, which includes an educational approach as well. These are generally residential programs in which group therapy is the primary treatment modality and family participation is actively sought. Discharge planning provides for continued support and structure, required attendance of NA meetings, urine screens to monitor possible drug usage, aftercare groups, and individual or family therapy when needed. This approach is thought to be most useful for addicts in the early stages of addiction who are motivated for change (Klein & Miller, 1986).

Other outpatient, drug-free programs provide various resocialization experiences, such as group discussions, assistance with social and vocational problems, and recreational activities. Some are organized along the lines of a daytime therapeutic community (Sells, 1979).

Psychotherapy. In spite of the widespread opinion that individual psychotherapy is ineffective with opiate addicts, there are several studies which indicate that professional psychotherapy can provide addicts additional benefits when combined with standard drug counseling services in a methadone-maintenance program (Resnick et al., 1981). Short-term interpersonal psychotherapy was found to be effective by Klerman, Dimascio, & Weissman (1974) and by Weissman et al. (1976), but not by Rounsaville et al. (1983). Supportive-expressive and cognitive-behavioral psychotherapies have also been reported to be useful within the context of a methadone program (Woody et al., 1983). Several studies have provided some evidence that psychodynamic (Willett, 1973), cognitive-behavioral (Abrahms, 1979), and implosive (Hirt & Greenfield, 1979) group therapies may be helpful for this population. Psychotherapy is particularly indicated in patients with psychiatric symptoms. Opiate addicts show a high degree of psychopathology, and addiction itself may often be viewed as self-medication to avoid depression, anxiety, and other dysphoric symptoms (Khantzian, Mack, & Schatzberg, 1974; Wurmser, 1979). Opiate addicts may require more intensive treatment than is typically offered in methadone programs (McLellan et al., 1979). For more detailed information about the use of psychotherapy in opiate abuse, the reader is referred to a review by Woody et al. (1986).

Psychopharmacotherapy. This may be indicated in addicts presenting serious psychiatric symptoms, and especially depression. In a placebo-controlled study of the effect of doxepin on depressed opiate addicts in a methadone program, doxepin was shown to produce substantially greater reduction of depressive symptoms (Woody, O'Brien & Rickels, 1975). On the other hand, a more recent placebo-controlled study using imipramine (Kleber et al., 1983) found that the two treatment groups showed equal improvement. Outcome studies of long-term treatment and rehabilitation programs show that methadone maintenance and therapeutic communities are the most successful approaches (Sells, 1979; Simpson, 1981).

HIV. Finally, one should recognize the possibility of HIV and other infections of intravenous drug users who share needles, and the continuing spread of Acquired Immune Deficiency Syndrome (AIDS) among them. Recent statistics show that 25% of approximately one million people exposed to HIV are intravenous drug users and that 40% of IV drug users tested are HIV seropositive (Fry, 1986).

304.10 Sedative, Hypnotic, or Anxiolytic Dependence
305.40 Sedative, Hypnotic, or Anxiolytic Abuse
This disorder is often iatrogenically initiated and/or maintained. Indiscriminate or poorly supervised prescription of hypnotics and anxiolytic drugs, especially in the elderly, is not an uncommon practice. Younger people abuse these drugs for their intoxicating effect, to enhance the euphoria of opioids, or to counteract the stimulant effects of cocaine and amphetamine. Benzodiazepines are the most commonly abused drugs.

Detoxification is a prerequisite of any treatment approach (see Withdrawal section in Chapter 12). Following detoxification, the patient should be evaluated to rule out primary psychopathology (e.g., Major Depression) and be given appropriate treatment if necessary.

There are no controlled studies on the efficacy of psychotherapy on this type of drug abuse. The few older studies available indicate poor outcome (Anderson et al., 1972; Tennant, 1979). It has been suggested that psychotherapy and group therapy may be useful in the patient with psychiatric illness (Liskow, 1982).

304.50 Hallucinogen Dependence
305.30 Hallucinogen Abuse
304.30 Cannabis Dependence
305.20 Cannabis Abuse
304.50 Phencyclidine (PCP) or Similarly Acting Arylcyclohexylamine Dependence
305.90 Phencyclidine (PCP) or Similarly Acting Arylcyclohexylamine Abuse

These classes of substances, commonly referred to as "soft drugs," are discussed together because they share common aspects of epidemiology and pattern of use. They are often used within the context of a characteristic drug subculture (Balis, 1974).

Severity of the disorder varies according to the type of substance used, degree of dependence, and concomitant psychopathology. Polydrug abuse often involves alcohol. Underlying psychopathology is a common problem, especially with the polydrug abuser, and usually involves depression, personality disorders, or both. Treatment of the underlying disorder is necessary for the long-term rehabilitation.

Detoxification is a prerequisite to treatment (see respective sections). Individual and/or group therapy are recommended for most patients, although its efficacy has not been established (Berger & Tinklenberg, 1979). Referral to drug-free outpatient programs and utilization of community support agencies are important. Unfortunately, most patients are not well motivated; the majority drop out early in treatment (Anderson, O'Malley, & Lazare, 1972).

Residential programs, especially therapeutic communities with rigorously structured resocialization programs, provide the greatest chance for success, particularly for the highly motivated or legally constrained individual (Sells, 1979). Generally, the longer a person stays in treatment, the more favorable the outcome (Simpson, 1981).

304.20 Cocaine Dependence
305.60 Cocaine Abuse

There is no consensus regarding optimal treatment for cocaine use disorder. In general, cocaine treatment programs use the methods of

Alcoholics Anonymous, contingency contracting, and urine monitoring. Hospitalization is necessary for those with chronic free-base or IV use, with medical or psychiatric complications, and/or with concurrent dependence on other drugs (Gold & Dackis, 1984).

"Contingency contracting" (Anker & Crowley, 1982) is based on the patient's agreement to participate in a urine-monitoring program and to accept an aversive contingency in the event of either a cocaine-positive urine or failure to produce a urine sample. Current treatments emphasize psychological strategies (individual, group, family therapy) aimed at modifying addictive behaviors, with reported success rates of psychotherapy in the range of 40%-45% for experienced programs (Anker & Crowley, 1982; Kleber & Gawin, 1984).

Pharmacological approaches to Cocaine Abuse and Cocaine Dependence have recently been introduced, with some promising results especially for tricyclic antidepressants. Desipramine was shown in an open clinical trial by Gawin and Kleber (1984) to be effective as adjunct to psychotherapy in decreasing craving and promoting abstinence, regardless of whether an affective disorder was also present. On the other hand, lithium was effective only in cyclothymic subjects.

In a subsequent double-blind, placebo-controlled study by Gawin, Byck, and Kleber (1985), desipramine facilitated abstinence in both depressed and nondepressed cocaine abusers. Similar results were reported by Giannini et al. (1986). Several larger-scale studies are currently under way (Gawin, 1986). Most recently, amantadine, a dopamine agonist, was reported to attenuate cocaine abuse in methadone maintenance patients at doses of 200 mg b.i.d. (Handelsman, 1987).

304.40 Amphetamine or Similarly Acting Sympathomimetic Dependence
305.70 Amphetamine or Similarly Acting Sympathomimetic Abuse

There are no established treatment guidelines for this class of psychoactive drugs. Treatment approaches are similar to the psychosocial methods described in Cocaine Abuse and Cocaine Dependence (see section on Organic Delusional Disorders in Chapter 11).

304.60 Inhalant Dependence
305.90 Inhalant Abuse

Once abstinence is achieved (see section on Intoxication in Chapter 12), psychosocial interventions are necessary to prevent recurrence (Westermeyer, 1987). Concomitant psychopathology needs to be recognized and treated accordingly. Various psychotherapies, sociodrama, and vocational rehabilitation have been used to treat adolescent abusers (Stybel, 1977). Family intervention and the mobilization of community resources are particularly important in an effort to improve family functioning and socioeconomic setting (Nurcombe et al., 1970). Various social approaches have been used during "epidemics" of inhalant abuse (Westermeyer, 1987). The syndrome is very difficult to treat.

305.10 Nicotine Dependence

In contrast to other substance use disorders, Nicotine Dependence alone is not associated with impairment in social or occupational functioning. There are numerous treatment methods, reporting varying rates of success. Behavioral and psychotherapeutic techniques include aversive conditioning, desensitization, symptom substitution, covert desensitization, hypnotherapy, group therapy, relaxation training, supportive therapy, and education therapy (Katz, 1980; Orleans et al., 1981). No one technique has proved superior to others, and none has consistently shown long-term success rates in excess of 20% (Mann, Johnson, & Levine, 1986). Several educational programs are available for smokers interested in giving up the habit.

The best results are seen in programs that combine education with group therapy and support. In spite of reported high rates of success for some programs, the majority of smokers relapse. Pharmacological methods using lobeline sulfate (a nicotine agonist), sedatives, or psychostimulants have not been proven effective (Hunt & Bespalec, 1974; Jaffe & Jarvik, 1978; Jarvik et al., 1977).

Nicotine chewing gum has had some limited success (Hjalmarson, 1984; Schneider et al., 1983); however, a large follow-up study showed that nicotine vs. placebo gum vs. advice booklets produced no significant improvement over physician advice, as measured by abstinence rates at one year (Thoracic Society, 1983). There is some evidence that subjects with high nicotine tolerance are more apt to benefit from the use of nicotine gum (Fagerstrom, 1982; Hall et al., 1985; Jarvik & Schneider, 1984).

Propranolol has been reported to be effective (Farebrother et al., 1980). Similarly, clonidine, an alpha noradrenergic blocker, was recently reported to reduce craving for cigarettes (Glassman et al., 1984). Abrupt abstinence when motivation is high may be the best method for most patients (Jarvik et al., 1977).

304.90 Polysubstance Dependence

According to new *DSM-III-R* criteria, this classification is used when there has been repeated use, for at least six months, of three or more categories of psychoactive substances (not including nicotine and caffeine), but no single drug has predominated. During this period, the criteria have been met for dependence on psychoactive substances as a group, but not for any specific substance. Many polysubstance abusers follow an indiscriminate use of multiple drugs, while others follow a characteristic pattern of alternating psychostimulant drugs with sedative, hypnotic, or anxiolytic drugs or alcohol.

Polydrug abusers are more likely to show significant psychopathology than single-substance abusers. Treatment of the concomitant psychiatric disorder is of major significance. Detoxification of patients with mixed drug dependence was discussed in the Treatment section on Withdrawal and Withdrawal Deliria in Chapter 12. There are no established specific guidelines for the long-term treatment and rehabilitation of the polysubstance abuser. In general, treatment approaches are similar to those described in single substance dependence.

304.90 Psychoactive Substance Dependence Not Otherwise Specified
305.90 Psychoactive Substance Abuse Not Otherwise Specified

These are residual categories and need not be discussed separately. The reader is referred to the previous sections on Psychoactive Substance Use Disorders.

References for Sections II and III

Abrahms, J. L.: A cognitive-behavioral versus nondirective group treatment program for opioid addicted persons: An adjunct to methadone maintainance. *International Journal of Addictions*, 14:503–511, 1979.

Adams, R. D.: Anxiety, depression, asthenia, and personality disorders. In R. G. Perrdord, R. D. Adams, et al. (Eds)., *Harrison's Principles of Internal Medicine* (10th ed.). New York: McGraw-Hill, 1983, pp. 68–75.

Amdurski, S., Radwan, M., Levi, A., et al.: A therapeutic trial of amantadine in haloperidol-induced malignant neuroleptic syndrome. *Current Therapy Research*, 33: 225–229, 1983.

Anderson, J. W.: Reactive hypoglycemia. In H. F. Conn (Ed.), *Current Therapy, 1979*. Philadelphia: W. B. Saunders Co, 1979, pp. 421–423.

Anderson, W., O'Malley, J. E., & Lazare, A.: Failure of outpatient treatment of drug abuse: Amphetamines, barbiturates, hallucinogens. *American Journal of Psychiatry*, 128:122–125, 1972.

Aniline, O., Allen, R. E., & Pitts, F. N.: Treatment of PCP intoxication and abuse. In *Syllabus and Scientific Proceedings*. Washington D.C.: American Psychiatric Association, 1981, p.31.

Anker, A. L., & Crowley, T. J.: Use of contingency in specialty clinics for cocaine abuse. In L. S. Harris (Ed.), *Problems of Drug Dependence, 1981*. NIDA Research Monograph series No. 41. Washington, D.C.: U.S. Government Printing Office, 1982.

Atsmon, A., & Blum, I.: The discovery. In E. Roberts & P. Amacher (Eds.), *Propranolol and Schizophrenia*. New York: Alan R. Liss, 1978, pp. 5–38.

Ausabel, D. P.: Methadone maintainance treatment: The other side of the coin. *International Journal of Addictions*, 18:851–862, 1983.

Ayd, F. J.: Haloperidol: Twenty years' clinical experience. *Journal of Clinical Psychiatry*, 39:807–814, 1978.

Balis, G. U.: Delirium and other states of altered consciousness. *The Practice of Medicine*, Volume 10. Hagerstown, MD: Harper & Row, 1970.

Balis, G. U.: The use of psychotomimetic and related consciousness-altering drugs. In S. Arieti (Ed.), *American Handbook of Psychiatry*, Volume 3. New York: Basic Books, 1974, pp. 404–445.

Balis, G. U.: Behavior disorders associated with epilepsy. In G. U. Balis, L. Wurmser, E. McDaniel, & R. G. Grenell (Eds.), *Clinical Psychopathology, Psychiatric Foundations of Medicine, Volume 4*, Boston: Butterworth, 1978, pp. 3–64.

Balis, G. U.: The effects of drugs in episodic dyscontrol disorders. In S. Fielding & R. C. Effland (Eds.), *New Frontiers in Psychotropic Drug Research*. New York: Futura Publishing Co., 1979, pp. 191–240.

Balis, G. U.: Criterion value of atypical drug responses in the diagnosis of atypical psychiatric disorders. *Journal of Nervous and Mental Disease*, 170(12):737–743, 1982.

Ban, T. A.: Vasodilators, stimulants and anabolic agents in the treatment of geropsychiatric patients. In M. A. Lipton, A. DiMascio, & K. F. Killam (Eds.), *Psychopharmacology: A Generation of Progress*. New York: Raven Press, 1978a.

Ban, T. A.: The treatment of depressed geriatric patients. *American Journal of Psychotherapy*, 32:93–104, 1978b.

Barnes, R., Veith, R., Okimoto, J., et al.: Efficacy of antipsychotic medications in behaviorally disturbed dementia patients. *American Journal of Psychiatry*, 139:1170–1174, 1982.

Bayne, J. R. D.: Management of confusion in elderly persons. *Canadian Medical Association Journal*, 118:139–141, 1978.

Bear, D., Freeman, R., Schiff, D., et al.: Interictal behavioral changes in patients with temporal lobe epilepsy. In R. E. Hales, & A. J. Frances (Eds.), *Annual Review*. Washington, D.C.: American Psychiatric Association, 1985, pp. 177–199.

Benson, D. F.: Amnesia. *South Medical Journal*, 71:1221–1227, 1978.

Benson, D. F., Marsden, D. C. & Meadows, J. C.: The amnestic syndrome of posterior cerebral artery occlusion. *Acta Neurologica Scandanavica*, 50:133–145, 1974.

Berger, P. A., & Tinklenberg, J. R.: Medical management of the drug abuser. In A. M. Freeman, R. L. Sack, & P. L. Berger (Eds.), *Psychiatry for the Primary Care Physician*. Baltimore: Williams & Wilkins, 1979, pp. 359–380.

Bigger, J. T., Kantor, S. J., Glassman, A. H., et al.: Cardiovascular effects of tricyclic antidepressant drugs. In M. A. Lipton, A. DiMascio, & K. F. Killam (Eds.), *Psychopharmacology: A Generation of Progress*. New York: Raven Press, 1978.

Bill, W.: The fellowship of Alcoholics Anonymous: In R. J. Cantanzaro (Ed.), *Alcoholism: The Total Treatment Approach*, Springfield, IL: Charles C Thomas, 1968.

Blitt, C. D. & Petty, W. C.: Reversal of lorazepam delirium by physostigmine. *Current Researches in Anesthesia and Analgesia*, 54:607–608, 1975.

Blumenthal, M. D., & Davie, J. W.: Dizziness and falling in elderly psychiatric outpatients. *American Journal of Psychiatry*, 137:203–206, 1980.

Blumer, D.: Temporal lobe epilepsy and its psychiatric significance. In D. Benson & D. Blumer (Eds.), *Psychiatric Aspects of Neurological Disease*. New York: Grune & Stratton, 1975.

Blumer, D.: Treatment of patients with seizure disorders referred because of psychiatric complications. *McLean Hospital Journal*, 53, June 1977.

Brady, J. P., Foulks, E. T., Childress, A. R., & Pertshuk, M.: The Michigan Alcoholism Screening Test as a survey instrument. *Journal of Operational Psychiatry*, 13:27–31, 1982.

Brodsky, L., Zuniga, J. S., Casenas, E. R., et al.: Refractory anxiety: A masked epileptiform disorder. *Psychiatric Journal of the University of Ottawa*, 8:42–45, 1983.

Brown, J., Lewis, V., Brown, M., et al.: A comparison between transient amnesias induced by two drugs (diazepam or lorazepam) and amnesia of organic origin. *Neuropsychology*, 20:55–70, 1982.

Burest, J. C. M., & Behemns, M. M.: "Release hallucinations" as the major symptom of posterior cerebral artery occlusion: A report of 2 cases. *Annals of Neurology*, 2:432–436, 1977.

Butler, R. W.: Psychotherapy of old age. In S. Arieti (Ed.), *American Handbook of Psychiatry, Volume 5*. New York: Basic Books, 1975, pp. 807–828.

Cade, J. F. J.: Massive thiamine dosage in the treatment of acute alcoholic psychosis. *Australia and New Zealand Journal of Psychiatry*, 6:222-230, 1970.

Caine, E. D.: Pseudodementia. *Archives of General Psychiatry*, 38:1359-1364, 1981.

Cami, J., Torres, S., San, L., et al.: Efficacy of clonidine and methadone in the rapid detoxification of patients dependent on heroin. *Clinical Pharmacology and Therapeutics*, 38:336-341, 1985.

Charney, D. S., Riordan, C. E., Kleber, H. D., et al.: Clonidine and naltrexone—A safe, effective, and rapid treatment of abrupt withdrawal from methadone therapy. *Archives of General Psychiatry*, 39:1327-1332, 1982.

Charney, D. S., Sternberg, D. E., Kleber, M. D., et al.: The clinical use of clonidine in abrupt withdrawal from methadone. *Archives of General Psychiatry*, 38:1273-1277, 1981.

Christie, J. E., Shering, A., Ferguson, J., et al.: Physostigmine and arecoline: Effects of intravenous infusions in Alzheimer's presenile dementia. *British Journal of Psychiatry*, 138:46-50, 1981.

Cohen, M. R., & Niska, R. W.: Localized right cerebral hemisphere dysfunction and recurrent mania. *American Journal of Psychiatry*, 137:847-848, 1980.

Cohn, C. K., Wright, J. R., & DeVaul, R. A.: Post head trauma syndrome in an adolescent treated with lithium carbonate—Case report. *Diseases of the Nervous System*, 38:630-631, 1977.

Cole, J. O., & Braconnier, M. A.: Drugs and senile dementia. In J. O. Cole (Ed.), *Psychopharmacology Update*. Lexington, MA: Collamore Press, 1980.

Coons, D. J., Hillman, F. J., & Marshall, R. W.: Treatment of neuroleptic malignant syndrome with dandrolene sodium: A case report. *American Journal of Psychiatry*, 139:944-945, 1982.

Cooper, D. S., Halpern, R., Wood, L. L., et al.: L-thyroxine therapy in subclinical hypothyroidism: A double-blind placebo-controlled trial. *Annals of Internal Medicine*, 101:18-24, 1984.

Cummings, J. L.: Organic delusions: phenomenology, anatomical correlations, and review. *British Journal of Psychiatry*, 146:184-197, 1985.

Cummings, J. L., Dementia syndromes: Neurobehavioral and neuropsychiatric features. *Journal of Clinical Psychiatry*, 48:3-8, 1987.

Cummings, J. L., Benson, D., & LoVerme, S.: Reversible dementias. *Journal of the American Medical Association*, 243:2434-2439, 1980.

Cummings, J. L., & Benson, D. F.: *Dementia: A Clinical Approach*. Boston: Butterworths, 1983.

Cummings, J. L., & Mendez, M. F.: Secondary amnesia with focal cerebrovascular lesions. *American Journal of Psychiatry*, 141:1084-1087, 1984.

Czechowicz, D.: *Detoxification Treatment Manual*. Rockville, MD: National Institute of Drug Abuse, U.S. Dept. of Health, Education, and Welfare, 1978.

Dackis, C. A., Goggams, F. C., Bloodworth, R., et al.: The prevalence of hypothyroidism in psychiatric populations. In *Abstracts of Scientific Proceedings* of the American Psychiatric Association Annual Meeting, New York, 1983.

Davies, P., & Maloney, A. J. F.: Selective loss of central cholinergic neurons in Alzheimer's disease. *Lancet*, ii:1403, 1976.

Davies, P., & Wolozin, B. L.: Recent advances in the neurochemistry of Alzheimer's disease. *Journal of Clinical Psychiatry*, 48:28-30, 1987.

Davies, R. K., Tucker, G. J., Harrow, M., et al.: Confusional episodes and antidepressant medication. *American Journal of Psychiatry*, 128:95-99, 1971.

Davis, J. M., & Benvenuto, J. A.: Acute reactions from drug abuse problems. In H. L. P. Resnick & H. L. Ruben (Eds.), *Emergency Psychiatric Care*. Bowie, MD: Charles Press, 1975, pp. 81-101.

Davis, J. M., Sekerke, J., & Janowsky, D.: Drug interactions involving drugs of abuse. In *National Commission on Marijuana and Drug Use, Drug Use in America: Problem in*

Perspective (Second Report of the National Commission on Marijuana and Drug Use). Washington, D.C.: U.S. Government Printing Office, 1973.

Davis, K. L., Mohs, R. C., & Tinklenberg, J. R.: Enhancement of memory processes in Alzheimer's disease with multiple-dose intravenous physostignomine. *American Journal of Psychiatry,* 139:1421–1424, 1982.

DeLeon, G.: The therapeutic community: status and evolution. *International Journal of the Addictions,* 20:823–844, 1985.

Denko, J. D., & Kaelbling, R.: The psychiatric aspects of hypoparathyroidism in psychiatric populations. *Acta Psychiatrica Scandinavica,* 38:7–70, 1962.

Dhib-Jalbut, S., Hesselbrock, R., Brott, T., et al.: Treatment of the neuroleptic malignant syndrome with bromocriptine. *Journal of the American Medical Association,* 250:484–485, 1983.

Diaz-Cabal, R., Pearlman, C., & Kawecki, A.: Hyperthyroidism in a patient with agitated depression: Resolution after electroconvulsive therapy. *Journal of Clinical Psychiatry,* 47:322–323, 1986.

Dole, V. P., & Nyswander, M.: Methadone maintainance treatment: A ten-year perspective. *Journal of the American Medical Association,* 235:2117–2119, 1976.

Dubovsky, S. L., & Weisberg, M. P.: *Clinical Psychiatry in Primary Care* (2nd Ed.). Baltimore, MD: Williams & Wilkins, 1982, pp. 102–103.

Eames, P., & Wood, R.: Rehabilitation after severe brain injury: A follow-up study of a behavior modification approach. *Journal of Neurology, Neurosurgery, Psychiatry,* 48:613–619, 1985.

Eisendrath, S. J., Goldman, B., Douglas, J., et al.: Meperidine-induced delirium. *American Journal of Psychiatry,* 145:1062–1065, 1987.

Ellinwood, E. H.: Amphetamines/anorectics. In R. I. DuPont, A. Goldstein, & J. O'Donnell (Eds.), *Handbook of Drug Abuse,* Washington, D.C.: U.S. Government Printing Office, National Institute on Drug Abuse, DHEW, 1979, pp. 221–231.

Elliott, F. A.: Propranolol for the control of belligerent behavior following acute brain damage. *Annuals of Neurology,* 1:489, 1977.

Elliott, F. P.: The episodic dyscontrol syndrome and aggression. *Neurological Clinics,* 2:113–125, 1984.

Emrick, C. D.: A review of psychologically oriented treatment of alcoholism: I. The use of and inter-relationship of outcome criteria and drinking behavior following treatment. *Journal of Studies on Alcohol,* 35:523–549, 1974.

Evans, D. L., & Nemeroff, C. B.: The dexamethasone suppression test in organic affective syndrome. *American Journal of Psychiatry,* 141:1465–1467, 1984.

Fagerstrom, K.: A comparison of psychological and pharmacological treatments in smoking cessation. *Journal of Behavioral Medicine,* 5:343–351, 1982.

Falk, W. E., Mahnke, M. W., & Poskanzer, D. C.: Lithium prophylaxis of cortico-tropin-induced psychosis. *Journal of the American Medical Association,* 241:1011–1012, 1979.

Farebrother, M., Pearce, S., Turner, P., et al.: Propranolol and giving up smoking. *British Journal of Diseases of the Chest,* 74:95–96, 1980.

Feibel, J. H., & Springer, C. J.: Depression and failure to resume social activities after stroke. *Archives of Physical Medicine and Rehabilitation,* 63:276–278, 1982.

Forrest, D. V.: Bipolar illness after right hemispherectomy. *Archives of General Psychiatry,* 31:817–819, 1982.

Francis, F. J., & Franklin, J. E., Jr.: Alcohol-induced organic mental disorders. In R. E. Hales & S. C. Yudolsky (Eds.), *Textbook of Neuropsychiatry.* Washington, D.C.,: American Psychiatric Press, 1987, pp. 141–156.

Fraser, J. F., Isbell, H., Eisenman, A. J., Wikler, A., & Pescor, F. T.: Chronic barbiturate intoxication: Further studies. *Archives of Internal Medicine,* 94:34–41, 1964.

Freinkel, N., & Arky, R. A.: Effects of alcohol on carbohydrate metabolism in man. *Psychosomatic Medicine,* 28:551–563, 1966.

Fricchione, G. L., Cassem, N. H., et al.: Intravenous lorazepam in neuroleptic-induced catatonia. *Journal of Clinical Psychopharmacology,* 3:334–338, 1983.

Fry, R. V.: Editor's introduction. *Journal of Psychoactive Drugs,* 18:191–197, 1986.

Gaitz, C. M., Varner, R. V., & Overall, J. E.: Pharmacotherapy for organic brain syndrome in late life. *Archives of General Psychiatry*, 34:839–845, 1977.

Gawin, F. H., New uses of antidepressants in cocaine abuse. *Psychosomatics*, 27 (Suppl., No. 11): 24–29, 1986.

Gawin, F. H., Byck, R., & Kleber, H. D.: Double-blind comparison of desipramine and placebo in chronic cocaine abusers. Paper presented at the 24th meeting, American College of Neuropharmacology, Kaanapoli, Hawaii, December 13, 1985.

Gawin, F. H., & Kleber, H. D.: Cocaine abuse treatment. *Archives of General Psychiatry*, 41:903–909, 1984.

Gelmers, H. J. Adverse side effects of metrizamide in myelography. *Neuroradiology*, 18:119–123, 1979.

Gerard, D. L., & Saenger, G.: *Outpatient Treatment of Alcoholism*. Toronto: University of Toronto Press, 1966.

Gerner, R., Estabrook, W., Stever, J., et al.: Treatment of geriatric depression with trazodone, imipramine, and placebo: A double-blind study. *Journal of Clinical Psychiatry*, 41:216–220, 1980.

Gershon, S. Neubauer, H., & Sundland, D. M.: Interaction between some anticholinergic agents and phenothiazines. *Clinical Pharmacology and Therapeutics*, 6:749–776, 1965.

Ghadirian, A. M., Gauthier, S., & Bertrand, S.: Anxiety attacks in a patient with a right temporal lobe meningioma. *Journal of Clinical Psychiatry*, 47:270–271, 1986.

Giannini, A. J., Malone, D. A., Giannini, M. C., et al.: Treatment of depression in chronic cocaine and phencyclidine abuse with desipramine. *Journal of Clinical Pharmacology*, 26:211–214, 1986.

Gillespie, L., Oates, J. A., Crout, J. R., et al.: Clinical and chemical studies with a methyldopa in patients with hypertension. *Circulation*, 25:281–291, 1967.

Glaser, G. H.: Psychotic reactions induced by corticotropin (ACTH) and cortisone. *Psychosomatic Medicine*, 15:689–693, 1953.

Glassman, A. H., Giardina, E. V., Perel, J. M., et al.: Clinical characteristics of imipramine-induced orthostatic hypotension. *Lancet*, i:468–472, 1979.

Glassman, A. H., Jackson, W. K., Walsh, B. T., et al.: Cigarette craving, smoking withdrawal, and clonidine. *Science*, 226:864–866, 1984.

Gloor, P., Quesney, L. F., et al.: The role of the limbic system in experiential phenomena of temporal lobe epilepsy. *Annals of Neurology*, 12:129–144, 1982.

Godwin, C. D.: Case report of tricyclic-induced delirium at a therapeutic drug concentration. *American Journal of Psychiatry*, 140:1517–1518, 1983.

Goekoop, J. G., & Carbaat, P. A. T.: Treatment of neuroleptic malignant syndrome with dantrolene. *Lancet*, ii:49–50, 1982.

Goggans, F. C., Allen, R. M., & Gold, M. S.: Primary hypothyroidism and its relationship to affective disorders. In I. Extein & M. S. Gold (Eds.), *Medical Mimics of Psychiatric Disorders*. Washington, D.C.: American Psychiatric Press, 1986, pp. 96–109.

Gold, M. S., & Dackis, C. A.: New insights and treatments: Opiate withdrawal and cocaine addiction. *Clinical Therapeutics*, 7:6–21, 1984.

Gold, M. S., & Pearsall, H.: Hypothyroidism—or is it depression? *Psychosomatics*, 24:646–656, 1983.

Gold, M. S., Pottash, A. C., & Extein, I.: Hypothyroidism and depression. *Journal of the American Medical Association*, 245:1919–1922, 1981.

Gold, M. S., Pottash, ALC, Sweeney, D. R., et al.: Opiate withdrawal using clonidine. A safe, effective, and rapid nonopiate treatment. *Journal of the American Medical Association*, 243:343–346, 1980.

Gold, M. S., Redmond, D. E., & Kleber, H. D.: Clonidine blocks acute opiate withdrawal symptoms. *Lancet*, ii:599–602, 1978.

Goldfrank, L., & Meliek, M.: Locoweed and other anticholinergics. *Hospital Physician*, 8:13–39, 1979.

Goldstein, A., & Judson, B. A.: Efficacy and side effects of three widely different methadone doses. In *Proceedings of the Fifth National Conference on Methadone Treatment*. New York: National Association for the Prevention of Addiction to Narcotics, 1973.

Goodman, W. K., Charney, D. S., Price, L. H., et al.: Ineffectiveness of clonidine in the treatment of the benzodiazepine withdrawal syndrome. Report of three cases. *American Journal of Psychiatry*, 143:900–903, 1986.

Goodwin, E. W.: Substance induced and substance use disorders: Alcohol. In J. H. Greist, J. W. Jefferson, & R. L. Spitzer (Eds.), *Treatment of Mental Disorders*. New York: Oxford University Press, 1982, pp. 44–61.

Granacher, R. P., Baldessarini, R. J., & Messner, E.: Physostigmine treatment of delirium induced by anticholinergics. *American Family Physician*, 13:99–103, 1976.

Granato, J. E., Stern, B. J., Ringel, A., et al.: Neuroleptic malignant syndrome: Successful treatment with dantrolene and bromocriptine. *Annals of Neurology*, 14:89–90, 1983.

Greden, J. F.: Caffeine and tobacco dependence. In H. I. Kaplan, A. M. Freedman, & B. J. Sadock (Eds.), *Comprehensive Textbook of Psychiatry, Volume 2*, Baltimore, MD: Williams & Wilkins, 1980, pp. 1645–1652.

Green, A. I., Meyer, R. E., & Shader, R. I.: Heroin and methadone abuse: Acute and chronic management. In R. I. Shader (Ed.), *Manual of Psychiatric Therapeutics: Practical Psychopharmacology and Psychiatry*. Boston: Little, Brown, 1975.

Greenblatt, D. J., & Shader, R. I.: Treatment of the alcoholic withdrawal syndrome. In R. I. Shader (Ed.), *Manual of Psychiatric Therapeutics: Practical Psychopharmacology and Psychiatry*. Boston: Little, Brown, 1975.

Greenstein, R. A., Evans, B. D., McLellan, A. T., et al.: Predictors of favorable outcome following naltrexone treatment. *Drug and Alcohol Dependence*, 12:173–180, 1983.

Hales, R. H., & Hershey, S. C.: Psychopharmacologic issues in the diagnosis and treatment of organic mental disorders. *Psychiatric Clinics of North America*, 7:817–829, 1984.

Hall, R. C. W., Gardner, E. R., Popkin, E. R., et al.: Unrecognized physical illness prompting psychiatric admission: A prospective study. *American Journal of Psychiatry*, 136:629, 1981.

Hall, R. W.: Psychiatric effects of thyroid hormone disturbance. *Psychosomatics*, 24:7–18, 1983.

Hall, S. M., Tunstall, C., Rugg, D., et al.: Nicotine gum and behavioral treatment in smoking cessations. *Journal of Counsulting and Clinical Psychology*, 53:256–258, 1985.

Hamilton, L. D.: Aged brain and the phenothiazines. *Geriatrics*, 21:131–138, 1966.

Handelsman, L.: Amantadine treatment of cocaine abuse. Abstract. In *New Research*, 140th Annual Meeting, American Psychiatric Association, Chicago, IL, May 9–14, 1987.

Haskett, R. F., & Rose, R. M.: Neuroendocrine disorders and psychopathology. *Psychiatric Clinics of North America*, 4:239–252, 1981.

Hass, W. K.: Acute ischemic cerebrovascular disease. In W. F. Conn (Ed.), *Current Therapy*, Philadelphia: W. B. Saunders, 1979, pp. 674–677.

Healey, M., Pickens, R., Meisch, R., et al.: Effects of clorazepate, diazepam, lorazepam and placebo on human memory. *Psychopharmacology*, 70:231–237, 1980.

Heizer, J. R., & Wilbert, D. E.: Reversal of delirium induced by tricyclic antidepressant drugs with physostigmine. *American Journal of Psychiatry*, 131:1275–1276, 1974.

Heston, L. L., Mastri, A. R., Anderson, E., et al.: Dementia of the Alzheimer type: Clinical genetics, natural history, and associated conditions. *Archives of General Psychiatry*, 38:1085–1090, 1981.

Hirt, M., & Greenfield, H.: Implosive therapy treatment of heroin addicts during methadone detoxification. *Journal of Consulting and Clinical Psychology*, 47:982–983, 1979.

Hjalmarson, A. I. M.: Effect of nicotine chewing gum in smoking cessation. A randomized, placebo-controlled, double-blind study. *Journal of the American Medical Association*, 252:2835–2838, 1984.

Hoffman, R. S.: Neuropsychiatric complications of AIDS. *Psychosomatics*, 25:393–400, 1984.

Hollister, L. E., Montzenbecker, R. P., & Degans, R. O.: Withdrawal reactions from chlordiazepoxide. *Psychopharmacologia*, 2:63–68, 1966.

Hrdina, P. D., Rovei, V., Henry, J. F., et al.: Comparison of single-dose pharmacokinetics of imipramine and maprotiline in the elderly. *Psychopharmacology*, 70:29–34, 1980.

Hunt, W. A., & Bespalec, D. A.: An evaluation of current methods of modifying smoking behavior. *Journal of Clinical Psychology*, 30:431–438, 1974.
Ifabumuyi, O. L., & Jeffries, J. J.: Treatment of drug-induced psychosis with diphenylhydantoin. *Canadian Psychiatric Association Journal*, 21:565–569, 1976.
Jaffe, J. H., & Jarvik, M. E.: Tobacco use and tobacco use disorder. In M. A. Lipton, A. DiMascio, & K. F. Killam (Eds.), *Psychopharmacology: A Generation of Progress*. New York: Raven Press, 1978, pp. 1665–1676.
Jamieson, R. C., & Wells, C. E.: Manic psychosis in a patient with multiple metastatic brain tumors. *Journal of Clinical Psychiatry*, 40:280–282, 1979.
Jampala, V. C., & Abrams, R.: Mania secondary to left and right hemisphere damage. *American Journal of Psychiatry*, 140:1197–1199, 1983.
Jarvik, M. E., Cullen, J. W., Gritz, E. R., Vogt, T. M., & West, L. J.: *Research on Smoking Behavior*. National Institute on Drug Abuse, Research Monograph Series #17, DHEW. Washington, D.C.: U.S. Government Printing Office, 1977.
Jarvik, M. E., & Schneider, N. G.: Degree of addiction and effectiveness of nicotine gum therapy for smoking. *American Journal of Psychiatry*, 141:790–791, 1984.
Jasinski, D. R., Johnson, R. E., & Kocher, T. R.: Clonidine in morphine withdrawal, *Archives of General Psychiatry*, 42:1063–1066, 1985.
Jenike, M. A.: Monoamine oxidase inhibitors in elderly depressed patients. *Journal of the American Geriatric Society*, 32:571–575, 1984.
Jenike, M. A.: Monoamine oxidase inhibitors as treatment for depressed patients with primary degenerative dementia (Alzheimer's disease). *American Journal of Psychiatry*, 142:763–764, 1985.
Jessee, S., & Anderson, G.: ECT in the neuroleptic malignant syndrome: Case report. *Journal of Clinical Psychiatry*, 44:186–188, 1983.
Judson, B. A., Goldstein, A., & Inturrisi, C. E.: Methadyl acetate (LAAM) in the treatment of heroin addicts. *Archives of General Psychiatry*, 40:834–840, 1983.
Kahn, A., Jaffe, J. H., Nelson, W. H., et al.: Resolution of neuroleptic malignant syndrome with dantrolene sodium: Case report. *Journal of Clinical Psychiatry*, 46:244–246, 1985.
Karoff, S. N.: The neuroleptic malignant syndrome. *Journal of Clinical Psychiatry*, 41:79–83, 1980.
Kathol, R. G., Turner, R., & Delahunt, J.: Depression and anxiety associated with hyperthyroidism: Response to antithyroid therapy. *Psychosomatics*, 27:501–505, 1986.
Katz, N. W.: Hypnosis and the addiction: A critical review. *Addictive Behaviors*, 5:41–47, 1980.
Kaufman, E.: Family systems and family therapy of substance abuse: An overview of two decades of research and clinical experience. *International Journal of the Addictions*, 20:897–916, 1985.
Khantzian, E. J., Mack, J. E., & Schatzberg, A. F.: Heroin use as an attempt to cope: Clinical observations. *American Journal of Psychiatry*, 131:160–164, 1974.
Khantzian, E. J., & McKenna, G. J.: Acute toxic and withdrawal reaction associated with drug use and abuse. *Annals of Internal Medicine*, 90:361–372, 1979.
Kissin, B., Lowinson, J. H., & Millman, R. B.: Recent developments in chemotherapy of narcotic addiction. *Annals of the New York Academy of Sciences*, Vol. 311, 1978.
Kleber, H. D., & Gawin, F. H.: The spectrum of cocaine abuse and its treatment. *Journal of Clinical Psychiatry*, 45:18–23, 1984.
Kleber, H. D., Weissman, M. M., Rounsaville, B. J., et al.: Imipramine as treatment for depression in addicts. *Archives of General Psychiatry*, 40:649–653, 1983.
Klein, J. M., & Miller, S. I.: Three approaches to the treatment of drug addiction. *Hospital & Community Psychiatry*, 37:1083–1085, 1986.
Kleist, K.: *Gehirnpathologie*. Leipzig: Barth, 1936.
Klerman, G. L., Dimascio, A., & Weissman, M. M.: Treatment of depression by drugs and psychotherapy. *American Journal of Psychiatry*, 131:186–191, 1974.
Krahn, D.: Affective disorder associated with subclinical hypothyroidism. *Psychosomatics*, 28:440–441, 1987.

Krauthammer, C., & Klerman, G. L.: Secondary mania: Manic syndromes associated with antecedent physical illness or drugs. *Archives of General Psychiatry*, 35:1333–1339, 1978.

Kuhn, R.: The psychotropic effect of carbamezepine in non-epileptic adults, with particular reference to the drug's possible mechanism of action. In W. Birkmayer (Ed.), *Epileptic Seizures-Behavior-Pain*. Baltimore, MD: University Park Press, 1976, pp. 268–271.

Kwentus, J. A., Hart, R. P., Peck, E. T., et al.: Psychiatric complications of closed-head trauma. *Psychosomatics*, 26:8–17, 1985.

Kwentus, J. A., Silverman, J. J., & Sprague, M.: Manic syndrome after metrizamide myelography. *American Journal of Psychiatry*, 141:700–702, 1984.

Lehman, H. E., & Ban, T. A.: Central nervous stimulants and anabolic substances in geropsychiatric therapy. In S. Gershon & A. Raskin (Eds.), *Aging, Volume 2: Genesis and Treatment of Psychologic Disorders in the Elderly*. New York: Raven Press, 1975.

Leigh, D.: Psychiatric aspects of head injury. *Psychiatry Digest*, 40:21, 1979.

Leigh, H. S., & Kramer, S. I.: *The 1984 Year Book*. New Haven, CT: Year Book Medical Publishers, 1984.

Lennard, H. L., Epstein, L. J., & Rosenthal, M. S.: The methadone illusion. *Science*, 176:881–884, 1972.

Levenson, J. L.: Neuroleptic malignant syndrome. *American Journal of Psychiatry*, 142:1137–1145, 1985.

Lewis, D. C., & Senay, E. C.: *Treatment of Drug and Alcohol Abuse*. Medical Monograph Series, Vol. II, No. 2, Career Teacher Center, State University of New York Downstate Medical Center, New York, 1981.

Lezak, M. D.: Living with the characterologically altered brain injured patient. *Journal of Clinical Psychiatry*, 39:592–598, 1978.

Ling, W., & Blaine, J. D.: The use of LAAM in treatment. In R. I. DuPont, A. Goldstein, & J. O'Donnell (Eds.), *Handbook on Drug Abuse*. Washington, D.C.: U.S. Government Printing Office, National Institute on Drug Abuse, DHEW, 1979, pp. 87–96.

Ling, M. H. M., Perry, P. J., & Tsuang, M. T.: Side effects of corticosteroid therapy: Psychiatric aspects. *Archives of General Psychiatry*, 38:471–477, 1981.

Lipowski, Z. J.: Organic brain syndromes: Overview and classification. In D. F. Benson & D. Blumer (Eds.), *Psychiatric Aspects of Neurologic Disease*. New York: Grune & Stratton, 1975, pp. 11–35.

Lipowski, Z. J.: Organic mental disorders: Introduction and review of syndromes. In H. I. Kaplan, A. M. Freedman, & B. J. Sadock (Eds.), *Comprehensive Textbook of Psychiatry*. Baltimore, MD: Williams & Wilkins, 1980a, pp. 1359–1392.

Lipowski, Z. J.: *Delirium. Acute Brain Failure in Man*. Springfield, IL: Charles C Thomas, 1980b.

Lipowski, Z. J.: Transient cognitive disorders (delirium, acute confusional states) in the elderly. *American Journal of Psychiatry*, 140:1426–1436, 1983.

Lipsey, J. R., Robinson, R. G., Perlson, G. D., et al.: Nortriptyline treatment of post-stroke depression: A double-blind treatment trial. *Lancet*, 1:297–300, 1984.

Liskow, B.: Substance-induced and substance use disorder: Barbiturates and similarly acting sedative hypnotics. In J. H. Greist, J. W. Jefferson, & R. L. Spitzer (Eds.), *Treatment of Mental Disorders*. New York: Oxford University Press, 1982.

Liston, E. H.: Delirium in the aged. *Psychiatric Clinics of North America*, 5:49–66, 1982.

MacKenzie, T. B., & Popkin, G. D.: Organic anxiety syndrome. *American Journal of Psychiatry*, 140:342–344, 1983.

Mair, R. G., & McEntee, W. J.: Cognitive enhancement in Korsakoff's psychosis by clonidine: A comparison with L-dopa and ephedrine. *Psychopharmacology* (Berlin), 88(3):374–380, 1986.

Mann, L. S., Johnson, R. W., & Levine, D. J.: Tobacco dependence: Psychology, biology, and treatment strategies. *Psychosomatics*, 27:713–718, 1986.

Marini, J. L., & Sheard, M. H.: Antiaggressive effect of lithium in man. *Acta Psychiatrica Scandinavica*, 55:269–286, 1977.

Martin, M. J., & Black, J. L.: Neuropsychiatric aspects of degenerative diseases. In R. E. Hales & S. C. Yudofsky (Eds.), *Textbook of Neuropsychiatry*. Washington, D.C.: American Psychiatric Press, 1987, pp. 257–286.
Mash, D. C., Flynn, D. D., & Potter, L. T.: Loss of M2 muscarinic receptors in the cerebral cortex in Alzheimer's disease and experimental cholinergic denervation. *Science*, 228:1115–1117, 1985.
Mathew, R. J., & Meyer, J. S.: Pathogenesis and natural history of transient global amnesia. *Stroke*, 5:303–311, 1974.
Mattes, J. A.: Metoprolol for intermittent explosive disorder. *American Journal of Psychiatry* 142:1108–1109, 1985.
May, D. C., Morris, S. W., Stewart, R. M., et al.: Neuroleptic malignant syndrome: Response to dantrolene sodium. *Annals of Internal Medicine*, 98:183–184, 1983.
McAllister, T. W., & Price, T. R. P.: Severe depressive pseudodementia with and without dementia. *American Journal of Psychiatry*, 139:626–629, 1982.
McCarron, M. M., Boettger, M. L., & Peck, J. J.: A case of neuroleptic malignant syndrome successfully treated with amantadine. *Journal of Clinical Psychiatry*, 43:381–382, 1982.
McElroy, S. L., Keck, P. E., & Pope, H. G., Jr.: Sodium valporate: Its use in primary psychiatric disorders. *Journal of Clinical Psychopharmacology*, 7:16–24, 1987.
McEntee, W. J., & Mair, R. G.: Memory enhancement in Korsakoff's psychosis by clonidine: Further evidence for a noradrenergic deficit. *Annals of Neurology*, 7(5):466–470, 1980.
McEvoy, J. P. Organic brain syndromes. *Annals of Internal Medicine*, 95:212–220, 1981.
McKay, A. C., & Dundee, J. W.: Effect of oral benzodiazepines on memory. *British Journal of Anesthesiology*, 52:1247–1257, 1980.
McKenna, P. J., Kane, J. M., & Parish, K.: Psychotic syndromes in epilepsy. *American Journal of Psychiatry*, 142:895–904, 1985.
McLellan, A. T., McGahan, J. A., & Druley, D. A.: Changes in drug abuse clients—1972–1978: Implications for revised treatment. *American Journal of Alcohol Abuse*, 6:151–162, 1979.
McMahon, T.: Bipolar affective symptoms associated with use of captopril and abrupt withdrawal of pargyline and propranolol. *American Journal of Psychiatry*, 142:759–760, 1985.
Mehr, J. J., & Holi, T. C.: Behavioral treatment for aggression in residents of institutions for the emotionally disturbed and the mentally retarded. In S. Saunders, A. M. Anderson, C. A. Hart, et al. (Eds.), *Violent Families and Individuals: A Handbook for Practitioners*. Springfield, IL: Charles C Thomas, 1984.
Mendelson, J. H.: Biologic concomitants of alcoholism. *New England Journal of Medicine*, 283:24–32, 1970.
Mirin, S. M., & Meyer, R. E.: Treatment of substance abusers. In W. G. Clark & J. Del Guidice (Eds.), *Principles of Psychopharmacology*. New York: Academic Press, 1978, pp. 701–720.
Mogelnicki, S. R., Waller, J. L., & Finlayson, D.C.: Physostigmine reversal of cimetidine-induced mental confusion. *Journal of the American Medical Association*, 241:826–827, 1979.
Mohr, J. P., Fisher, C. M., & Adams, R. D.: Cerebrovascular diseases. In Thorn, G. W., Adams, R. D., et. al. (Eds.), *Harrison's Principles of Internal Medicine*. New York: McGraw-Hill, 1977, pp. 1832–1868.
Mohs, R. C., Davis, B. M., Johns, C. A., et al.: Oral physostigmine treatment of patients with Alzheimer's disease. *American Journal of Psychiatry*, 142:28–33, 1985.
Monroe, R. R.: Anticonvulsants in the treatment of aggression. *Journal of Nervous and Mental Disease*, 1960:119–126, 1975.
Moore, D. P.: Rapid treatment of delirium in critically ill patients. *American Journal of Psychiatry*, 134:1431–1432, 1977.
Mueller, P. S., Vester, J. W., & Fermaglich, J.: Neuroleptic malignant syndrome: Successful treatment with bromocriptine. *Journal of the American Medical Association*, 249:386–388, 1983.

Murray, G. B., Shea, V., & Conn, D. K.: Electroconvulsive therapy for poststroke depression. *Journal of Clinical Psychiatry*, 47:258–260, 1986.
Nelson, T. E., & Flewellen, E. H.: The malignant hyperthermia syndrome. *New England Journal of Medicine*, 309:416–418, 1983.
Nichols, S. E., & Ostrow, D. G. (Eds.): *Psychiatric Implications of the Acquired Immune Deficiency Syndrome.* Washington, D.C.: American Psychiatric Press, 1984.
Nurcombe, B., Bianchi, G., Money, J., et al.: A hunger for stimuli: The psychosocial background of petrol inhalation. *British Journal of Medical Psychology*, 43:367–382, 1970.
O'Donnell, J. A.: *Narcotic Addicts in Kentucky.* (U.S. Public Health Service Publication No. 1881). Washington, D.C.: U.S. Government Printing Office, 1969.
Ogata, M., Mendelson, J., & Mello, N.: Electrolytes and osmolarity in alcoholics during experimental intoxication. *Psychosomatic Medicine*, 30:463–488, 1968.
Okada, F.: Depression after treatment with thiazide diuretics for hypertension. *American Journal of Psychiatry*, 142:1101–1102, 1985.
Orleans, C. T., Shipley, R. H., Williams, C., et al.: Behavioral approaches to smoking cessation. I. A decade of research progress, 1969–1979. *Journal of Behavior Therapy and Experimental Psychiatry*, 12:125–129, 1981.
Oyewumi, L. K., & Lapierre, Y. D.: Efficacy of lithium in treating mood disorder occurring after brainstem injury. *American Journal of Psychiatry*, 138:110–112, 1981.
Patten, B. M.: Modality-specific memory disorders in man. *Acta Neurologica Scandinavica*, 48:69–86, 1972.
Pattison, E. M.: Clinical approaches to the alcoholic patient. *Psychosomatics*, 27:262–270, 1986.
Perry, E. K., Perry, R. H., Blessed, G., et al.: Necropsy evidence of central cholinergic deficits in senile dementia. *Lancet*, i:189, 1977.
Perry, S.: Substance-induced-organic Mental Disorders. In R. E. Hales & S. C. Yudofsky (Eds.), *Textbook of Neuropsychiatry.* Washington, D.C.: American Psychiatric Press, 1987, pp. 157–176.
Peters, B. H., & Levin, H. S.: Memory enhancement after physostigmine treatment in the amnestic syndrome. *Archives of Neurology*, 34:215–219, 1977.
Peterson, P.: Psychiatric disorders in primary hyperparathyroidism. *Journal of Clinical Endocrinology*, 28:1491–1495, 1968.
Petrie, W. M., Ban, T. A., Berney, S., et al.: Loxapine in psychogeriatrics: A placebo- and standard-controlled clinical investigation. *Journal of Clinical Psychopharmacology*, 2:122–126, 1982.
Plutzky, M.: Principles of psychiatric management of chronic brain syndrome. *Geriatrics*, 29:120–127, 1974.
Preskorn, S. H., & Simpson, S.: Tricyclic-antidepressant-induced delirium and plasma drug concentration. *American Journal of Psychiatry*, 139:822–823, 1982.
Prichard, B. N. C., Johnston, A. W., Hill, D., et al.: Bethanidine, guanethidine and methyldopa in treatment of hypertension: A within-patient comparison. *British Medical Journal*, 1:135–144, 1968.
Puente, R. M.: The use of carbamazepine in the treatment of behavioral disorders in children. In W. Birkmeyer (Ed.), *Epileptic Seizures-Behavior-Pain.* Baltimore, MD: University Park Press, 1976, pp. 243–247.
Rada, R., & Kellner, R.: Thiothixene in treatment of geriatric patients with chronic organic brain syndrome. *Journal of the American Geriatric Society*, 24:105–109, 1976.
Raskind, M. A., & Risse, S. C.: Antipsychotic drugs and the elderly. *Journal of Clinical Psychiatry*, 47:17–22, 1986.
Ratey, J. J., Morril, R., & Oxenkrug, G.: Use of propranolol for provoked and unprovoked episodes of rage. *American Journal of Psychiatry*, 140:1356–1357, 1983.
Reisberg, B.: Office management and treatment of primary degenerative dementia. *Psychiatric Annals*, 12:631–642, 1982.
Reisberg, B., Borenstein, J., Salob, S. P., et al.: Behavioral symptoms in Alzheimer's disease: Phenomenology and treatment. *Journal of Clinical Psychiatry*, 48:9–15, 1987.

Reisberg, B., Ferris, S. H., Anand, R., et al.: Effects of naloxone in senile dementia: A double-blind trial (letter). *New England Journal of Medicine*, 308:165–173, 1982.

Reisberg, B., Ferris, S. H., & Gershon, S.: An overview of pharmacologic treatment of cognitive decline in the aged. *American Journal of Psychiatry*, 138:593–600, 1981.

Resnick, R. B., Schuyton-Resnick, E. S., & Washton, A. M.: Treatment of opioid dependence with narcotic antagonists: A review and commentary. In R. I. DuPont, A. Goldstein, & J. O'Donnell (Eds.), *Handbook on Drug Abuse*. Washington, D.C.: U.S. Government Printing Office, National Institute on Drug Abuse, DHEW, 1979, pp. 97–104.

Resnick, R. B., Washton, A. M., Stone-Washton, N., et al.: Psychotherapy and naltrexone in opioid dependence. In L. S. Harris (Ed.), *Problems of Drug Dependence, 1981*. NIDA Research Monograph series No 34. Washington, D.C.: U.S. Government Printing Office, 1981.

Reus, V. I., & Berlant, J. R.: Behavioral disturbances associated with disorders of the hypothalamic-pituitary-adrenal system. In I. Extein, & M. S. Gold (Eds.), *Medical Mimics of Psychiatric Disorders*. Washington, D.C.: American Psychiatric Press, 1986, pp. 111–130.

Robinson, D. S.: Age-related factors affecting antidepressant drug metabolism and clinical response. In K. Nancy (Ed.), *Geriatric Psychopharmacology*. New York: Elsevier/North Holland, 1979.

Robinson, R. G., Kubos, K. L., Starr, L. B., et al.: Mood disorders in stroke patients: Importance of location of lesions. *Brain*, 107:81–93, 1984.

Robinson, R. G., Lipsey, J. R., & Price, T. R.: Diagnosis and clinical management of post-stroke depression. *Psychosomatics*, 26:769–778, 1985.

Robinson, R. G., Starr, K. L., et al.: A two year longitudinal study of post-stroke mood disorders: Findings during the initial evaluation. *Stroke*, 14:736–741, 1983.

Romand, A., Forrest, C., & Kleber, H. D.: Follow-up of participants in a drug dependence therapeutic community. *Archives of General Psychiatry*, 32:369–374, 1975.

Roose, S., Glassman, A. H., Siris, S., et al.: Comparison of imipramine and nortriptyline induced orthostatic hypotension: A meaningful difference. *Journal of Clinical Psychopharmacology*, 1:316–321, 1981.

Rosenbaum, A. H., & Barry, M. J.: Positive therapeutic response to lithium in hypomania secondary to organic brain syndrome. *American Journal of Psychiatry*, 132:1072–1073, 1975.

Rothstein, E., Cobble, J. C., & Sampson, N.: Chlordiazepoxide: Long-term use in alcoholism. *Annals of the New York Academy of Sciences*, 273:381–384, 1976.

Rounsaville, B. J., Glazer, W., Wilber, C. H., et al.: Short-term interpersonal psychotherapy in methadone-maintained opiate addicts. *Archives of General Psychiatry*, 40:629–636, 1983.

Rundall, J. R., Wise, M. G., & Ursano, R. J.: Three cases of AIDS-related psychiatric disorders. *American Journal of Psychiatry* 143:777–778, 1986.

Sakles, C. J., & Balis, G. U.: Acute brain syndromes. In G. U. Balis, L. Wurmser, E. McDaniel, & R. G. Grenell (Eds.), *Clinical Psychopathology, The Psychiatric Foundations of Medicine, Volume 4*. Boston: Butterworths, 1978, pp. 65–86.

Salzman, C.: Electroconvulsive therapy. In R. I. Shader (Ed.), *Manual of Practical Psychopharmacology and Psychiatric Therapeutics*. Boston: Little, Brown, 1975.

Salzman, C.: Update on geriatric psychopharmacology. *Geriatrics*, 34:87–90, 1979.

Salzman, C.: A primer on geriatric psychopharmacology. *American Journal of Psychiatry*, 139:67–74, 1982.

Salzman, C.: Treatment of the elderly agitated patient. *Journal of Clinical Psychiatry*, 48 (5, suppl):19–22, 1987.

Salzman, C., Shader, R. I., & Pearlman, M.: Psychopharmacology and the elderly. In R. I. Shader & A. DiMascio (Eds.), *Psychotropic Drug Side Effects*. Baltimore, MD: Williams & Wilkins, 1970.

Scarlett, J. D., Zimmerman, R., & Berkovic, S. F.: Neuroleptic malignant syndrome. *Australian New Zealand Journal of Medicine*, 13:70–73, 1983.

Scharf, M. B., Khosha, N., Brocker, N., et al.: Differential amnestic properties of short and long acting benzodiazepines. *Journal of Clinical Psychiatry*, 45:51–53, 1984.

Schneider, N. G., Jarvik, M. E., Forsyth, A. B., et al.: Nicotine gum in smoking cessation: A placebo-controlled double-blind trial. *Addictive Behaviors*, 8:253–261, 1983.

Schottenfeed, R. S., & Cullen, M. R.: Organic affective illness associated with lead intoxication. *American Journal of Psychiatry*, 141:1423–1426, 1984.

Schreier, H. A.: Use of propranolol in the treatment of post encephalitic psychosis. *American Journal of Psychiatry*, 136:840–841, 1979.

Sellers, E. M., & Kalant, H.: Alcohol intoxication and withdrawal. *New England Journal of Medicine*, 294:757–762, 1976.

Sells, S. B.: Treatment effectiveness. In R. I. DuPont, A. Goldstein, & J. O'Donnell (Eds.), *Handbook on Drug Abuse*. Washington, D.C.: U.S. Government Printing Office, National Institute on Drug Abuse, DHEW, 1979, pp. 105–118.

Selzer, M. L.: Alcoholism and alcoholic psychosis. In H. I. Kaplan, A. M. Freedman, & B. J. Sadock (Eds.), *Comprehensive Textbook of Psychiatry, III*. BBaltimore, MD: Williams & Wilkins, 1980, pp. 1629–1645.

Selzer, M. L., Vinokur, A., & Von Rooijen, L. A.: A self-administered short Michigan Alcoholism Screening Test (MAST). *Journal of Studies on Alcohol*, 36:117–126, 1975.

Sergent, J. S., Lockshin, M. D., Klempner, M. S., et al.: Central nervous system disease in systemic lupus erythematosus. *American Journal of Medicine*, 58:644–654, 1975.

Seymour, D. G., Henschke, P. J., Cape, R. D. T., et al.: Acute confusional states and dementia in the elderly: The role of dehydration/volume depletion, physical illness and age. *Age and Aging*, 9:137–146, 1980.

Sheard, M. H.: The effect of lithium in the treatment of aggression. *Journal of Nervous and Mental Disease*, 160:108–118, 1975.

Sheard, M. H., Marini, J. L., Bridges, C. K., et al.: The effect of lithium on impulsive aggressive behavior in man. *American Journal of Psychiatry*, 133:1409–1413, 1976.

Simpson, D. D.: Treatment for drug abuse. *Archives of General Psychiatry*, 38:875–880, 1981.

Simpson, F. O., & Waal-Manning, H. J.: Hypertension and depression. *Journal of the Royal College of Physicians London*, 6:14–24, 1971.

Sluping, J. R., Rollinson, R. D., & Toole, J. F.: Transient global amensia. *Annals of Neurology*, 7:281–285, 1980.

Smego, R. A., & Durack, D. T.: The neuroleptic malignant syndrome. *Archives of Internal Medicine*, 142:1183–1185, 1982.

Smith, D. L., & Wesson, D. R.: A new method of treatment of barbiturate dependence. *JAMA*, 2:294–295, 1970.

Solursh, L. P., & Clement, W. R.: Hallucinogenic drug abuse: Manifestations and management. *Canadian Medical Association Journal*, 98:407–410, 1968.

Sorensen, J. L., Hargreaves, A., & Weinberg, J. A.: Withdrawal from heroin in three to six weeks. *Archives of General Psychiatry*, 39:167–171, 1982.

Steele, C., Lucas, M. J., & Tune, L.: Haloperidol versus thioidazine in the treatment of behavioral symptoms in senile dementia of the Alzheimer type: Preliminary findings. *Journal of Clinical Psychiatry*, 47:310–312, 1986.

Stending-Lindberg, G.: Hypomagnesemia in alcohol encephalopathies. *Acta Psychiatrica Scandinavica*, 50:465–480, 1974.

Sterman, A. B., & Coyle, P. K.: Anxiety attacks present as focal neurologic disturbances: A new clinical association. *Neurology (Abstracts)*, 34 (Suppl. 1), 1984.

Stern, M.: Office management of organic mental disorders. *Psychiatric Annals*, 12:618–630, 1982.

Storey, P. B.: Brain damage and personality change after subarachnoid hemorrhage. *British Journal of Psychiatry*, 117:129–142, 1970.

Stoudemire, A., & Thompson, T. L. II: Recognizing and treating dementia. *Geriatrics*, 136:112–120, 1981.

Strub, R. L., & Black, F. W.: *Organic Brain Syndromes.* Philadelphia, PA: F. A. Davis, 1981, p. 384.

Stybel, L. J.: Psychotherapeutic options in the treatment of child and adolescent hydrocarbon inhalers. *American Journal of Psychotherapy,* 31:525–532, 1977.

Summers, W. K., Majovski, L. V., Marsh, G. M., et al.: Oral tetrahydro-aminoacridine in long-term treatment of senile dementia, Alzheimer type. *New England Journal of Medicine,* 315:1241–1245, 1986.

Targum, S. D., Greenberg, R. D., Harmon, R. L., et al.: Thyroid hormone and the TRH stimulation test in refractory depression. *Journal of Clinical Psychiatry,* 45:345–346, 1984.

Taylor, R. L., Maurer, J. I., & Tinklenberg, J. R.: Management of "bad trips" in an evolving drug scene. In C. P. Rosenbaum & J. E. Beebe (Eds.), *Psychiatric Treatment.* New York: McGraw-Hill, 1975, pp. 155–160.

Tennant, F. S.: Outpatient treatment and outcome of prescription drug abuse. *Archives of Internal Medicine,* 139:154–156, 1979.

Thal, L. J., Rosen, W., Sharpless, N. S., et al.: Choline chloride fails to improve cognition in Alzheimer's disease. *Neurobiology of Aging,* 2:205–208, 1981.

The Medical Letter, Vol. 23 (3) (Issue 576), February 6, 1981.

Thoracic Society: Comparison of four methods of smoking withdrawal in patients with smoking-related diseases: Report by a subcommittee of the research committee of the British Thoracic Society. *British Medical Journal,* 286:595–597, 1983.

Troupin, A. S.: Carbamazepine in epilepsy. In H. L. Klawans (Ed.), *Clinical Neuropharmacology, Volume 3.* New York: Raven Press, 1978.

Tunks, E. R., & Dermer, S. W.: Carbamazepine in the dyscontrol syndrome associated with limbic system dysfunction. *Journal of Nervous and Mental Disease,* 164:56–63, 1977.

Tupin, J. P.: Usefulness of lithium for aggressiveness (letter to the Editor). *American Journal of Psychiatry,* 135:1118, 1978.

Varney, N. R., Alexander, B., & MacIndoe, J. H.: Reversible steroid dementia in patients without steroid psychosis. *American Journal of Psychiatry,* 141:369–377, 1984.

Victor, M., & Adams, R. D.: The effect of alcohol on the nervous system. In *Proceedings of the Association for Research in Nervous and Mental Disease.* Baltimore, MD: Williams & Wilkins, 1953.

Victor, M., Adams, R. D., & Collins, G. H.: *The Wernicke-Korsakoff Syndrome.* Philadelphia: F. A. Davis, 1971.

vonLoveren-Huyben, C. M. S., Engelaar, H. F. W. J., Hermans, N. B. M., et. al.: Double-blind clinical and psychologic study of ergoloid mesylates (Hydergine) in subjects with senile mental deterioration. *Journal of the American Geriatric Society,* 32:584–588, 1984.

Washton, A. M., & Resnick, R. B.: Clonidine in opiate withdrawal: Review and appraisal of clinical findings. *Pharmacotherapy,* 1:140–146, 1981.

Weil, A. A.: Ictal emotions occurring in temporal lobe dysfunction. *Archives of Neurology,* 1:101–111, 1959.

Weissman, M. M., Klerman, G. L., Prusoff, B. A., et al.: Depressed outpatients one year after treatment with drugs and/or interpersonal psychotherapy (IPT). *Archives of General Psychiatry,* 133:1434–1438, 1976.

Wells, C. E.: Pseudodementia. *American Journal of Psychiatry,* 136:895–900, 1979.

Wells, C. E.: Other organic brain syndromes. In H. I. Kaplan & B. J. Sadock (Eds.), *Comprehensive Textbook of Psychiatry, Volume 1* (4th ed.). Baltimore: Williams & Wilkins, 1985, pp. 873–882.

Westermeyer, J.: *Primer on Chemical Dependence.* Baltimore, MD: Williams & Wilkins, 1976.

Westermeyer, J.: The psychiatrist and solvent-inhalant abuse: Recognition, assessment, and treatment. *American Journal of Psychiatry,* 144:903–907, 1987.

White, N. J. Complex visual hallucinations in partial blindness due to eye disease. *British Journal of Psychiatry*, 136:284–286, 1980.

Whitehouse, P. J., Price, D. L., Struble, R. G., et al.: Alzheimer's disease and senile dementia: Loss of neurons in the basal forebrain. *Science*, 215:1235–1239, 1982.

Whitlock, F. A.: *Symptomatic Affective Disorders*. New York: Academic Press, 1982.

Whitlock, F. A., & Evans, L. E. J.: Drugs and depression. *Drugs*, 15:53–71, 1978.

Willett, E. A. Group therapy in a methadone treatment program: An evaluation of changes in interpersonal behavior. *Internation Journal of Addictions*, 8:33–39, 1973.

Williams, D., Mehl, R., Yudofsky, S., et al.: The effect of propranolol on uncontrolled rage outbursts in children and adolescents with organic brain dysfunction. *Journal of the American Academy Child Psychiatry*, 21:129–135, 1982.

Wolanin, M. O., & Phillips, L. R. F.: *Confusion*. St. Louis: C. V. Mosby Co., 1981.

Wolozin, B. L., Bruncnicki, A., Dickson, D. W., et al.: A neuronal antigen in the brains of patients with Alzheimer's disease. *Science*, 232:648–650, 1986.

Woody, G. E., Luborsky, L., McLellan, A. T., et al.: Psychotherapy for opiate addicts. *Archives of General Psychiatry*, 40:639–645, 1983.

Woody, G. E., McLellan, A. T., Lubursky, L., & O'Brian, C. P.: Psychotherapy for substance abuse. *Psychiatric Clinics of North America*, 9:547–562, 1986.

Woody, G. E., O'Brien, B. P., & Rickels, K.: Depression and anxiety in heroin addicts: A placebo controlled study of doxepin in combination with methadone. *American Journal of Psychiatry*, 132:447–450, 1975.

Wulff, M. H.: The barbiturate withdrawal syndrome: A clinical and electroencephalographic study. *Electroencephalographic Clinical Neurophysiology* (Suppl.), 14:1–173, 1959.

Wurmser, L.: *The Hidden Dimension: Psychotherapy of Compulsive Drug Use*. New York: Jason Aronson, 1979.

Yesavage, J. A., Tinklenberg, J. R., Hollister, L. E., et al.: Vasodilators in senile dementia: A review of the literature. *Archives of General Psychiatry*, 36:220–223, 1979.

Yudofsky, S., Williams, D., & Gounan, J.: Propranolol in the treatment of rage and violent behavior in patients with chronic brain syndromes. *American Journal of Psychiatry*, 138:218–220, 1981.

Yudofsky, S. C., Stevens, L., Silver, J., et al.: Propranolol in the treatment of violent behavior associated with Korsakoff's psychosis. *American Journal of Psychiatry*, 141:114–115, 1984.

Zubenko, G., & Pope, H. G., Jr.: Management of a case of neuroleptic malignant syndrome with bromocriptine. *American Journal of Psychiatry*, 140:1619–1620, 1983.

Zubenko, G. S., & Nixon, R. A.: Mood-elevating effect of captopril in depressed patients. *American Journal of Psychiatry*, 141:110–111, 1984.

Section IV
Other Adult Disorders

by

William H. Reid, M.D., M.P.H.

Chapter 14

Schizophrenia

295.1x   Schizophrenia, Disorganized
295.2x   Schizophrenia, Catatonic
295.3x   Schizophrenia, Paranoid
295.9x   Schizophrenia, Undifferentiated

Although research continues into the neurochemical substrates of schizophrenic subtypes, the general treatment for each of the first four listed schizophrenic disorders (Disorganized, Catatonic, Paranoid, Undifferentiated) is similar. Presentation, treatment motivation, treatment acceptance, community adaptation, and prognosis may vary; however, the principles of psychiatric intervention do not.

The treatment of acute exacerbations of schizophrenic psychosis is similar to that of Schizophreniform Disorder (295.40) (see page 201) and Brief Reactive Psychosis (298.80) (see page 200).

Acute Exacerbation. After appropriate examination, observation, protection from self-destructive or aggressive behaviors, and the ruling out of contraindications to biological treatments, pharmacologic and milieu treatment should begin. There is little controversy about the need for antipsychotic medication. Two general treatment schedules may be employed. The clinician may choose either, depending on the patient's discomfort, his or her tolerance for the medication used, and the need for rapid alleviation of psychotic symptoms.

"Rapid neuroleptization." A number of antipsychotic medications* have established efficacy in high-dose, intensive treatment schedules, although rapid neuroleptization is less commonly recommended than

---
*The reader is referred to **Appendix B** for generic and trade names of medications.

a few years ago. Donlon and colleagues (1980) were among the first to show the effectiveness of treatment of this type, which may be preferable when there is an emergency that preempts issues of patient control, invasiveness, feelings of assault, and potential for future noncompliance. Haloperidol, fluphenazine, thiothixene, and others may be given in tablet or liquid form. Intramuscular medication is commonly used, however, and provides rapid absorption and peak serum concentration.

A common schedule is haloperidol 5–10 mg, IM or PO, every 60 minutes until symptoms improve, sedation intervenes, medical complications (e.g., hypotension) arise, or the total dose over 12 hours approaches 100 mg. Most patients require far less in order to reestablish control and contact with their environment. The less potent neuroleptics, such as chlorpromazine, prematurely sedate the patient and may in some instances be more uncomfortable.

It should be noted that the rapid neuroleptization schedule is not primarily a sedating or "snowing" measure, but actually addresses the patient's psychosis (although sedation often occurs).

Neborsky et al. (1981) found that the amount of medication in rapid IM neuroleptization may be less important than frequency of injection and intensive treatment milieu. In their study, patients receiving 2 mg injections improved as rapidly as those receiving 10 mg injections, with no significant differences in side effects. Lower doses are now routine, and hourly medication is less common than a few years ago.

Sedation and extrapyramidal symptoms (EPS) are the most common early side effects. The sedation is likely to be welcomed by the physician and hospital staff, although it may be distressing to the patient or his family. It is rarely lasting.

EPS should, with a few exceptions, be treated only if they arise, since virtually all of the antiparkinsonism agents (benztropine, trihexyphenidyl, amantidine, and others) used to treat them may lower available serum or platelet levels of the antipsychotic medication and add to their frequent anticholinergic effects. Some clinicians use diphenhydramine (an anticholinergic) or benzodiazepines in low doses for this purpose.

If the patient is at risk for significant EPS (e.g., has exhibited them in the past) or is a young male (and thus prone to dystonia), preventive doses of the antiparkinsonism drug may be indicated. Many clinicians choose to try to prevent EPS, rather than waiting for them to arise, since they are uncomfortable for the patient and may interfere with future treatment compliance. Some patients who state that they are "allergic" to one or more antipsychotic agents have actually only had severe EPS at some point.

Tardive dyskinesia, which must be discussed with patients and families before *chronic* neuroleptic medication is begun, should not be a consideration in the alleviation of the acute psychosis. Indeed, it is often countertherapeutic to suggest tardive dyskinesia to the acutely psychotic patient as the somewhat frightening topic may interfere with his or her ability to make an adequate judgment about consenting to medication. Other side effects, such as anticholinergia, are generally mild at this point in treatment, although some patients become quite constipated, and older males may have difficulty urinating.

Acute dystonia, which may include painful muscle spasms, torsion of the trunk, and/or oculogyric crisis, should be treated at once with intramuscular or intravenous medication. Diphenhydramine 5–10 mg may be given IV, as may biperiden 2.5 to 5 mg. Benztropine, 1–2 mg IM, is as rapidly effective as the IV route. Short-acting barbiturates and benzodiazepines may also be used; however, their sedative effect may not be wanted. Other EPS, such as akathisia and "parkinsonian" symptoms, may be treated with a variety of antiparkinsonian drugs and other medications (see section on Side Effects and Adverse Effects on p. 175).

Other approaches to rapid cessation of psychotic symptoms include single moderately large doses of high potency neuroleptics (e.g., 25–40 mg of haloperidol orally or intramuscularly) and large doses of sedative neuroleptics such as chlorpromazine. In general, the chlorpromazine-like drugs lead to oversedation and tend to produce more hypotension than the better-tolerated high potency medications; however, the high-potency drugs are more likely to produce dystonia. As mentioned earlier, large-dose approaches to early acute treatment appear to be yielding to lower-dose regimens in many clinical communities.

A few recent articles imply that the *benzodiazepines* may have a place in the treatment of acute psychosis, although this is far from proved. Nestoros et al. (1982) carried out a double-blind, placebo-controlled study in which very high doses of diazepam, up to 400 mg per day, relieved both positive and negative schizophrenic symptoms in five of six patients within a few hours to a few days.

Salzman et al. (1987) and Modell, Lenox, and Weiner (1985) are among those who have shown that intramuscular benzodiazepines, given with low doses of high-potency IM neuroleptics, can provide a better, safer control of acute agitation in schizophrenics than the neuroleptic alone. The data suggest that particularly lorazepam, 1–2 mg IM, may be helpful in the early stages of treatment.

There is some indication that *catatonic schizophrenia* (295.2x), particularly syndromes with catatonic stupor, rigidity, or posturing, may have neurochemical complications not found in other schizophrenic syndromes (Sheline & Miller, 1986; Trabert, von Blohm, & Gawlitza, 1986). Diazepam has been used intravenously or orally to relieve acute, sometimes life-threatening catatonic symptoms in schizophrenics (McEvoy & Lohr, 1984), as has lorazepam. Lithium may be tried, added to neuroleptics (Climo, 1985; Weizsacker, Woller, & Tegeler, 1984). Acute or life-threatening, treatment-resistant catatonia is also considered an indication for electroconvulsive therapy (ECT).

Rough comparisons of effective oral doses of several common antipsychotic drugs are given in Table 3. One should remember that there are significant differences among these medications, especially those in different chemical groups (e.g., phenothiazine, thioxanthene). In many ways, then, they are not "equivalent."

Treatment setting. Patients who are well-known to the treating physician, and who may be experiencing a relapse of psychosis without a need for any inpatient milieu, may be treated outside traditional inpatient settings. Some emergency rooms are equipped to observe such patients for several hours. Some facilities have beds and nursing care available without complete admission to the hospital. This may be useful in situations in which the patient has a sophisticated and supportive environment to which he can return. Nevertheless, the overall treatment of acute schizophrenia usually requires a multifaceted approach (see following pages), and the need for medical monitoring of the patient during and shortly after this intensive treatment program

TABLE 3
Equivalent Doses of Neuroleptics
Approximate Antipsychotic Effect of Oral Dose

Chlorpromazine	100mg
Chlorprothixene	40mg
Fluphenazine	2mg
Haloperidol	2mg
Loxapine	15mg
Mesoridazine	60mg
Molindone	10mg
Thioridazine	100mg
Thiothixene	5mg
Trifluoperazine	5mg

should be obvious. Inpatient treatment, preferably with a psychiatrically experienced nursing staff, is recommended. Less experienced nursing staff, such as that found on a nonpsychiatric ward in a general hospital or nursing home, may misinterpret (or not recognize) the effects of treatment, particularly mistaking sedation for antipsychotic response.

Electroconvulsive therapy (ECT). ECT can be helpful in the emergency treatment of some intractably psychotic patients, but probably does not change the course of the illness (Koehler & Sauer, 1983; Richelson, 1986; Taylor & Fleminger, 1980). Patients with severe affective complements, intractable withdrawal, or "malignant catatonia" may benefit.

Consent. The issue of consent to acute treatment when the patient is clearly psychotic is an important one, but should not be allowed to interfere with rapid treatment of this painful, potentially dangerous situation. Some clinicians or hospital staffs balk at the use of intramuscular medication. One may discuss at great length whether or not the patient is able to truly understand the nature of the treatment, appreciate the risks and benefits, or otherwise competently consent to or refuse treatment. In the majority of cases, however, the physician or other staff should explain the need for treatment to the patient and, if available, his family. Then, in the absence of explicit refusal, proceed with treatment.

If the patient specifically refuses treatment, then a judgment should be made as to the extent of the crisis or emergency at hand, followed by a medical decision to treat immediately; to seek substitute consent from family, judge, and so forth; or to abandon this particular treatment modality (perhaps offering an alternative if feasible). A psychotic patient is not necessarily "incompetent," and is not *legally* incompetent unless a judge has so ruled. Nevertheless, a physician acting in the patient's best interests, and documenting his or her rationale for crisis or emergency intervention, is far less likely to be criticized later than is one who hesitates or abandons reasonable treatment efforts.

Conservative Treatment of Acute Schizophreniform Psychosis. The mere presence of a stable, consistent, protective inpatient milieu which is structurally different from the patient's community living situation may serve to calm some agitated schizophrenic patients. Although many patients who respond dramatically to environmental change will later be found to have some diagnosis other than schizophrenia, the idea that the patient deserves an opportunity to improve before "rapid neuroleptization" is attractive to many psychiatrists. The psychiatric inpatient ward is usually a place that can tolerate moderate agitation and inappropriate behavior, thus lessening the level of "crisis" often felt by family and nonpsychiatric professionals.

If the patient is not too uncomfortable, one may have the luxury of a day or two of observation without drugs; however, most schizophrenic patients will already have shown a need for maintenance medication (although they may have stopped taking it). The physician may then either restart the medication at or above the previous maintenance dose, or may start with lower doses of medication, increasing it every few days until an antipsychotic effect is clear.

There is increasing recent evidence that low doses act as rapidly as high ones to eliminate psychotic symptoms and signs (Allen, Davis & Davis, 1987). Unless rapid control with sedation is an issue, one may wish to consider the long-term psychosocial benefits of lower doses. The eventual dose of medication necessary to stabilize the acute condition may be considerably less than that used in the rapid treatment modalities, and the patient may be more amenable to individual, group, and milieu psychotherapy.

Acute agitation, aggressive behavior, or sleeplessness may be treated separately from the target psychosis. If sedation is needed, for example, sedative drugs may be added to the antipsychotic regimen in such a way that physiologic REM cycles are conserved. The wrenching anxiety often seen in acutely ill patients can be treated with any of several short-acting benzodiazepines. Although these may alter the bioavailability of the neuroleptic, the advantage of symptom-specificity may be worth the compromise.

Nonpharmacologic means of protecting the patient or others should also be considered, including a locked ward, close observation by staff, restraint, or seclusion. These are discussed in more detail below.

Brief Hospital Treatment. The inpatient milieu for early or brief hospital treatment of the schizophrenias should include a therapeutic combination of *architecture, staffing, programs, social structure, respite* and *patient participation.* Each has a place in a dynamic inpatient experience which will lead to successful transition either to outpatient care or to extended residential treatment.

Architectural requirements vary with clinical philosophy and the needs of the usual patient population. Persons treated under court order or involuntary commitment may require a closed unit, although reasons for locked doors may be more administrative, legal, or political than therapeutic. Modern treatment environments combine patient and staff safety with pleasing design, using durable materials to provide warmth, color, texture, adequate illumination, and communication within the unit. Most licensing and accrediting agencies provide for group and individual areas, with space for gathering together as well as for patient privacy. The need to observe patients—for evaluation and protection—should be tempered to avoid the feeling of being in a "fish bowl."

Nursing stations should be highly accessible, not hidden away where they are likely to be used as retreats by some staff. The glassed-in style of nursing station is a countertherapeutic anachronism which should be avoided on all but the "intensive care" ward. It combines the worst aspects of the "fish bowl," "us vs. them," and tempting staff retreat.

Access to other aspects of the treatment program, such as dining facilities, group therapy, occupational therapy, and recreation should be as open as is feasible. For example, meals should be served in an ordinary cafeteria or dining room setting, avoiding regressive in-room meal service whenever possible.

Staffing should reflect the number and variety of mental health professionals needed to effect the various tasks of medical, social, and educational treatment; administration; ward maintenance; and the like. Cost-saving efforts in the public sector and profit considerations in the private sector have unfortunately led to a substitution of architecture for staff in many hospitals. Adequate staffing ratios vary with patient care needs; however, a quality inpatient environment will not need to substitute locked doors, extra seclusion rooms, highly regimented activities, or other barriers for individual observation and care by staff.

Each staff member should be competent in his or her particular field and sensitive to the needs of the patient with acutely disturbed thought process. Sometimes these needs are for intervention or redirection; sometimes they are for intrusive presence. Staff's sex, age, or cultural background may be relevant to some treatment issues. Both the administrative hierarchy and the attending physicians and professionals should support the ward staff, and express their support through mutual respect, professional use of the staff members' expertise, opportunity for additional education and training, and fair compensation.

One must take care to recognize and deal with the staff member who is exploiting, hostile, or otherwise nonprofessional in the care of patients. By the same token, the hospital should be alert to the toll taken on the staff by continuous work with difficult, sometimes frustrating patients.

The active inpatient area should contain *therapeutic programs,* some required or encouraged and some elective, during most of the patient's waking hours. At least several hours of organized activity should be available each day, including therapeutically oriented ward meetings or group therapy. In other activities, organization is evident but the structure less pronounced, such as in occupational therapy (OT), recreational therapy (RT), or at meal time. Even completely "free" periods may have some semblance of structure, by virtue of the fact that they are scheduled or because of optional alternatives.

Programs should allow for individual needs and preferences, rather than assuming a sameness among all patients. They should be neither intrusive nor overstimulating, but rather provide an atmosphere of security and consistency, in which the patient's world is one of predictability, caring, and growth.

The brief treatment unit must provide a therapeutic and *socializing* environment which is dynamic, not static. Although medication and simple shelter from the outside world will often lead to improvement, the patient should not be expected merely to remain here while the medication does its work or the psychosis remits of its own accord. In the best of circumstances, the patient is engaged in a multimodal environment from which he or she emerges as either an outpatient or an extended-stay patient with the best possible opportunity for continued improvement.

This implies that discharge planning should begin early, within the first few days of hospitalization. The projected length of stay for acute schizophrenic or schizophreniform psychosis should be between seven and 30 days. Although the patient should not be pushed to return to the outside world prematurely, the physician and ward staff should have a knowledge of the expected post-hospital environment in order to prepare him or her eventually to leave, and to prepare the family and community to receive and work with the patient. Family visits and meetings, practical counseling, and realistic transition plans are important parts of the treatment program. Extensive or exploratory psychotherapy, individually or within groups, should not be started except on units specializing in this form of treatment. Relationships formed with staff and other patients are important, but should be pursued as relationships which may soon be broken. Encouragement of reintegration into the family and/or community should begin soon after the psychosis abates, with appropriate attention to how forbidding or nontherapeutic the outside world may seem.

Transition to outpatient care should be done with meticulous attention to detail. The patient and others should clearly understand all aspects of follow-up. Often, there is an aftercare group or program in which the patient may work with staff and/or patients from the inpatient milieu. Whenever possible, community plans should begin early, with patient participation, and the future physician, psychotherapist, or clinic should contact the patient before actual discharge from the hospital.

The *respite* function of brief hospitalization is often overlooked in descriptions of clinical milieus. When patients respond to the shelter or protective setting in which the reorganization and healing process can occur, we sometimes accuse them of being "dependent." However, a significant component of the patient's psychotic symptoms may be related to special stresses, sometimes from the environment but more often from a combination of idiosyncratic internal and external conflict. It is reasonable for the clinician to accept, and make use of, ways in which the hospital can be protective. Careful attention to the discharge or transition process becomes all the more important in this regard.

The patient is expected to be an active *participant* in hospital treatment. The dynamic inpatient milieu has certain expectations of even the most disorganized schizophrenic patient. At the least, he or she is expected to behave within broad human guidelines, dressing rather than remaining naked, refraining from striking others, and the like. These are not always within the control of the most acutely disturbed patients, but denying basic responsibilities over long periods of time because of his or her "illness" may usurp many of the patient's human rights, and communicate the expectation that he or she will remain sick.

One cannot endanger the safety of others while expecting an agitated patient to contain himself; however, there must be a basic implication that the patient is a legitimate part of the ward environment, with its reassuring consistency and rules. Although he, other patients, and staff will be protected as necessary, his responsibilities, insofar as possible, are those of an adult. He is not patronized nor treated as a child, but is expected to participate in and be responsible for his care to whatever extent is possible.

A differentiation among acute-care treatment settings, inpatient environments, intensive partial hospital, and outpatient and "rehabilitative" settings is outlined in the 1987 American Psychiatric Association's *Psychiatry Update* (Klar, 1987). Klar feels that long-term inpatient rehabilitation, as opposed to acute or chronic treatment, should not take place in hospitals, because of the "clinical, economic and ethical dilemmas for both clinician and patient" (p. 344). He points out, however, that the great strides some patients can make in the more intensive hospital setting may be worth the possibility of creating "institutionalism" for patients with previously good functioning and poor adaptation to outpatient rehabilitation.

Psychopharmacology in Early and Brief Hospitalization. For almost all schizophrenic patients, the use of antipsychotic medication is the clinician's most effective means to alleviate or attenuate symptoms and shorten the hospital stay. Adequate drug treatment during hospitalization helps promote social adjustment after discharge and increases the patient's potential for continued remission during outpatient care (May et al., 1981).

Assuming that one draws from the large number of effective antipsychotic drugs currently available, the particular choice is generally less important than proper, consistent administration and appropriate monitoring for drug response and side effects. Drugs of the phenothiazine, butyrophenone, and thioxanthene classes have all been shown to be effective. Molindone is probably effective, but has not gained much popularity in the United States, and has not shown any therapeutic advantage over the more established medications.

In spite of the large number of sophisticated studies that compare the relative efficacy of various phenothiazine, butyrophenone, and thioxanthene medications, and/or that try to establish subtypes of schizophrenia for which a particular medication may be more effective, most clinicians do not have the sophisticated laboratory diagnostic methodology, carefully chosen patient subtypes, or the time needed to make practical use of these early data.

Several other classes of drugs are being studied with mixed success, including calcium channel blockers such as verapamil (Pickar et al., 1987), benzamides such as remoxipride (den Boer, Verhoeven, & Westenberg, 1986), propranolol (Manchanda & Hirsch, 1986), dopamine agonists (Del Zompo et al., 1986), and gamma-endorphins (van Ree et al., 1986). Many others are being studied for chronic and recurrent schizophrenic symptoms.

Most clinicians prefer "high-potency" neuroleptic drugs for most of their patients. The sedative and other side effects of medications such as chlorpromazine, which require doses of several hundred milligrams, make them second choices during acute treatment.

Three issues seem of overriding importance to practical prescribing for schizophrenic patients:

1. If possible, choose a medication to which the patient or a close family member has responded successfully in the past, and which he or she has tolerated reasonably well.
2. In the absence of a clinical reason to do otherwise, the psychiatrist should choose from among those medications with which he is most familiar.

3. The patient may have specific symptoms or sensitivities which suggest treatment with particular medications.

The therapy of schizophrenic or schizophreniform psychoses takes time and patience. Once one has reached a dose that is likely to be effective, it is important to continue the medication for several weeks, if necessary, to assess its effect accurately. Although the patient may at times need additional, or different, treatment temporarily, and although the patient, his family, and sometimes the ward staff may press for a change in treatment, clinical experience and the available literature are both quite clear that frequent medication changes, use of multiple drugs from similar classes, and premature stopping of a potentially successful medication usually confuse treatment rather than help it (Nurnberg & Levine, 1986).

"Positive symptoms" of schizophrenia are more likely to respond quickly to pharmacology treatment than are "negative symptoms." Patients with relatively shorter durations of illness may have broader improvement. Some new classes of neuroleptics, such as the diphenylbutylpiperidines may address negative symptoms more specifically. The addition of L-dopa to the neuroleptic regimen may be helpful as well (Meltzer, Sommers, & Luchins, 1986).

Once emergency treatment, described above, has taken place, the drug initially used to control the acute psychosis may be continued for intermediate treatment (unless side effects are poorly tolerated). Initial dosage levels can often be reduced up to 50% once the patient has been stabilized.

Oral administration of antipsychotic medication is preferable for most patients. Intramuscular injection carries with it a number of countertherapeutic connotations, including those of penetration, assault, and infantilization. Depot preparations such as fluphenazine decanoate or haloperidol decanoate should be used with caution at this stage of treatment, since their effects are not reversed as easily as those of other dosage forms, and side effects or adverse effects may be difficult to control. The convenience of the depot preparation often does not outweigh the disadvantages.

Surreptitious administration, for example in fruit juice without informing the patient, usually leads to more problems than solutions. The familiar "odorless, tasteless" preparations advertised for acute patients belie a basic atmosphere of manipulation and distrust. It is usually better to deal directly with an issue of medication refusal, and address the reasons for it, than to circumvent the problem. Given openly, however, the liquid form of antipsychotic medication may be preferred early in treatment, since it is difficult for the patient to "cheek" or spit out without the staff's knowledge.

Although virtually all of the common antipsychotic medications can be given once daily, and although there are psychotherapeutic as well as convenience reasons for doing this, it is often best to begin treatment with divided doses. This allows for better monitoring of the patient's immediate response, may alleviate some side effects (such as late evening akathisia), especially in older patients, and may result in better bioavailability for some patients. When the response has stabilized, the physician and/or patient may choose the daily dosage schedule which is most convenient.

Fixed-dose combinations. This author strongly recommends against the use of fixed-dose drug combinations. Currently in the United States at least two antipsychotic-plus-antidepressant combinations are marketed (Triavil and Etrafon), as well as one antipsychotic-plus-anxiolytic (Limbitrol). If one's patient requires two kinds of psychotropic drug therapy, it is important to retain the flexibility of drug, dose, and dosage schedule which is not possible with fixed-dose combinations.

Predicting response. "Challenge doses" and other methods of predicting dosage or therapeutic response have not been shown accurate or effective enough for general clinical use with neuroleptics. At this writing, plasma levels of antipsychotic drugs, although advertised as available to clinicians, appear to be neither reliable nor valid as practical predictors of bioavailability or therapeutic response (Faraone, Brown, & Laughren, 1987; Volavka & Cooper, 1987).

"Therapeutic windows" have not been helpful thus far in routine clinical practice; however, haloperidol has shown some promise in this respect. Although higher levels are often effective for some refractory patients, 5–15 nm/ml may be optimal for most patients, assuming a treatment setting with sophisticated laboratory resources (Smith et al., 1982). Poor serum levels are reasonably associated with lack of therapeutic response (Tune et al., 1980).

Red blood cell levels, certain computed ratios, and more sophisticated research tools such as cerebrospinal fluid indices, serum prolactin, and so forth are useful research tools; clinical application of such research data is not yet feasible for the majority of patients (Faraone et al., 1986). The dexamethasone suppression test (DMST) has had little success as a predictive vehicle in schizophrenia (Wik et al., 1986).

All major classes of antipsychotic drugs stimulate prolactin secretion. These prolactin-stimulating effects are correlated with clinical effectiveness and binding affinity to dopamine receptors. Maximum prolactin-stimulating response increases with dose, to a point, generally reaching maximum at the equivalent of 500–700 mg of chlorpromazine per day (Allen, Davis, & Davis, 1987). This lends support to current findings that high or very high doses of antipsychotic medication are, except for extraordinary patients, no more clinically effective than medium doses in the long run.

Side effects and adverse effects of antipsychotic medications must be understood by the clinician before the drugs are prescribed. (See *Side Effects and Adverse Effects of Antipsychotic Drugs* below.) The ward staff should be trained in the recognition of these, and of signs of toxicity. Fortunately, most side effects of antipsychotic medications are benign and little more than inconvenience for the patient. However, some (such as dystonia) can be quite painful, and many others may be frightening or misunderstood by the patient and his family. Without attention by the physician and ward staff, any side effect can become a part of some patients' rationalization for stopping the medication, not cooperating with treatment, or severing the doctor-patient relationship.

Most common side effects can be controlled by either titrating the dosage of the drug or additional medication (see below). When additional medication is added, one must bear in mind that a number of clinical considerations are added as well, including new side effects (such as anticholinergic effects of many antiparkinsonian drugs), drug–drug interactions (including lessened bioavailability of the antipsychotic medication), other alterations of clinical response to the antipsychotic, and the patient's psychological reaction to the change in treatment.

Side Effects and Adverse Effects of Antipsychotic Drugs. Neurologic and nonneurologic side effects and adverse effects will be discussed briefly. So-called "neuroleptic malignant syndrome" and tardive dyskinesia will be presented in more detail at the end of this section.

Sedation. This is a common side effect, even with the so-called nonsedating neuroleptics. It dissipates after a few days or weeks, as tolerance (to the effect, not the antipsychotic action) develops. This side effect is often used as a substitute for a hypnotic agent, although it does not provide physiologically useful sleep (with regular REM and non-REM cycles, etc.)

Autonomic effects. Those not mentioned elsewhere in this section are most commonly represented by postural hypotension. Most are dose-related. Both orthostatic and persistent hypotension are more common with the low-potency neuroleptics, although geriatric patients in particular may have difficulties with haloperidol and other high potency drugs as well (Petrie et al., 1982).

Anticholinergic effects. Since the antipsychotic, antidepressant, and antiparkinsonian drugs all have anticholinergic effects, and since two or more may be prescribed together, considerations of dose and additive effects are important. For most patients, these represent only an inconvenience such as dry mouth or mild constipation. For some, such as middle aged or older men they may be significant (e.g., prostate enlargement). Blurry vision related to problems with accommodation is common, but should not be confused with exacerbation of glaucoma (see p. 178). Serious symptoms, including anticholinergic delirium which may be confused with functional psychosis, are often related more to antiparkinsonian drugs than to the neuroleptics themselves.

Severe syndromes, such as those related to overdose or (rarely) abuse of antiparkinsonian agents, can easily be treated with physostigmine 0.5–2.0 mg every 15 to 30 minutes, IM or *slow* IV, until CNS or cardiac symptoms abate. Because physostigmine is rapidly metabolized, the patient should be closely observed and the dose repeated as needed to maintain improvement until the anticholinergic medications have been metabolized. If a trial of physostigmine at the above doses does not have a positive effect, other sources for the patient's symptoms, including stroke or neuroleptic malignant syndrome, should be strongly considered.

Neuroleptic-induced pseudoparkinsonism. This is similar to Parkinson's disease. It generally begins within a few weeks of the onset of treatment. The akinetic symptoms may be mistaken for depression, and include shuffling gait, flattening of expression, and general psychomotor retardation. Severe rigidity may be confused with catatonia, and may eventually lead to muscle damage, difficulty breathing, or difficulty eating. Pill-rolling and intention tremors are common.

Oral antiparkinsonian (benztropine, trihexyphenidyl, etc.) or anticholinergic (diphenhydramine, etc.) drugs are the primary treatment; amantadine works as well. Intramuscular anticholinergic agents are generally quite effective for acute discomfort, but if they are not, dopamine agonists such as bromocriptine may be used (Levinson & Simpson, 1987). Thioridazine has few extrapyramidal side effects.

The "rabbit syndrome," with rapid lip twitches, is a very unusual form of EPS, and should not be confused with tardive dyskinesia. It will usually respond to antiparkinsonian drugs.

Akathisia. This can easily be mistaken for anxiety or worsened psychosis. Restlessness is generally felt primarily in the legs, or as difficulty sitting still. It is a major source of discomfort, and should be treated. When found in the absence of pseudoparkinsonism, it may respond poorly to the usual antiparkinsonian, anticholinergic, or antihistaminic preparations, but often yields to benzodiazepines.

Acute dystonia. The majority of acute dystonic reactions occur within 24 hours of treatment, 90% by the third day (Sranek et al., 1986). They are painful and frightening, and often include torsion of the trunk and oculogyric crisis. They are more common in young males. Dystonic reactions (and other side effects as well) are often confused by the patient with "allergy." Patients who say they are "allergic" or "hypersensitive" to neuroleptics should be carefully questioned, since these effects are easily preventable in most cases and there are few alternatives for antipsychotic treatment.

Symptoms should be treated immediately with IM or IV medication. Benztropine, 1–2 mg IM, is usually sufficient, and about as rapidly acting as IV injection. Diphenhydramine (5–10 mg IV) or biperiden (2.5–5 mg IV) is effective as well. Oral antiparkinsonian drugs are preventive, and should be considered in young male patients both to prevent the dystonia and to enhance medication compliance.

Endocrine abnormalities. Many patients taking antipsychotics for long periods gain modest amounts of weight, and sometimes develop a fuller facies. Some of these effects, particularly in men, are probably related to increased prolactin levels, which in turn may lead to gynecomastia and/or lactation. Thioridazine is the neuroleptic most commonly associated with sexual dysfunction, including occasional impotence or retrograde ejaculation.

Increased seizure potential. This is frequently a concern in patients taking neuroleptic drugs, particularly the low-potency ones and promazine (rarely psychiatrically prescribed). In actual practice, seizures are very rare with proper medication dosage; however, patients with seizure disorders should be monitored until their stability is established. Patients who have taken overdoses or very large amounts of neuroleptics should be considered at risk.

ECG changes. The antipsychotic drug most likely to the alter the electrocardiogram is thioridazine (Mellaril). Serious arrhythmias are quite unusual, although a pretreatment ECG may be advisable when high doses are anticipated, or in patients at cardiac risk.

Ophthalmic effects. As already mentioned, anticholinergic effects frequently cause mild accommodation problems, particularly in the elderly. Thioridazine is associated with a well-known, serious retinopathy, almost always in doses above 800 mg per day. Small deposits of melanin in the lens or cornea, usually of no clinical significance, may appear with any of the phenothiazines, but are uncommon in other neuroleptics. Glaucoma is listed as a possible side effect for most of these drugs, primarily because of the anticholinergic effects and the theoretical vulnerability to narrow-angle disease. This potential has probably been considerably overstated in the literature (Reid, Blouin, & Schermer, 1976).

Photosensitivity and other skin reactions. Patients taking neuroleptics, particularly chlorpromazine, are often vulnerable to sunburn (which may exacerbate other temperature-regulation problems). Sunscreens are recommended. Inconvenient rashes, usually maculopapular, are common. Although these may represent real allergies or hypersensitivities, their importance should not be overplayed to the patient. An antihistamine (e.g., diphenhydramine) is usually effective, as is switching to another medication. If the rash continues, a clinical decision can be made as to whether treatment of the psychosis is more important than the dermatitis.

Liver toxicity. Because all of the neuroleptics are metabolized through the liver, most with some difficulty, it is important to establish baseline liver function levels and to be alert for clinical signs of hepatotoxicity. Mild elevations of liver enzymes are generally not contraindications for neuroleptic use. The phenothiazines are the most likely offenders, and should probably not be used in patients with significant cholestasis (Dossing & Andreasen, 1982; Simpson, Pi, & Sramek, 1984).

Agranulocytosis. Most cases of this rare adverse effect are related to chlorpromazine use, probably because of its high dose and low potency. Onset is usually within three months of the beginning of drug therapy, and most often involves high doses. Death is unusual, with recovery following standard supportive and antibiotic treatment for one to three weeks. Suddenness of onset precludes the effectiveness of serial monitoring of the white blood count; however, a baseline CBC is prudent. Patients frequently relapse if the phenothiazine is reinstituted; switching to a non-phenothiazine antipsychotic is recommended.

Tardive dystonia. This refers to the rare, rapid onset of abnormal movements similar to those seen in tardive dyskinesia, but more rapidly disabling, after even brief prescription of antipsychotic medication. Treatment is unclear. Very high doses of antiparkinsonism medications (e.g., 60 mg/day of trihexyphenidyl may be helpful for some patients. Stereotaxic surgery may be helpful in extreme cases (Goldman et al., 1985).

Neuroloptic-induced catatonia. This is an unusual syndrome which is difficult to differentiate from schizophrenic symptoms. A change of neuroleptic or prescription of amantadine is the accepted treatment.

Neuroleptics in pregnancy or during lactation. There is probably little risk in becoming pregnant while taking therapeutic doses of neuroleptics, although a few cases of congenital malformation possibly related to antipsychotic drugs have been reported. It is probably prudent to postpone drug treatment until the second trimester when clinically feasible; however, no definitive studies regarding the pros and cons of this practice have been done. Postnatal syndromes may be prevented by discontinuing medication at least 10 days before delivery. Since antipsychotic drugs enter breast milk, breast feeding should be discouraged.

Drug-drug interactions. As implied above, neuroleptics add to the sedative, CNS depressant, and anticholinergic effects of other drugs. They probably decrease blood levels of tricyclic antidepressants, and may decrease either the blood level or the anticonvulsant effect of phenytoin. The interactions of neuroleptics with cardiac preparations or pressor drugs must be considered for the individual agents involved. They probably increase the analgesic effects of pain relievers, including narcotics, either through drug interaction or through their own pain-dulling effects (see **Appendix A**).

Tardive Dyskinesia. Tardive dyskinesia (TD) is a serious adverse effect of all of the commonly prescribed antipsychotic medications. It is clear that not all patients—and perhaps not even most—will develop TD, even if taking neuroleptics for many years. Gardos and Casey (1984) describe the appearance of dyskinetic symptoms in 3%-4% of patients per year during the first five years of treatment, with older women perhaps being at greater risk. A very few patients develop lasting dyskinesia early in treatment.

Kane and Smith (1982) report an increasing incidence of TD, probably due primarily to recognition of the disorder. They suggest that about 15% of the patients chronically taking neuroleptics will develop the syndrome in some form; however, other studies have suggested higher rates. In any given year, roughly 4% of a neuroleptic-treated population of chronic patients develop dyskinetic symptoms (Kane et al., 1984).

The point-prevalence of persistent dyskinesia, based on a stable British cohort of schizophrenics, is about 12%. There is some indication that dyskinesia is only a transient feature for some patients, since at any particular time 41% of chronic schizophrenic patients in that cohort had some symptoms (Robinson & McCreadie, 1986).

Although there is little risk that the disorder will occur during brief hospitalization early in the course of drug therapy, successful prescribing of antipsychotic drugs often leads to a recommendation for months or years of similar treatment. The patient and his or her family should be given clear, accurate information about TD, its persistent nature, and the risks and benefits of accepting neuroleptic therapy. For the great majority of schizophrenic patients, the benefits of antipsychotic medication are significant. It should be carefully explained that TD almost always begins slowly, with symptoms that can be recognized early. At that point, a decision concerning treatment can be made, with the expectation that mild, early symptoms will probably remit if the medication is discontinued.

Dyskinetic symptoms frequently become temporarily worse after the medication is discontinued, and sometimes do not appear until that time. In the past, some authorities recommended masking these symptoms with increased neuroleptics; however, this practice is largely in disrepute.

Not all dyskinesia seen in psychiatric patients is related to antipsychotic medication. There is a natural rate of occurrence which may approach 5% in some populations without neuroleptics.

The cumulative dose of antipsychotic medication may be related to eventual development of dyskinesia; however, most recent evidence indicates that the total time the patient is on such drugs is probably the most important factor. "Drug holidays," changing neuroleptics, adding or not adding antiparkinsonism drugs, and so forth have not been consistently shown to prevent, or lessen the incidence of, this condition. Molindone may be less predisposing to tardive dyskinesia than other antipsychotic drugs; however, this has not been proved, and the therapeutic activity of molindone is probably less than that of the more established medications.

Symptoms. The patient should be examined for signs and symptoms of TD before and early in treatment, and at least every several months thereafter so long as the medication is prescribed.

Early symptoms of TD include mild, vermicular tongue movements, smacking of the lips, pressing the tongue against the cheeks, and chewing movements. Frequent examination for such movements should be carried out with the patient's mouth open and relaxed, while he or she is doing something distracting such as tapping the foot. Symptoms should be differentiated from other sources of mouth movements such as ill-fitting dentures; however, such movements should not be blamed on benign causes until TD has been ruled out. All dyskinetic movements can increase with various forms of stress and decrease when a patient is sedated. They generally disappear during sleep. Many patients deny that the movements are present, even while they are occurring.

The abnormal involuntary movement scale (AIMS) (see below) is a commonly used, rapid means of screening patients. It can be administered by trained, nonphysician personnel, but results should be reviewed by a psychiatrist or neurologist.

Abnormal Involuntary Movement Scale (AIMS)

- Have the patient sit in a hard chair without arms. Remove dental appliances, gum. Ask about dental or mouth problems.
- Observe and rate on the following scale: *0=no abnormality evident; 1=minimal abnormality; 2=mild; 3=moderate; 4=severe.*
- Record *individual and total ratings* for future comparisons.

    ____1. *Muscles of Facial Expression* (forehead, eyebrows, periorbit, cheeks; involuntary frowning, blinking, smiling, grimacing)
    ____2. *Perioral Muscles* (lip puckering, pouting, smacking)
    ____3. *Jaw* (biting, clenching, chewing, opening, lateral movements)
    ____4. *Tongue* (increased or vermiform movements)—Observe at rest in the mouth and when protruded; repeat.

___5. *Upper Extremities* (choreoathetoid movements)—Observe with hands hanging freely; omit tremors.
___6. *Lower Extremities* (choreathetoid movements, foot tapping, lateral knee movements)—Observe; may "activate" by distracting patient with finger exercises such as tapping fingers against thumb.
___7. *Neck, Trunk* (squirming, twisting, gyrating, rocking)—Observe sitting quietly, standing, standing with arms forward and palms down.
___8. *Overall Severity of Abnormal Movements*
___9. *Patient's Incapacity Due to Abnormal Movements*
___10. *Patient's Awareness of Abnormal Movements* (0=unaware . . . 4=aware and severely distressed by movements)
___11. *Current Dental Problems?* (0=no, 1=yes)
___12. *Usual Presence of Dental Appliances* (0=no, 1=yes)

Treatment of tardive dyskinesia is, at this point, entirely palliative and largely unsuccessful. There are a few patients who appear to respond to one of several different therapies (and a few whose symptoms remit spontaneously); however, none is broadly useful. Should symptoms be persistent or serious, neurological consultation is indicated.

Neuroleptic Malignant Syndrome. Neuroleptic malignant syndrome (NMS) is the most serious acute adverse effect of antipsychotic medications. Although rare, it is regularly reported in the literature, and has been seen at least a few times by most experienced clinicians. It affects all age groups, and, depending upon early recognition and treatment, may have a mortality of up to 20%. Significant mortality or morbidity is almost always associated with medical complications. Patients treated rapidly for their extrapyramidal symptoms, and promptly supported medically, are very likely to survive. Levinson and Simpson (1986) suggest naming the syndrome "EPS with fever" rather than "neuroleptic malignant syndrome."

At least 10%, and probably over 25%, of cases of NMS are probably related to nonneuroleptic causes (Levinson & Simpson, 1986). In some cases, severe EPS's interact with a medical condition to increase vulnerability. Perhaps only 20%–35% of apparent NMS appears in previously healthy patients.

Symptoms include rapid rise in body temperature, up to 105–107°F, severe EPS, muscle rigidity, elevated creatinine phosphokinase (CPK), and elevated white count. Although the condition appears to be related to basal ganglionic dysfunction, the actual mechanisms for the hyperthermia and rapidly altered sensorium are not entirely clear. Similar syndromes have occurred in patients on neuroleptics exposed to extreme heat or sunburn. The condition may recur in the same patient, making a change of medication and careful consideration of whether or not to continue neuroleptic therapy important concerns for the psychiatrist. Although molindone has been said to have a lowered risk of this and similar syndromes, cases of massive, life-threatening rhabdomyolysis with hyperthermia have been reported following its administration (Johnson et al., 1986).

Treatment of neuroleptic malignant syndrome. Treatment is fairly straightforward, and often successful. Neuroleptics should be discontinued and the patient immediately treated with bromocriptine, a dopamine agonist, orally 25–60 mg/day in divided doses (every three to four hours) (Rampertaat, 1986); amantadine orally 200–300 mg per day; or carbidopa/L-dopa orally up to 50/200 mg q.i.d. Bromocriptine is the most direct of these therapies. Muscle relaxant therapy such as dantrolene sodium 0.8–1.25 mg/kg IV or 50–200 mg/day orally (Lesser et al., 1986), or lorazepam 1.5–2.0 mg IV to start has also been effective. Support and cooling must accompany any of the above.

Other Drugs. *Lithium carbonate* is another nonneuroleptic drug sometimes used in schizophrenia. Although lithium may be a helpful adjunct to antipsychotic medication, and may address specific symptoms such as episodic violence or mood swings, it is not considered adequate treatment alone. Some patients with labile affective components of schizophrenic pathology, or patients who have been misdiagnosed as schizophrenic in the first place, may respond, however. "Schizophrenic" patients with affective or vacillating symptoms who have not responded well to neuroleptics should receive an adequate trial of lithium while continuing the antipsychotic regimen. The routine use of lithium to decrease aggressive or agitated behavior in schizophrenics is probably not warranted.

Judicious use of lithium and antipsychotic drugs together is not particularly dangerous, as was once thought. This is especially true if the lithium is added to a stable dose of an antipsychotic drug, and lithium levels are monitored appropriately. More detailed information may be found in Jefferson, Greist, and Ackerman (1983).

Naloxone has been carefully studied, but recent work indicates it is ineffective when prescribed alone for schizophrenia (Pickard Bartanian et al., 1982). The *benzodiazepines*, cited earlier for control of refractory acute psychosis, should not be considered adequate for ongoing antipsychotic treatment in schizophrenic disorders.

Pharmacologic milieu. As is the case for all other psychotropic medications, antipsychotic drugs should not be given in a therapeutic vacuum. The appropriate inpatient milieu for acute treatment has already been briefly outlined. In addition, the patient should understand the characteristics of his or her medication, its uses, its drawbacks, and its important place in the overall treatment plan.

Failure to continue needed medication is the single most common reason for relapse in discharged schizophrenic patients. The individual who understands his drug treatment, and who feels support from the psychiatrist, other psychotherapists, or family, is far more likely to feel he is an active participant in his treatment. This in turn may provide less need to manipulate the medication, less fear of its effects, a feeling of more control, greater optimism about one's destiny, and better understanding of the medication's role in rehabilitation.

Other Forms of Acute and Intermediate Antipsychotic Treatment. In addition to the pharmacologic approaches mentioned above, and expanded below for the treatment for refractory chronic patients, several other biologic, psychotherapeutic, special milieu, and dietary treatments have been tested during the past two decades.

Although *electroconvulsive therapy (ECT)* is useful for several types of acute schizophrenic episodes, most clinicians feel that pharmacologic treatment is preferable at all stages. It is unusual to see ECT used for routine treatment of schizophrenic patients in the United States or Canada (Salzman, 1980). If ECT is considered, one should adhere to the modern standards of practice described elsewhere in this text with regard to pretreatment protocol, consent, electrode placement, stimulus waveform, stimulus intensity, and number of treatments (Martin, 1986).

The possibility that dietary gluten may cause or affect schizophrenic symptoms has not been well proved in studies of *gluten-free diets* for schizophrenic patients. Most serious studies find little or no effect (Osborne et al., 1982; Potkin et al., 1981; Storms, Clopton, & Wright, 1982). Vlissides, Venulet, and Jenner (1986) carried out a 14-week double-blind trial of gluten-free diet in a psychiatric environment. They felt that most positive changes in their 27 subjects could be attributed to the attention they received; however, two patients did improve during the gluten-free period who relapsed when the gluten-containing diet was reintroduced.

Hemodialysis has been similarly disappointing in carefully controlled studies (Fogelson, Marder, & van Putten, 1980). *Luekotomy* is rarely used today except in the most intractable cases; however, at least one long-term follow-up suggests that carefully controlled psychosurgery may have been effective in the past in some patients, and probably led to less morbidity than is commonly assumed (Benson et al., 1981).

Outcome and Prognosis After Acute Treatment. Once the psychosis has remitted and reasonable psychosocial adaptation has occurred, the prognosis for many patients with schizophrenic, schizophreniform, and brief reactive psychoses is fair. In one study, over 70% of schizophrenic patients remained in remission at one-year follow-up (Rabiner, Wegner, & Kane, 1986). Premorbid factors such as inadequate social adjustment and longer duration of illness are correlated with poorer outcome. Three factors that appear to be very important to a good prognosis and that are under at least partial control of the psychiatrist are:

1. adequate intensity of hospital treatment
2. careful preparation for and transition to outpatient status
3. appropriate maintenance medication

The addition of paranoid psychosis to the schizophrenic syndrome complicates treatment and worsens the prognosis for most patients. The doctor–patient relationship is often strained, and the patient's paranoia interferes with his motivation for treatment compliance. Family and social adjustment tends to be poorer on average (Jorgensen, 1985). This may be because paranoid symptoms stand out in the community and are often more unsettling for others than are those of simple psychosis or psychotic withdrawal. It may also stem from our experience that paranoid delusions and hallucinations are more difficult to treat successfully. Review of the literature suggests that paranoid schizophrenics are commonly among those chosen for special "last resort" treatments for "intractable" or "treatment-resistant" patients (Brizer et al., 1985; Frances & Carpenter, 1983).

It is important to understand that although outward psychotic symptoms may rapidly remit during the first few weeks of hospital treatment, this does not necessarily indicate alleviation of all signs of the schizophrenic disorder itself, or of the depression and anxiety that accompany a psychotic break. One must focus treatment and follow-up on these aspects of care as well, and not merely upon the more visible psychotic signs (Szymanski, Simon, & Gutterman, 1983).

Work with the *families* of schizophrenic patients is important for preventing relapse, in part by helping the families develop the skills necessary to solve the many problems associated with schizophrenia, and in part by tempering some of the negative communication and relating among family members and the schizophrenic patient (Doane et al., 1986). Education about the illness, and particularly about maintenance medication, probably prevents or delays rehospitalization (Hogarty et al., 1986).

Supportive care in the *community*, including special clinics, social support networks, and short-term dynamic day hospital programs (defined separately from those for chronic patients) appear to increase quality of life and decrease use of both psychiatric and nonpsychiatric medical services (Glick et al, 1986; Schwartz et al, 1986; Vidalis & Baker, 1986).

One sometimes encounters efforts to incorporate meditative or "holistic" programs into the treatment milieu. Although patients may respond favorably during hospitalization, there is little information to indicate that such programs accelerate improvement, or that they have any positive effects on relapse rate, especially for chronic patients (Lukoff et al., 1986).

Suicide in Schizophrenia. The risk of completed suicide in schizophrenia is significant. The addition of an acute or subacute psychosis to the affective component sometimes seen in schizophrenic patients makes suicide attempts likely. At the same time, psychotic thinking makes attempts less predictable by clinicians or families, less organized, more impulsive, and sometimes more likely to be lethal.

Hopelessness concerning one's disease or social adaptation can be a contributing factor. Most schizophrenics are aware of their illness and of the fact that it may respond incompletely to medication. Withdrawal and ostracism by the community often lead to isolation. Suicide should be considered a possibility for all patients, and a probability for those who are particularly withdrawn or hopeless, or have a history of previous attempts. The "gesture"-like quality—or even bizarre nature—of previous attempts should not decrease one's caution about the seriousness of the patient's impulses. Schizophrenics may confuse self-directed and other-directed aggressive impulses, with a concomitant danger to others, particularly during acute psychosis. Drake, Gates, and Cotton (1986) feel that schizophrenics who have completed suicide may be distinct in many ways from the larger group of those who have attempted; however, they also advise caution because of the lower predictability of this group, compared to patients with affective disorders.

Chronic Schizophrenia

Outpatient Care. As noted above, the quality of the patient's transition from acute treatment to outpatient management has considerable bearing on adaptation and prognosis. Although patients differ, length and quality of remission are favorably affected by continuing medication in adequate doses and by consistent clinical follow-up.

Medication. Antipsychotic medication does not cure schizophrenia; it suppresses the symptoms. For patients whose diagnosis is Brief Reactive Psychosis (298.80) and who thus have specific stressors and time-limited psychoses, medication can usually be tapered and discontinued. Such tapering should be done with close monitoring by the psychiatrist, generally over several months, since tapering of the actual serum level does not closely follow decreases in dose, and the patient is in an environment quite different from that in which he or she received acute inpatient care (and often the same environment which precipitated the psychosis in the first place).

For those with Schizophreniform Disorder (295.40), the possibility of chronic schizophrenia is high. Drugs should be only cautiously tapered and discontinued, although such patients deserve at least one trial at being free of medication.

For patients with documented schizophrenic disorders or other psychoses which require continued antipsychotic medication, a decrease to maintenance dosage levels is recommended. This often decreases side effects and minimizes the total dose of neuroleptic received over the years during which the patient is likely to require such treatment. It is important, however, to wait until the patient's social situation has stabilized, with return to the family, establishment of office or clinic visits, return to work or school, and so forth, before changing the prescription significantly. Once this transition is complete, most patients can be maintained on as little as half or less of their acute treatment dosage.

The popularity of depot-injected medications for chronic schizophrenic patients is perhaps more related to marketing and pseudo-common sense than to any consistent recognition of its greater efficacy over other dosage forms and schedules. Several studies indicate that groups of patients receiving, for example, fluphenazine decanoate differ little from those taking oral fluphenazine at the same effective dose, although at least one large study (Babiker, 1987) indicates a slight—but statistically significant—lowering of rehospitalization rate among patients on the depot preparations. Interestingly, the highest rehospitalization rate in the Babiker study was found for patients taking both depot and oral antipsychotics.

Haloperidol decanoate has recently been introduced in the United States. It is said to have a slightly longer half-life than fluphenazine decanoate (up to four or five weeks), and is probably slightly less potent. There are few differences in side-effect profiles between fluphenazine and haloperidol, and any therapeutic differences may only be related to how often injections are given (and thus perhaps to bioavailability) (Wistedt, 1986). Other depot neuroleptics, such as zuclopenthixol decanoate (Kazi, 1986) and pipothiazine palmitate (Schmidt, 1986) are not yet available in the U.S. Some oral medications, such as pimozide, have long plasma half-lives and are effective when given less than once a day (McCreadie et al., 1982); however, most are not available in the United States.

The apparent advantages of depot medication are obvious: greater clinician control over patient compliance (and thus, apparently, over bioavailability), patient convenience in some cases, and assurance to the family and community (sometimes important in cases of committed or recently discharged violent patients) that drug treatment is continuing. Some of the *detriments* include the patient's feeling of lessened control over his or her care; misperceptions related to assault, penetration, or physical control by the caregiver; infantilization; limited choice of medication and side effect profile; and inability to rapidly discontinue the medication should serious side effects or adverse effects appear. No depot medication should be given without initial trials of nondepot preparations of the same active drug.

Medication compliance. Enlisting the active, positive participation of schizophrenic outpatients in their drug treatment draws upon the highest art of medicine. Many of the same issues mentioned under depot neuroleptic treatment must be frequently addressed. Each time the patient takes his or her medication, there is an opportunity for lowered self-image, frustration with the chronic illness, denial of need for the medication, rationalization for discontinuing it, and acting out within the therapeutic relationship.

If a previously stable patient begins to deteriorate or show early psychotic symptoms, the first thought should be related to whether or not he or she has taken his medication. Although one should not discourage patients' independence and autonomy, the use of family members, roommates, or even close friends as supports to help the patient make positive decisions about his or her treatment is recommended.

Deterioration does not always mean noncompliance, however. A number of factors may either decrease the bioavailability of antipsychotic medication or increase the patient's vulnerability to relapse. Some have to do with weakening of internal defenses. Intercurrent physical illness is a common source of deterioration. Even such simple things as cigarette smoking can significantly lower plasma neuroleptic concentrations (Jann et al., 1986).

The addition of other medications can either raise or lower (e.g., in the case of antiparkinsonian drugs) plasma levels through a variety of mechanisms. Assaying neuroleptic blood levels may help establish gross deficiencies for chronic outpatients or inpatients who have not responded after several weeks or whose response has markedly changed; however, such levels should not be used to titrate response (Faraone, Brown, & Laughren, 1987; Volavka & Cooper, 1987).

"Drug holidays"—which decrease total dose and perhaps the chance for tardive dyskinesia—have been suggested for many chronic patients. However, recent work by McMillan et al. (1986) indicates that even a two-day drug holiday may decrease serum levels of haloperidol by up to 40%. This probably does not correlate directly with CNS bioavailability; however, it may be a consideration in patients particularly prone to relapse or erratic drug response.

Intermittent medication. An alternative to simple maintenance of low dose antipsychotic medications for the chronic schizophrenic patient has been suggested by Marder and colleagues (1984), Carpenter and Heinrichs (1984), and others. Their approach recommends medication only when symptoms of psychosis or developing psychosis appear in the patient, reducing the neuroleptic dose considerably when the patient shows no psychotic symptoms. *This requires much closer monitoring* of chronic patients than is possible in many current social and treatment settings. This "intermittent" medication approach may also adversely affect treatment compliance for schizophrenic patients in general, since it may support denial and rationalizations for stopping medication when not recommended.

Chronic schizophrenic patients, particularly those refractory to traditional medication regimens, often deserve carefully monitored *pharmacological adjuncts* to their neuroleptic medication in order to reverse firmly entrenched symptoms or maximize improvement. In some cases, simply switching to a different class of antipsychotic may be helpful (sometimes because of enhanced bioavailability or selective receptor blockade): for example, changing from long-chain phenothiazines to mesoridazine or thioridazine (Vital-Herne et al., 1986).

Pharmacological adjuncts to continuing antipsychotic medication include the benzopyrones (Casley-Smith et al., 1986), reserpine (Berlant, 1986), thyrotropin-releasing hormone (TRH), and vasopressin (Branbilla et al., 1986). The benzopyrones were associated with statistically significant improvement in 16 clinic schizophrenic subjects treated for three months. The effect appeared to begin at about two weeks.

Reserpine, which has been associated with iatrogenic depression when prescribed for hypertension, has recently been associated with a moderate to dramatic response rate in 50% of 36 chronically disabled psychotic patients (Berlant, 1986). TRH (in doses of 600 micrograms IV every other day) and vasopressin (EDAVP) (4 micrograms IV every other day) were associated with improvement particularly in negative symptoms and memory of 23 chronic, undifferentiated schizophrenics who had responded poorly to neuroleptics alone. TRH treatment produced transient mild hyperthyroidism after about two weeks of treatment (Branbilla et al., 1986).

The "negative" symptoms of schizophrenia tend to be more troublesome than acute hallucinations or delusions. The addition of monoamine oxidase inhibitors (MAOIs) to neuroleptic therapy has been helpful in some treatment-resistant patients, and is considered safe when carefully monitored by the clinician (Bucci, 1987). Pipothiazine is a neuroleptic which may be particularly helpful for negative and affective symptoms (Schmidt, 1986).

Community Resources for the Chronic Patient. Available data indicate that some 75% of the primarily schizophrenic, chronically mentally ill lead lives with inadequate social adjustment. Talbott (1982) feels that no more than 25% of these patients get acceptable aftercare in addition to medication. He reports that housing is the most critical need for these patients, and reminds us that the incidence of medical illness for this group is roughly three times that of the general population.

Continuity of care is reasonably available to some patient groups, particularly in public sector settings such as the Veterans Administration hospital system. Mere availability of programs of social skills, education, and modification of disturbing behaviors does not, however, guarantee that patients will know about them, that they will be available in a practical sense (e.g., that appropriate transportation will be available), or that patients or families will want to take advantage of them. In spite of evidence that very active community support programs may reduce rehospitalization rates by up to 80% over rates seen with medication-oriented aftercare, both public and private payers, such as insurance companies or health maintenance organizations (HMOs), rarely fund such care.

Self-help groups can be enormously useful for many patients. There are now organized groups such as Recovery, Inc., the National Alliance for the Mentally Ill, and smaller groups devoted to particular disorders (such as the Depression and Manic–Depressive Association) in most large cities. Clinicians, particularly physicians, sometimes complain that information disseminated by self-help groups is inaccurate, or that patients' association with such groups can promote treatment noncompliance. One should learn about the quality and availability of self-help groups in one's own community, and then should offer lay-oriented information and guidance.

Chronic Hospital or Residential Settings. Return to the community is not possible for all chronic schizophrenic patients. Some maintenance treatment programs must take place in residential settings such as mental hospitals or nursing homes. Adequate psychiatric and other medical care, along with appropriate housing, educational and vocational opportunity, social skills training and recreation, should be provided. The concept of milieu or community should be at its best in the chronic-care institution. Nursing-home-like facilities tend to be inadequate substitutes, but are necessary in many locales.

The inpatient therapeutic setting should provide goals that are modest rather than far-reaching, and gentle support rather than intense or overstimulating settings. Unless the facility and its staff are equipped to deal with the regression and patient frustration that arise when treatment goals are overwhelming, the milieu should focus upon long-term adjustment as well as symptom removal (Drake & Sederer, 1986a).

There are a few hospitals in which long-term care is also considered acute treatment. In such highly specialized settings, the patient receives appropriate pharmacological treatment, becomes involved in an intensive attempt to bolster needed defenses and, to some extent, restructures portions of the personality that can become foundations for more effective adaptation.

These approaches are generally psychoanalytically oriented, although they may also follow learning theory approaches, and require great investments of energy, time, and money on the part of the patient and the clinical staff. For selected patients, the results are often better than those expected for those receiving only brief hospitalization and community follow-up or ordinary institutional care. The expertise and resources necessary for this work are unavailable to most patients, however, and may not be appropriate for many, provided good brief hospitalization and biopsychosocial follow-up are available.

A final long-term treatment modality, which should be mentioned but has not proved itself, is the community residential facility which encourages patients to view their psychotic episodes as useful life events or learning experiences. Such programs, sometimes supported by psychiatrists, appear to work well for a small subset of patients, perhaps those who would have done well in any event (and may not, in retrospect, have been schizophrenic). The environment is extremely accepting, usually homelike, with great support and encouragement to experience psychotic symptoms without anxiety, as a sort of temporary phase of life.

There is a difference between the above, global approach to schizophrenic illness and supportive psychotherapy for patients who are experiencing frightening delusions or hallucinations. Alleviating the anxiety associated with psychosis is an important, kind thing for the clinician to do. It may be done psychotherapeutically with support and reassurance, pharmacologically, or, for some patients, with insight. (See also the section on Psychotherapy of Schizophrenia, p. 194.)

Prognosis. Ratey, Sands, and O'Driscoll (1986) have recently written an interesting paper on the phenomenology of recovery for these patients. Outcome studies which in the past indicated that about one-third of schizophrenic patients returned to near-baseline emotional and social functioning after their first psychotic episode, with another third faring quite poorly, were often based on diagnostic criteria which today are felt to be overly broad, and probably included many patients with brief reactive psychoses.

Thirty-eight-year follow-up of a rural British cohort indicated complete recovery for almost 30%, with permanent disability in about 35% (Watts, 1985). An important German study indicated that about 22% of schizophrenics demonstrated complete recovery, with 56% "socially recovered." About two-thirds of the patients regained their level of premorbid functioning after acute episodes. This study separated several subtypes of psychosis, including schizoaffective, and found the schizophrenic population to contain several types. About one-quarter had a very unfavorable prognosis (Gross & Huber, 1986).

A complete discussion of social outcome and utilization of medical services in a European cohort is found in Biehl and colleagues (1986). A Japanese study, which may not represent the behavior of similar patients in western cultures, nonetheless gives international corroboration to the general medical finding that earlier onset, longer duration of prodromal signs, and longer time periods between onset and first clinical presentation, predict poor psychosocial outcome (Inoue, Nakajima, & Kato, 1986).

Paranoid schizophrenics appear to respond better to acute treatment with the phenothiazines or other neuroleptics than nonparanoid schizophrenics. Individual and group psychotherapy, as well as milieu therapy, are generally supported in the literature; however, they have not been systematically evaluated. There is a greater likelihood of relapse for patients with paranoid symptoms, when compared with nonparanoid schizophrenics, when remission occurs without chronic deterioration. In general, paranoid patients tend to have better recovery of social function, in spite of the poor prognosis for full remission of symptoms. Premorbid adjustment is an important predictor of remission (Ritzler, 1981).

There is no doubt that the attitudes of patient and family contribute to the substrate of schizophrenic illness and help determine the level of recovery for individual patients. A combination of education and support is useful. Community supports, including day hospitals, appear to be beneficial for many patients, not just those who have few other social resources (Vidalis & Baker, 1986).

Many clinicians and social scientists feel that the biologic and social resources available for helping the chronic schizophrenic are, at least for the time being, largely exhausted. Gralnick (1986), for example, points to increasingly brief hospital stays (largely for financial reasons) focused on medication as the primary form of treatment, and burgeoning numbers of severely disabled, socially bereft patients. Many community alternatives need not be nearly so expensive as "back ward" care for the seriously disabled chronic patient and may be clinically preferable (Dickey et al., 1986).

Psychotherapy of Schizophrenia

Psychotherapy as a Primary Treatment. There are a number of psychotherapists and psychoanalysts who treat subacute schizophrenic illness with psychodynamic psychotherapy (with or without medication). This approach cannot be recommended to all clinicians, since the psychotherapy of severe emotional disorders, particularly those involving thought disorder, should be viewed as a subspecialty requiring particular training, skill, and experience. A number of principles for the psychotherapy of schizophrenia have been outlined by Arieti (1980):

1. The therapist should attempt to cause little or no anxiety early in treatment, and should try to diminish anxiety which is already present.
2. The therapist should not wish merely to return the patient to his or her premorbid condition.
3. The therapist must be able to provide and tolerate a delicate balance within the patient, sometimes for several years, before independence from therapy can be achieved.
4. Treatment must be seen as a way in which the patient proceeds toward gradual acceptance of the self.

The first two of these are quite different from psychotherapy of the healthier or "neurotic" patient. This treatment approach is an arduous task for all concerned; both therapist and patient must understand the requirements of time and energy involved.

Psychotherapy as Adjunct to Medication and Milieu. Carpenter, Heinrichs, and Hanlon (1986) have recently reviewed several approaches to interpersonal treatment of schizophrenia. D'Angelo and Wolowitz (1986) summarize the generally held suggestion of two distinct styles of recovery from schizophrenic episodes: *integration* and *sealing over*. It may be that patients able to integrate psychotic experiences have less primitive characters or defensive systems than those who deny or repress ("seal over") such experiences. On the other hand, the "integrators" may represent a separate diagnostic group.

The potential adverse effects of intensive milieu or psychotherapeutic treatment have been described in this chapter and in additional work by Drake and Sederer (1986b). McGlashan (1983) provides another review of intensive individual psychotherapeutic treatments.

The presence of a family into which the patient can be reintegrated is important; many therapists emphasize the family as a major part of restoration of the patient. Although the therapist may recognize serious pathology in the family, which may have victimized or scapegoated the patient, focusing intently on these problems and refusing to support the family until they are solved may interfere with the patient's reintegration.

Group psychotherapy with schizophrenics should be practical, be oriented toward support and social skills, and promote the beginning or sustaining of interpersonal relationships. Groups whose primary goal is facilitation of insight tend to be unsuccessful in ordinary inpatient or outpatient treatment settings (Mosher & Keith, 1979). Johnson et al. (1986) discussed the "pairing group." Groups that focus on day-to-day issues of community within structured inpatient, day hospital, or outpatient settings appear to be very helpful and gratifying for patients in these environments.

Tardive Dyskinesia and the Chronic Schizophrenic Patient

In a number of patients, symptoms of tardive dyskinesia will appear after several years of neuroleptic medication. In some others, symptoms may appear when antipsychotic drugs are discontinued, and may be confused with the more benign "withdrawal–emergent dyskinesia."

Since there is at present no treatment approach which is accepted as effective, the prospect of tardive dyskinesia is truly upsetting for patients and clinicians alike. The benefits of appropriate neuroleptic treatment for chronic schizophrenic patients generally outweigh the risks of developing a serious movement disorder, however. This is especially true when one considers the tremendous morbidity of schizophrenic illness, our increasing diagnostic accuracy, the probability that medications will be found in the future that either do not induce tardive dyskinesia or can be used to treat it effectively, and the fact that the dyskinesias almost always develop slowly and are often not permanent in the early stages. There is time for complex treatment decisions when and if symptoms first appear. (See pp. 180–181 for a more complete discussion of recognition and management.)

When stopping medication after several years of neuroleptic therapy, one may wish to carefully taper the antipsychotic to allow (in theory) dopamine receptors to become less hypersensitive. This does not always protect the patient against the exacerbation of dyskinetic symptoms, however. In those cases in which the physician decides that a neuroleptic should be used to mask dyskinetic effects—cases that should be quite rare—Branchy, Branchy, and Richardson (1981) report that a dose of approximately one-eighth of the maintenance dose is generally sufficient for the masking purpose.

295.6x Schizophrenia, Residual

The treatment of residual schizophrenia largely parallels that of maintenance treatment for the other forms of schizophrenia. Because of the prominence of social and "negative" symptoms rather than acute psychosis, one may wish particularly to focus on those sections of the foregoing chapter that address interpersonal and social functioning, and pharmacologic attempts to restore appropriate affect and demeanor.

Chapter 15

Delusional (Paranoid) Disorder

297.10   Delusional (Paranoid) Disorder
         Erotomanic Type
         Grandiose Type
         Jealous Type
         Persecutory Type
         Somatic Type
         Unspecified Type

Acute Treatment. Acute psychotic presentation of Delusional (Paranoid) Disorder, differentiated from schizophreniform illness, affective illness, organically induced paranoia, or paranoid personality, is unusual. The literature reflects a number of case reports and studies of paranoid disorders which eventually show themselves to be related to schizophrenia, or which follow a deteriorating course.

These are not the topic of this brief chapter, but are best treated with careful medical and psychiatric evaluation, antipsychotic medication, and follow-up similar to that of Brief Reactive Psychosis or Schizophreniform Disorder. They are sometimes confused with paraphrenia, a late-onset form of schizophrenia (Bridge & Wyatt, 1980; Jorgensen & Munk-Jorgensen, 1985; Varner & Gaitz, 1982). Some atypical paranoid psychoses respond to antidepressant pharmacotherapy, with or without neuroleptics (Akiskal et al., 1983).

Because of the generally normal vocational functioning but possibly deteriorating social or marital functioning in Paranoid (Delusional) Disorder, and the absence of hallucinations or evidence of acute psychosis or organic disorder, the initial setting for evaluation or treatment is likely to be the psychiatrist's office (sometimes a forensic psychiatrist, for persons whose delusions have begun to impinge upon the rights of others). If the presentation is such that others appear to be in danger (e.g., the patient seems about to take action based upon delusions of persecution or jealousy), then physical management such as hospitalization may be indicated. For those patients who have evidenced dangerousness, a secure facility or referral to a law enforcement agency may be the best course.

A number of physical and environmental influences may precipitate paranoid delusions. Deafness, for example, particularly in the elderly, may be a treatable cause of the delusions and may cause one to change the diagnosis. Persons recently separated from distant cultures, particularly eastern cultures, may respond either to understanding or, in some cases, to return to that culture (Waynik, 1985). Much of the literature focuses upon patients who are elderly or medically ill; these cases are most often related to dementia, other organic causes, or environmental deprivation.

A few studies indicate that pure paranoia is not well treated with antipsychotic medications or ECT (Astrup, 1984). Most patients are reluctant to take neuroleptics, although they are effective in some cases.

The author has seen several cases of paranoia, with and without delusions, related to vitamin absorption syndromes such as pernicious anemia (Zucker et al., 1981). Even when no anemia can be found, a trial of intramuscular vitamin B-12 is inexpensive and easily accepted by the patient.

In general, the longer the symptoms have been present, the more refractory they are to simple treatment such as explanation, education, or medication. Some culturally induced syndromes may respond to relocation, even if they have taken months to come to clinical attention, however.

Psychotherapy, when accepted, tends to be the treatment of choice, and should be begun in such a way that the patient is likely to see some benefit from it and some support from the therapist. The therapist should be alert for the appearance of other sources for the paranoia and should be qualified to evaluate them as they arise. There is some evidence that systematic desensitization may be effective in reducing delusional behavior; however, generalization to other parts of the patient's life is limited (Ritzler, 1981).

The patient is often quite uncomfortable, particularly in situations of persecutory, somatic, or even erotomanic delusions. A good therapeutic relationship may at least prevent the patient from taking action which might be destructive to himself or others, and may help with family relationships. Counseling for family members is usually welcomed.

Chapter 16

Psychotic Disorders Not Elsewhere Classified

298.80 Brief Reactive Psychosis
Remembering the caveat *primum no nocere*, it is often prudent to allow the acutely psychotic patient about whom little is known to go without neuroleptic or thymoleptic medication for a few hours (or even a few days), provided he or she is not extremely uncomfortable or threatening to others. Placing the patient in a protected environment, away from possible psychosocial or chemical sources of his or her psychosis (e.g., great stress, drug or chemical exposures) will often allow the symptoms to clear, sometimes completely. Psychoses related to, for example, unusual reactions to incarceration (e.g., the dissociative "Ganser syndrome"), sleep deprivation, chemical exposure in the workplace, surreptitious drug abuse, intentional or accidental poisoning, and the like should clear with simple medical support. Neuroleptics, with their long durations of action and many side effects, can significantly cloud the diagnostic picture and have been responsible for more than a few patients' appearing to be psychotic long after the initial source of the symptoms was gone.

When early, acute restraint or sedation is necessary to protect the patient or to make him comfortable, short-acting barbiturates or short-acting benzodiazepine anxiolytics are usually sufficient. Humane physical restraint or seclusion may be preferable to medicating a patient whose history is unclear during the first few hours of treatment.

In many cases, of course, antipsychotic drugs will be needed. They should be prescribed using the guidelines for emergency and acute treatment in Chapter 14.

After the acute psychosis has abated, more complete recovery may take considerable time. The person's emotional vulnerability to psychosis, presence of precipitating factors in the home or work environment, history of illness and prescribed or nonprescribed drugs, and so forth must all be evaluated. Treatment should continue, on an open psychiatric unit if possible, until the patient is ready to return to the outpatient setting. The transition from the hospital should be certain to include at least some outpatient contact which focuses on support and reorganization, and efforts to prevent future problems.

295.40 Schizophreniform Disorder

Since this disorder meets virtually all criteria for schizophrenia except that of symptom duration, treatment of the acute, early, and even some maintenance stages are essentially as described in the chapter on schizophrenia (Chapter 14). The possibility that the patient has schizophrenia should be carefully considered, although the diagnostic label should be avoided until it is clear. The symptoms of thought disorder should be carefully monitored after discharge from acute hospitalization. As with brief reactive psychosis, one should carefully consider whether any continuing symptoms are related to the illness, or to medication that is being prescribed.

Although schizophrenia may be diagnosed later, a number of patients with Schizophreniform Disorder will remain free of psychosis on little or no medication. The clinician should cautiously decrease maintenance medication and attempt to discontinue drugs in those patients whose symptoms are in good remission. Frequent monitoring with brief office visits and/or family contact for a few months after the psychosis has abated is good practice, and is usually appreciated by patients and their families.

295.70 Schizoaffective Disorder

Because of the poorly defined, "residual" nature of the *DSM-III-R* category, Schizoaffective Disorder, no specific treatment is recommended. Primary treatment should be provided for the particular clinical form taken by the disorder. That is, if a patient exhibits schizophreniform symptoms, treatments similar to those recommended for the schizophrenias (Chapter 14) should be one's first choice. Conversely, if the symptoms of thought disorder seem secondary to marked affective characteristics, such as depression, hypomania, or lability of mood, then lithium and/or antidepressant regimens should be considered in much the same way as is described in the chapter on Mood Disorders (Chapter 17).

There is no reason not to consider a combination of neuroleptic and thymoleptic (antidepressant) medication. The first—neuroleptic or thymoleptic—should be stabilized before the second is added. The patient may respond favorably and obviate any need for additional drugs. Fixed-dose combination preparations should be avoided. As previously stressed, the nonpharmacological components in treatment of both schizophrenic and affective disorders should receive careful consideration in the overall care of the patient.

Among the types listed in the *DSM-III-R* (bipolar or depressive), treatment of the depressive patient without clear psychotic or manic symptoms, but with symptoms similar to the "negative" symptoms of schizophrenia, is probably more difficult than treatment of other types. It should be remembered that the antidepressants of choice are likely to take at least three or four weeks to show their effect, and that the patient's response (or apparent response) may be delayed by schizophreniform symptoms. As is the case with other severely depressed or suicidal patients, serious suicide risk, morbid withdrawal, or manic or catatonic agitation unresponsive to medication are all indications for electroconvulsive therapy. The course of this disorder is not well known, largely because of its diagnostic vagaries and the probability that the patient later will be shown to have either a thought disorder or an affective disorder. There is some evidence that maintenance antipsychotic medication should not be used for as long a period as for schizophrenic patients.

Finally, one should note that dysphoria is a common symptom in schizophrenia. Drug-induced or post-psychotic depressions are common. These and akinetic effects of antipsychotic drugs may be mistaken for schizoaffective withdrawal and psychomotor retardation.

297.30 Induced Psychotic Disorder

In Induced Psychotic Disorder, or similar disorders with other names (shared paranoid disorder, *folie à deux*), many clinicians recommend separation of the persons involved. The secondary patient, whose delusions began after those of the person with a primary disorder, may particularly respond to such separation. This is especially true if the patient is the child of a psychotic "primary." Hospitalization should be considered in order to provide a supportive environment in which the patient's loss can be resolved and more productive defenses strengthened. Medication may be necessary either for psychosis or for the affective symptoms that may develop.

Confrontation alone, sometimes attempted when the "secondary" patient merely appears to be immature, should be avoided unless a more complete therapeutic context can be offered. Although the patient may not wish vigorous treatment, and may avoid it, the clinician should remember that sooner or later the patient will separate from the "primary," perhaps, for example, through the death of a psychotic parent. Preparation for this event, and support when it occurs, may prevent further decompensation.

298.90 Psychotic Disorder Not Otherwise Specified (Atypical Psychosis)

Atypical psychoses should by and large be treated symptomatically, using the principles outlined for more specific disorders elsewhere in this book. Early treatment should always include careful evaluation for organic, environmental, or other psychosocial causes of the psychosis that might lead one toward or away from certain interventions.

When rapid control of acute agitation is imperative for complete evaluation, in order to implement necessary medical treatment, or to prevent damage to the patient or others, short-acting barbiturates may be useful without masking important symptoms. Low doses of haloperidol or other potent antipsychotics are safe and may be effective. Neither should be given before evaluating the medical status of the patient.

Chapter 17

Mood Disorders

17A BIPOLAR DISORDERS
(Note: See Chapter 14 for more detailed descriptions of inpatient setting and milieu. See p. 219 for discussion of antidepressants.)

296.4x Bipolar Disorder, Manic
296.6x Bipolar Disorder, Mixed, Manic Phase

Emergency Treatment. Acute mania should be considered a medical emergency. It can result in severe physical decompensation or death if not treated properly. Although the *DSM-III-R* allows for mild or moderate manic episodes, the paragraphs below refer to patients who are in a state of marked physical and mental stimulation, who often have not slept for at least 24 hours, and whose exertion may exceed safe limits.

The first goal of treatment is rapid, safe calming of the patient within a medically supervised setting. Sedation with antipsychotic medication,* IM if necessary initially, is one treatment choice. Some clinicians prefer the "rapid neuroleptization schedule" described in Chapter 14. Others prefer more sedative drugs, such as chlorpromazine. In either case, one should expect the patient to require larger amounts than similar patients with other kinds of neuroleptic-responsive psychosis (e.g., schizophreniform psychosis), and should plan to use the neuroleptic for only a short time. Monitoring of medical status, particularly

---
*The reader is referred to **Appendix B** for generic and trade names of medications.

blood pressure, is necessary. Medication side effects such as dystonia, tremor, or anticholinergic effects may appear and should be promptly treated.

The use of short-acting barbiturates is highly recommended for simple sedation of patients with acute psychotic agitation. These have the advantage of controlling the physical dangers without most neuroleptic side effects, and mask fewer symptoms of psychiatric or medical illness. ECT has been recommended for life-threatening mania, unless or until pharmacologic regimens can take effect. The course of ECT should be routine, rather than only two or three treatments to control immediate symptoms.

Post-Emergency Acute Treatment. Most patients present for treatment with moderate mania or hypomania. The clinician should determine whether the patient has previously responded to a particular drug regimen which has been discontinued, and which could be reinstituted with probable success. The patient should be hospitalized during this time, for continuing evaluation, monitoring of response, assuring compliance with treatment, and psychosocial preparation to return to the community.

If the patient is unfamiliar to the clinician or has just received emergency treatment for mania, the pharmacologic aspects of the treatment plan should include starting oral lithium carbonate, with initial control of symptoms using neuroleptic medication. One should expect the lithium to take effect within one to one-and-a-half weeks of reaching an appropriate serum level.

Pre-lithium workup. Healthy patients under 40 years of age can safely be started on lithium after a routine medical history; physical exam; and laboratory determination of normal CBC, electrolytes, kidney function, and thyroid function. Patients over 40 (or those with histories of heart disease) should receive an electrocardiogram. If there is any suspicion of compromised renal function, then creatinine clearance, urine concentrating ability, and urine output should be evaluated. After therapeutic levels have been stable for a few weeks, the blood chemistries should be repeated.

Although many psychiatrists occasionally start lithium treatment on an outpatient basis, inpatient treatment is prudent, particularly for patients whose psychiatric problems make compliance difficult, patients who might take an overdose of the medication, or those requiring close medical monitoring. Most patients discussed in this section will be hospitalized for 10 to 30 days.

Dose. Lithium carbonate should be begun at 600–900 mg per day in divided doses of 300 mg each. The sustained-release preparations (e.g., Eskalith CR, Lithobid) should not be used at this stage of treatment, although they may be more convenient for maintenance. A liquid form, lithium citrate, is also available.

Serum lithium levels should be checked twice a week after beginning treatment, and the dose increased every few days until about 0.7–1.2 mEq per liter is attained. Lithium levels should be obtained in the morning, before the first dose (and at least 10 hours after the last dose).

Although there is some variability in patient response, serum lithium levels below 0.7 mEq/l are unlikely to be helpful in acute stages. Levels above 1.2 mEq/l and up to 1.5 mEq/l may be needed in treatment of acute mania; however, many patients develop toxic signs at this dose. Levels should not be allowed to exceed 1.5 mEq/l. Most patients will reach therapeutic serum levels at 900–1800 mg of lithium carbonate ($LiCO_3$) per day.

One may slowly increase the lithium over one or two weeks to the dose that results in therapeutic levels, but several other ways of predicting the eventual lithium dose have been reported. These generally suggest a loading dose followed by serial lithium levels over 24 hours. Zetin et al. (1986) have developed a "mathematical alternative" to the loading-dose method. At this time, the trial-and-error method seems easy and quite satisfactory in most settings.

Combining lithium with neuroleptic medication is considered safe and clinically appropriate for many manic patients who do not respond to lithium alone. The patient should be monitored closely, however, and significant increases in the dose of either drug should be followed by monitoring of the lithium level (e.g., at three days and 10 days post-increase). If a severe adverse reaction should occur, both drugs should be stopped, medical support promptly initiated, electrolytes closely monitored, and the patient treated as one would treat neuroleptic malignant syndrome (q.v.) until clinical condition dictates otherwise.

Lithium side effects. Mild tremor, mild gastric upset, and increased thirst (accompanied by appropriately increased urinary output) are the most common side effects. They may be seen in patients whose lithium levels are well below the toxic range. The dose may be adjusted to decrease side effects while retaining therapeutic effect. Extrapyramidal symptoms occasionally occur. A few patients complain of memory problems. Weight gain is not unusual, whether from increased appetite (perhaps because of the patient's improved psychiatric condition) or lithium-induced edema. Temporary hypothyroidism is routine and should not be treated unless clinical symptoms occur. Thyroid supplements can usually be discontinued after a few weeks, if they are needed in the first place.

In spite of traditional concerns about combining lithium with thiazide diuretics, cautious addition of a thiazide diuretic to control benign polyuria can allow some patients who truly need lithium treatment to continue it safely. When this is done, *the lithium dose should be decreased by 50%, and the lithium level restabilized.* The clinician must remember that lithium is a salt whose concentration and bioavailability is closely linked to that of sodium (and to some extent potassium) (see Patient Instructions, p. 208).

Other side effects, mostly rare, include benign skin rashes (which may disappear if the brand is changed), exacerbation of psoriasis, altered glucose tolerance test (Shah et al., 1986), Graves' disease (or the masking of Graves' disease) (Thompson & Baylis, 1986), self-limited alopecia (Ghadirian & Lalinec-Michaud, 1986), and a variety of benign renal effects (see below) (Vaamonde et al., 1986).

Serious adverse effects of lithium are almost always related to toxicity. Although the toxic level for this drug is quite close to the therapeutic level, serum levels tend to be stable, with the following exceptions:

1. Acute electrolyte imbalance, usually caused by significant vomiting, diarrhea, or other fluid loss, rapidly increasing the serum lithium level.
2. Ingestion of medications, almost always physician-prescribed, which alter electrolyte balance. Diuretics are the most obvious offenders; however, ibuprofen (Ragheb, 1987) and other drugs increase lithium levels to a variable extent in many patients.
3. Anything that decreases glomerular filtration rates and lithium clearance through the kidney, increasing serum lithium levels. Some examples are found in elderly patients (Greil et al., 1985; Vestergaard & Schou, 1984) and pregnant patients (Kaufman & Okeya, 1985)
4. Dietary salt restriction. Patients should be cautioned to include normal amounts of salt in their daily diets. Although no added

salt is necessary, patients beginning low-or no-salt diets (or unusual or "fad" diets) should have their lithium levels restabilized.

Early reports of *renal* damage from chronic lithium prescription have been replaced by many studies that indicate little or no danger of irreversible renal impairment (e.g., glomerular damage) (DePaulo, Correau, & Sapir, 1986; Vaamonde et al., 1986). Because of effects on *thyroid* function, a few studies have been done that indicate possible fluctuations in thyroid immune status on chronic lithium carbonate therapy (Lazarus et al., 1986). There is a small but measurable rate of development of persistent *tardive dyskinesia* in bipolar patients. Most such cases involve patients who have taken neuroleptics at some point (Mukherjee et al., 1986; Perenyi, Szuchs, & Frecska, 1984). This danger is not felt to be significant enough to warrant specific warnings to patients receiving lithium alone.

Lithium therapy should be continued only with caution in *pregnant patients*, particularly in the first trimester. The risk:benefit ratio may be acceptable for many patients, since symptomatic bipolar illness can be dangerous to both the woman and the fetus. The many physiological changes of pregnancy make close monitoring and restabilization of the lithium level necessary. Lithium should be discontinued well before delivery (Jefferson, Greist, & Ackerman, 1983). Breast-feeding should be discouraged, since lithium easily passes into breast milk.

Treatment of lithium toxicity and overdose. Ordinary toxicity is treated very simply, by withholding one or more doses of the drug. In the absence of renal complications, it is rapidly cleared. Serious toxicity, such as that associated with overdose (which may produce acute renal failure) can be treated with hemodialysis, over several days if necessary (Fenves, Emmettt, & White, 1984; Jaeger et al., 1985).

Patient instructions. Patients should be carefully told, orally and in writing, about the special characteristics of lithium carbonate, especially compared to other commonly prescribed psychotropic drugs. Patients are often accustomed to medications whose blood levels are not closely monitored, and whose therapeutic-to-toxic-level ratio is fairly low. There are a number of patient information sheets commercially available, including one from the American Medical Association.

The patient should be cautioned not to alter the dose, to maintain a normal dietary salt intake, to report for scheduled lithium level monitoring, to communicate to other physicians that he or she is taking lithium (and tell the psychiatrist if other drugs are prescribed), and to call the psychiatrist if serious vomiting, diarrhea, or other fluid loss occurs. The patient should be instructed to skip a lithium dose if toxic signs arise or fluid or electrolyte loss occurs, especially if he or she is unable to contact the doctor or clinic.

Patients with Manic or Mixed Bipolar Disorder are often concerned about how their treatment will affect the feelings of well-being, creativity, or social and professional success that have often been present for many years before their first "break." It is useful to tell them that, unlike some of the medications used for serious psychiatric illness, lithium is not an emotional "downer," nor is it known to affect normal energy or creativity. The lay impression of lithium as a "mood stabilizer" is a useful one, implying that the patient remains free to experience the normal emotions of life, but is protected from destructive or bizarre swings of mood.

Acute hospital settings. Although the patient may not appear amenable to logic or verbal approaches, a structured setting is important. The staff should be familiar with treatment methods for agitated or highly active patients, as well as with signs of lithium toxicity.

As the acute symptoms subside, discharge plans should be formulated which stress the biological, psychological, and social needs of the patient. Education of the patient and significant others about the special characteristics of bipolar illness (in addition to the characteristics of lithium carbonate, mentioned above) is important, since relapse of hypomania or mania is not usually associated with dysphoric warning signs.

Maintenance Treatment. Careful discharge planning and attention to the transition from inpatient to outpatient care are the keys to lasting psychiatric and social post-hospital success. Care should be taken to help the patient with his or her first contact with the outpatient environment: for example, providing for visits from the therapist (or visits to the outpatient clinic) while the patient is still in the hospital. At the least, the name and location of the follow-up therapist, a scheduled appointment, and a written description of medications and dosages should be in the patient's hands before he or she leaves the hospital.

Most bipolar patients do not require chronic medication other than lithium to remain in remission. Neuroleptics can usually be discontinued before the patient leaves the hospital, or soon thereafter. It is poor practice to discontinue the neuroleptic just as the patient is discharged (or, for that matter, to make any major changes in the medication regimen during this transition period). Even if it is pharmacologically unnecessary, one should wait until the outpatient situation is stabilized before proceeding to discontinue the neuroleptic.

The lithium itself is crucial to preventing relapse. It should not be discontinued without careful supervision. Most patients require treatment for an indefinite period.

Patients on maintenance lithium may be able to remain in remission at serum levels below those required for acute treatment. Most clinicians prefer serum levels above about 0.6 mEq/l (Maj et al., 1986). There are patients who can remain in remission at levels as low as 0.4 mEq/l; however, it seems imprudent to allow this in the absence of unusual dose-related side effects.

Prognosis and Outcome. The prognosis for lithium-responding manic or mixed bipolar patients is generally good, provided they remain in treatment and lithium levels can be reasonably monitored (at least every three months once the patient is completely stable). A large collaborative study (Prien et al., 1984) showed no advantage of drug combinations over lithium carbonate alone in maintenance treatment.

Relapse rate is correlated with a number of clinical factors. Goodnick and colleagues (1987) found response to lithium prophylaxis largely determined by frequency of manic or depressive episodes and duration of lithium treatment. Others find few predictors of outcome based upon clinical factors alone (Mander, 1986). Keller and colleagues (1986) found that bipolar manic patients were considerably more likely to remain free of illness after treatment than either mixed or purely depressed patients. Finally, a Danish population study followed bipolar and unipolar "manic depressive" patients and compared them with the general population, finding that all patients with the "manic depressive" illness had increased mortality by suicide and accidents, and that the bipolar group had a higher mortality from nonviolent causes than the unipolar group (Weeke & Vaeth, 1986).

Alternative Biological Therapies. Refractory manic psychosis or rapid cycling of manic–depressive psychosis can often be successfully treated with *ECT* (Berman & Wolpert, 1987). (Guidelines are summarized on pp. 234–237)

Folic acid supplements, up to 200 mcg per day, may add to the ability of lithium to prevent return of affective illness. In one study, patients for whom this supplement actually increased plasma folate to 13 ng/ml or above had significant reduction in affective morbidity. Some authors suggest a daily supplement of 300–400 mcg (Coppen, Chaudhry, & Swade, 1986).

The use of *depot neuroleptics* in patients with poor lithium prophylaxis or psychotic symptoms between manic episodes has been recommended by several authors (Lowe & Batchelor, 1986). Both fluphenazine decanoate and haloperidol decanoate have been used. The doses are usually about the same as, or lower than, doses required for control of schizophrenia. Maintenance should be at the lowest effective dose, since affective illness has been associated with increased risk of tardive dyskinesia in patients taking neuroleptics.

Adding *carbamazepine* to the lithium regimen has often been found superior to lithium alone or combinations of lithium and neuroleptics, particularly in maintenance treatment (Shukla, Cook, & Miller, 1985). Carbamazepine alone also has an antimanic effect and some ability to prevent recurrent depression (Lerer et al., 1987; Stromgren & Boller, 1985). The clinician should be familiar with the prescription information and cautions regarding blood count before proceeding.

The calcium channel blocker *verapamil* has also been studied and found to have some antimanic activity. When available, it may be useful for patients unable to take lithium (Dubovsky et al., 1986; Solomon & Williamson, 1986). When verapamil is given with lithium, there is apparently increased danger of neurotoxicity (Price & Giannini, 1986). *Sodium valproate* has both an acute antimanic effect and prophylactic action, as does *oxcarbazepine*, a relative of carbamazepine (Emrich, Dose, & von Zerssen, 1985). Of all these alternatives to lithium, carbamazepine is felt to be the most reliable (Lerer, 1985).

Finally, acute treatment of manic agitation with *lorazepam* (Lenox, Modell, & Weiner, 1986) and other benzodiazepines may have not only a sedative, but also an antipsychotic effect. These medications are generally quite safe, rarely mask other symptoms, and act rapidly; however, they should not be considered for definitive treatment or prophylaxis of mania.

Psychosocial Treatments in Manic and Mixed Bipolar Disorder. Even in highly medical settings, combined psychopharmacologic and psychodynamic therapies are more useful in the long run than biological therapies alone. The "biopsychosocial" approach is too often overlooked by psychiatrists, particularly in academic or busy clinical settings. Personality characteristics of recovered patients, for example, differ substantially from the general population, particularly in measures of emotional growth (Hirschfeld et al., 1986). Social support has been strongly correlated with good clinical outcome (O'Connell et al., 1985).

296.5x Bipolar Disorder, Depressed.

The treatment of acute and subacute recurrent depressive episodes, whether part of Bipolar Disorder, Depressed or Bipolar Disorder, Mixed, is essentially similar to that of Major Depression (which is often recurrent as well). This is addressed beginning on page 214.

Lithium carbonate is not the initial treatment choice for acute depression, even when related to bipolar disorder. Similarly, antipsychotic agents are not usually helpful except for the treatment of specific psychotic symptoms.

Induction of a manic or hypomanic episode is a concern when treating any patient with bipolar disorder and depressed symptoms. Treatment of such episodes, which can occur with virtually any of the antidepressant medications or ECT, is generally the same as that for any other acute manic episode. For patients known to be vulnerable to rapid mood swings, the addition of lithium carbonate to acute antidepressant treatment may be preventive (Lewis & Winokur, 1982).

Once the depression has been successfully treated, its return may be prevented—or made less likely—in a number of ways. Lithium carbonate at doses consistent with therapeutic serum lithium levels will prevent recurrence of depression in most bipolar patients. This is true whether the acute treatment was pharmacologic or with ECT (Coppen et al., 1981). Lithium workup, instigation of treatment, and continued monitoring are all described previously under Bipolar Disorder, Manic. Patients with bipolar depressed illness may be more motivated for treatment because of the marked dysphoria they experience. On the other hand, their depression may produce apathy and withdrawal from treatment.

As with any depression, *suicide* remains a serious risk during acute phases of the illness, *as well as early in recovery*, when increased activity and cognitive ability may increase the likelihood of the patient's being able to act on self-destructive impulses.

Maintenance Treatment. Principles of clinical maintenance are taken from those already discussed for the manic and mixed bipolar patient, and for Major Depression (see p. 215). Conditions of follow-up are similar. Prognosis for bipolar mixed patients is probably slightly worse than that of either the bipolar manic or bipolar depressed patient.

For bipolar mixed patients, the addition of tricyclic antidepressants to the lithium regimen generally provides no advantage over lithium alone (although it may with unipolar patients) (Prien et al., 1984). Preliminary work with monoamine oxidase inhibitors indicates that they may augment the stabilizing effects of lithium. The addition of augmenting medications to antidepressants (e.g., L-triiodothyronine) increases the possibility of induction of mania, probably because of the antidepressant effect and not any particular pharmacologic property of the adjunctive drug (Evans et al., 1986).

296.6x Bipolar Disorder, Mixed
(See earlier sections of this chapter.)

Acute treatment should be consistent with the patient's presentation, either manic or severely depressed. Occasionally, patients will refer themselves when between mood swings, this being the period of better judgment and some ability to reflect upon the damage done by their symptoms. In such cases, lithium carbonate should be begun at once. When patients are quite stable, lithium treatment may be begun outside the hospital, although the author prefers an inpatient evaluation, pre-lithium workup, stabilization of the medication, and education of the patient and others.

301.13 Cyclothymia
If the relatively mild mood swings of chronic Cyclothymia are considered a phenotypic variant or attenuated form of Bipolar Disorder, then lithium is a logical treatment. The same considerations of pre-lithium workup, patient instructions, attaining therapeutic levels, and monitoring during maintenance already discussed should be observed. The patient may be more able to participate in his or her own care, because the mood swings do not, by definition, lead to deep depressions or the extremely poor judgment of hypomania or mania. Lithium should not be given as a first choice for the depressive phase of cyclothymia, but rather for the times of increased emotional activity or to prevent mood swings once the patient is stabilized. Unfortunately, controlled research with lithium in specifically diagnosed cases of Cyclothymia is either lacking or difficult to evaluate.

In depressed phases, one may try tricyclics (and watch for induction of mania or hypomania); however, they are usually ineffective. Small doses of MAOI or carbamazepine have been successful for some patients with this diagnosis.

A number of authors consider cyclothymic patients to be suffering more from character pathology, suggesting borderline, narcissistic, or histrionic traits, than from a primary affective disorder. Patients with character pathology may present mood swings as well. On the other hand, some patients with rapid changes in mood and behavior, without obvious "illness," may appear merely eccentric.

If the mood swings appear to be reactive (i.e., responsive to changes in a patient's physical or emotional environment), psychotherapy or environmental manipulation may be helpful. Antianxiety medications, including alprazolam, may make the patient feel better at times, but are not to be considered long-term treatments of choice.

296.70 Bipolar Disorder Not Otherwise Specified
Once organic etiology and/or influence has been ruled out, it is prudent to treat bipolar disorders for which specific diagnoses cannot be made in much the same ways as described above. A conservative approach is recommended, with psychotherapy or environmental manipulation, or the use of only one medication (especially lithium) suggested until the need for more vigorous medical intervention has been established. Assuming a patient who is able to participate responsibly in his or her own care, and/or one who can be treated in a supervised setting, a trial of lithium is generally indicated since it may have a dramatic positive effect, the incidence of serious side effects or adverse effects is quite low, and the patient's response can usually be seen within several weeks.

17b DEPRESSIVE DISORDERS
Although depressions not related to medical illness or specific loss are often considered to exist on a common "continuum," this text will treat Major Depression separately from Dysthymia.

296.2x   Major Depression, Single Episode
296.3x   Major Depression, Recurrent

Diagnostic Concepts Critical to Treatment Choice. Although not as physically disabling as acute mania, the pain and clouded judgment of acute Major Depression make rapid treatment imperative. Initial goals must include evaluation and management of suicide potential. Hospitalization, even against the patient's will, may be life-saving. Even if the patient has not volunteered information about a history of suicidal ideation or attempt, hospitalization may be imperative if suicide predictors are present.

Evaluation of suicide potential should be done by the most qualified mental health professional present. Concepts such as "suicidal gesture," "self-destructive acting out," suicidal talk or action to "get attention," or a "cry for help" are clever catch words; however, *they must not diminish one's caution.* Even if the chance of death or serious injury is low, the stakes are very high. Persons with suicidal behavior—even "gestures"—have high probabilities of eventually dying by their own hands.

Once the psychiatrist has made a judgment of suicidal danger, he or she must not shrink from the actions that necessarily follow. Protecting the patient through hospitalization, close personal monitoring, and emergency treatment must be attempted, even over the objections of the patient or family. At this point, lethally suicidal patients may appear "normal," may "promise" not to harm themselves, may plead that hospitalization will ruin their jobs and reputations and thus make them more depressed, and so forth. It is difficult, if not impossible, to tell whether the patient is being truthful, or whether he has made a decision to die. It should particularly be pointed out that the patient's family or friends, while helpful in evaluating him or her, are not qualified to make the clinical decisions involved.

Precautions against suicide do not always mean admission to a locked unit, but rather to a unit staffed by persons familiar with the protection and treatment of acutely depressed patients. The goal is early alleviation of the tremendous psychic pain found in severe depression.

Although antipsychotic medication may be helpful for some aspects of depressive psychosis, treatment with antidepressants should begin as soon as possible. When rapid lifting of the depression is necessary to prevent suicide or alleviate severe discomfort, electroconvulsive therapy (ECT) may be a treatment of choice; most antidepressants take several weeks to attain maximum effect (although some symptoms, such as sleeplessness, may respond earlier). Alprazolam has rapid antianxiety effects which may alleviate some symptoms and sleeplessness; however, its ability to relieve deep depressions is questionable. There are many other considerations involved in selecting an antidepressant; these are described in the section on Antidepressant Medications (p. 219).

Since all known treatments for major depression require at least days, and often weeks, before the depression has significantly lifted, attention to nonbiological components of treatment is vital. Clinical reassurance and understanding from the physician are important to both the patient and his family. The psychiatrist should be able to communicate to everyone that the situation is far from being as hopeless as the patient feels it is. He or she can share the clinical optimism that although depression is among the most painful of illnesses, it is also one of psychiatry's "success stories," with well over 75% of patients who comply with therapy finding considerable relief. The patient, in the cognitive deficit and hopelessness of depression, may not be able to respond fully; however, it is not uncommon to hear several weeks later that this conversation with the doctor was reassuring.

As mentioned above, the clinician should take a firm, unambivalent position with respect to treatment recommendations for severe depression, rather than waiting for the patient, whose judgment is significantly clouded by the depression, to ruminate upon the best course of action. Within the hospital, initial contacts should reflect support and structure, discouraging withdrawal and encouraging adherence to an active milieu program and treatment regimen. During this acute phase, psychodynamic psychotherapy or any of the several cognitive or behavioral approaches (which may be quite useful later in treatment) are by themselves insufficient.

Treatment Choice. The treatments for single episodes of Major Depression (296.2x) and exacerbations of recurrent Major Depression (296.3x) are essentially identical. Treatment of recurrent episodes is in some ways easier, since the patient may already have shown an ability to respond to a particular treatment regimen, and/or may have revealed particular sensitivities to side effects or adverse effects of others. We now know that there are a number of common courses of serious depression. Clinical presentations of acute episodes are similar; considerations for maintenance treatment, prognosis, and outcome are covered in the next section (p. 217).

Although biological treatment, particularly tricyclic antidepressants or ECT, is an important part of first-line intervention, the psychosocial aspects of care must not be omitted or underestimated. Many of the aspects of hospitalization discussed earlier in this text have applications for the severely depressed patient, whether psychotic or not. The hospital milieu should be structured and supportive, and should discourage withdrawal, apathy, or other kinds of regression.

An atmosphere of "firm kindness" presses the patient toward physical and emotional activity while providing needed support. Staff should be experienced in the treatment of depressed patients, and should be aware that the frustrating passivity, dependency, and "manipulation" that one often sees in such patients is related to the depressive illness—and is thus temporary—and not usually related to a dependent, antisocial, or "borderline" character style.

Hospitalization should be considered a form of respite for the patient, although not merely a "rest." Many stresses and burdens of life outside the hospital, whether real or imagined, can be lifted from the patient's shoulders upon admission, with the understanding and expectation that within a few weeks he will be ready to accept them in a more realistic, hopeful light and return to his family and the community. The patient should feel that he is entering the hospital to perform needed emotional work and get some deserved help. Hospitalization should not add to burdens or unrealistic guilts about job or family problems. Support and "permission" from family and employers for the patient's taking time and spending money for inpatient treatment can be a strong factor in treatment compliance and eventual success.

Biological Treatments for Affective Disorders

Biological Predictors of Treatment Response. The dexamethasone suppression test (DMST), the TRH stimulation test, and measurements of urinary 3-methoxy, 4-hydroxyphenylglycol (MHPG) have all been used to predict therapeutic response to antidepressants and ECT. Polysomnograms to determine sleep latency, total sleep time, REM latency, REM time, and other sleep characteristics have also been explored (Dietzel et al., 1986) to distinguish patients with "major depression" or bipolar disorders, and their likelihood of response to biological intervention. Most authors agree that none of these provides a very accurate individual predictor—at least not sufficiently accurate to overrule clinical judgment—although both the DMST and the TRH stimulation test may support or refute clinical decisions in complex cases.

DMST. The procedure for the DMST involves measurement of baseline plasma cortisol, administration of 1.0 mg of oral dexamethasone late at night (11:00 p.m.–midnight), then measurement of hypothalamic–pituitary–adrenal reaction via plasma cortisol the next day. Plasma cortisols should be obtained several times following dexamethasone administration, with three (8:00 a.m., noon, 4:00 p.m.) considered a minimum and four (8:00 a.m., noon, 4:00 p.m., and 11:00 p.m.–midnight) optimal for establishing presence or absence of nonsuppression.

Most studies accept levels of 5 mcg/100 ml or below *at every sampling point for 24 hours after dexamethasone ingestion* as evidence of suppression (normal response of the hypothalamic–pituitary–adrenal axis). Any post-dexamethasone cortisol level above 5 mcg/100 ml implies nonsuppression.

A more cautious version of the test compares several baseline levels with post-dexamethasone levels (necessitating six or eight venipunctures). This usually does not yield enough additional information to justify the additional patient discomfort and expense.

The extent to which the DMST predicts response to biological treatments has been debated. It is clear that a positive test is highly correlated with response to either antidepressant medication or ECT; however, a number of endocrine conditions and medications can cause nonsuppression. At least one DMST study has indicated no relationship between nonsuppression and response to antidepressant medication (Ames et al., 1984). False–negative results are common enough that patients with serious depressive symptoms should not be deprived of biological treatments—at least ordinary tricyclic medications—on the basis of DMST results alone.

The use of a DMST to select specific drugs, once a decision has been made to use antidepressant medication, has been attempted (e.g., Rihmer et al., 1985); however, it is not generally accepted clinical practice.

TRH stimulation test. The procedure for the thyrotropin-releasing-hormone (TRH) stimulation test involves placing an indwelling venous catheter in a resting patient who has fasted overnight, taking a blood sample for baseline thyroid stimulating hormone (TSH), administering 500 mcg of synthetic TRH, and then sampling for RIA TSH determination at 15, 30, 60, and 90 minutes after TRH administration (Pottash, Gold, & Extein, 1986).

The *maximum* difference found between *any* of the four post-baseline samples and the baseline TSH level is the "delta TSH." TSH levels are normally increased by more than 7.0 micro-International-Units (micro-IU) after the TRH infusion. Major affective disorder and unipolar patients often—but not uniformly—show a delta TSH of 7.0 or less, implying decreased or "blunted" TRH stimulation of TSH production. Dysthymic and schizophrenic patients routinely have normal responses (delta TSH above 7.0 micro-IU). Responses in schizoaffective and bipolar (manic or depressed) patients are mixed, and thus less reliable for differentiating diagnoses.

Delta TSH is an unreliable indicator in a number of medical conditions, especially thyroid disease and alcoholism, in older males and in patients taking steroids or carbamazepine. Most antidepressant, antianxiety, and antipsychotic medications do not affect the test.

Monitoring of clinical response and estimation of the point at which maximum antidepressant response has been obtained are another use of the DMST, TRH stimulation test, and other biochemical markers. Normalization of a nonsuppressing DMST, for example, after outward signs that a depression has lifted, is evidence that a particular depressive episode is well controlled. It is not considered evidence that the episode has run its course and/or that medication can be discontinued. Increases in plasma prolactin levels, although not at this point clinically useful, are also associated with symptomatic recovery (Lisansky et al., 1984).

Antidepressant Medications

Prescribing Techniques. (See also the Side Effects and Adverse Effects section that follows.)

A note about using side-effects profiles. Side effects are an important consideration in choosing a medication. In some cases, it may appear that convenient side-effects profiles are used as excuses, even *apologia*, for using second-choice drugs. Although every effort should be made to help the patient tolerate a few side effects in the service of future improvement, there is sometimes reason to choose drugs with less clinical efficacy. No medication is effective if it is not ingested in the first place.

Tricyclic Antidepressants (TCAs). Given a physically healthy patient, not in extreme danger of suicide, treatment should be begun with a tricyclic antidepressant. If there is a history of good response to a specific antidepressant, either in the patient or a family member, then that agent should be tried first. Without such a predictive history, the clinician may choose a primarily noradrenergic tricyclic (e.g., desipramine), a primarily serotonergic one (e.g., amitriptyline), or one with elements of both (e.g., imipramine). Neurochemical methods of predicting which may be best for a given patient have been explored, but have not been found useful for most clinical settings.

The tricyclics are the most commonly used antidepressant medication in the psychiatric formulary. They are also among the most commonly misused, particularly by nonpsychiatric physicians. The touchstones for prescribing them, particularly as the first-choice treatments for many major affective disorders, are similar to the basic principles of neuroleptic therapy:

1. Choose a drug with which you are clinically familiar.
2. If possible, choose a drug to which the patient or a close member of his or her family has responded well in the past.
3. Give *enough* of the drug for an appropriate duration.
4. Caution patient and family about the potential lethality of overdose, and evaluate the patient for suicide potential before allowing him or her to control the medication.
5. If good clinical response does not occur in three to four weeks, consider obtaining a TCA blood level.

If the patient is able and willing to tolerate the significant anticholinergic effects that will occur, most tricyclics should be begun in doses of about half the expected maintenance dose and increased over three to seven days. Older patients or those for whom anticholinergic effects are likely to be a problem should be given less, perhaps as little as 25 mg per day to start. Except for patients whose hepatic metabolic pathways are compromised, it is unusual to reach therapeutic blood levels and obtain clinical response (with the exception of placebo response or response of syndromes not directly related to major affective disorder) in less than two to three weeks.

Maintenance doses of roughly 100-250 mg per day should be expected for most of the tricyclics, including imipramine, desipramine, amitriptyline, trimipramine, and doxepin. Nortriptyline should be used in slightly lower doses, with a maximum of around 150 mg per day. Protriptyline is significantly more potent, with effective response likely in the dosage range of 50-60 mg per day.

It is commonly accepted that once the blood level has stabilized, any of the tricyclics may be given in a once-daily dose. "Sustained release" preparations such as Tofranil PM are unnecessary. Some patients do not respond well to single daily doses, however, and many patients experience fewer side effects with divided daily doses. It is often helpful to let the patient dictate the daily schedule, so long as the required amount is ingested.

Many of the common tricyclic antidepressants have generic equivalents available in the U.S. market. Although this may represent considerable cost savings to the patient, and some payers (such as the Veterans Administration) will not honor brand-name prescriptions, this author has seen a number of patients who appeared to have higher, or more consistent, blood levels when taking brand-name tricyclics.

Therapeutic windows have been hypothesized for several of the TCAs. It is clear that nortriptyline, at least, is ineffective when the plasma level (see *therapeutic plasma levels* below) is either above or below the therapeutic range (50–150 ng/ml). Thus, if the patient is taking a significant amount of TCA—perhaps close to the maximum daily dosage—for several weeks without response, it is prudent either to measure the blood level (particularly of imipramine or desipramine, for which the most drug level experience is established) or to lower the dose and observe the clinical response over the next two weeks.

Speed of response to tricyclic and tetracyclic antidepressants (see below) may be predicted by pretreatment measurement of urinary MHPG; however, the meaning of research in this area is still unclear, and such measurements are unavailable to many patients or clinicians. Other methods of predicting the eventually effective dose, including "loading dose" methods, have been less than successful.

Duration of antidepressant therapy is difficult to predict for individual patients. There is considerable indication that almost all major affective disorders (but probably not simple dysthymia) are cyclic in nature. There is some support for the notion that the clinician can calculate when the next depressive episode is likely to occur and, if it is several months or years away, stop the medication for a while. In individual patients, however, return of symptoms is difficult to predict.

Some studies suggest maintenance for up to one or two years (Prien et al., 1984). On the other hand, it is fairly easy to taper the antidepressant slowly once or twice a year while monitoring for relapse. Since depression is a painful illness, with obvious symptoms for most patients, the patient, the family, or the clinician can usually recognize early signs and reinstate drug treatment with the expectation of rapid remission.

Patients often ask about addictive or abuse potential of antidepressant medications. Even if the patient does not inquire, it is good practice to anticipate such concerns, reassure the patient that these medications are not "uppers" or addictive, and at the same time tell the patient and family not to anticipate rapid or striking relief. This last communication is particularly important, since many patients are accustomed to alleviating physical discomfort within hours or days, and may become frustrated, even hopeless, as they wait weeks for relief of depression.

Therapeutic plasma levels of TCAs vary considerably. Adequate levels must be attained for assessment of response, although direct correlation of response with plasma level is poor for individual patients. The most reliable laboratory measurements are those for imipramine or desipramine, commonly said to have a therapeutic range of 150–300 ng/ml. This value is the *total concentration of active drug* (imipramine-plus-desmethylimipramine for imipramine; amitriptyline-plus-nortriptyline for amitriptyline, etc.). The psychiatrist should be aware of the clinical norms for his or her laboratory, and should consider occasionally sending samples to two labs, or sending split samples to the same lab, to test reliability. Although validity and reliability of drug level testing has improved considerably in recent years, the methodology is not yet perfected, despite claims by some laboratories.

Plasma levels of imipramine plus desipramine (or desipramine alone) above about 300 ng/ml are usually superfluous. There is no indication of additional clinical effectiveness and there is considerable opportunity for increased side effects or toxic effects. Thus, a basic principle for all tricyclic antidepressants is: in the face of apparent poor response after sufficient time at a clinically appropriate dose, it is often as wise to decrease the dose as it is to increase it. Toxic effects, including anticholinergic delirium, are often mistaken for nonresponse.

Tricyclic levels for the most commonly prescribed drugs are generally available from regional laboratories within a few days. Although not directly correlated with response, they do provide information about whether one is well below or well above an acceptable range. Plasma ranges for different drugs are different and are better established for some than for others.

Nortriptyline is the only antidepressant for which a highly specific target (50–150ng/ml) can reliably be sought at this time. Minimum therapeutic plasma level ranges have been suggested for *imipramine, desipramine, amitriptyline, and doxepin*, however (100–150 ng/ml). *Protriptyline* may be effective as lower levels, 75–100 ng/ml, but probably is also effective up to 250–300 ng/ml. Therapeutic ranges for nontricyclic antidepressants are either unknown or unclear for use in routine clinical settings.

Blood levels of tricyclics should be determined from samples drawn at least eight hours after the patient's last dose of medication, and should not be considered valid until the drug has been given at the same dose for about five to seven days. It is very important to note the wide range of individual blood levels that may be obtained in patients given identical oral doses of TCAs. Patients taking the same oral dose commonly differ in plasma level (and, by extrapolation, bioavailability) by 500%. Even broader differences are found among children, the elderly, and patients with liver, gastrointestinal, or plasma-binding abnormalities.

Changing medications. Patients who do not show a significant response to TCAs or tetracyclics at appropriate doses may be treated in several ways. Many depressions respond to a change of medication, even within the same general drug family (e.g., TCAs). Beneficial changes are often those which shift from a noradrenergic drug (desipramine, protriptyline, maprotiline) to a serotonergic one (e.g., amitriptyline). Drug changes within the TCA group may be made rapidly; however, changes between groups—especially the tricyclics and MAO inhibitors (see below)—should be carried out according to the protocols described later in this section.

Discontinuing TCAs. The tricyclics should be tapered over several weeks, if therapeutic blood levels have been reached. Most withdrawal symptoms appear to be related to rebound phenomena after discontinuing the anticholinergic drugs. Blackwell recommends substituting other anticholinergic drugs, such as atropine, if rapid cessation of TCA's is medically required (Blackwell, 1987).

Monoamine Oxidase Inhibitors (MAOIs). Although once a mainstay of antidepressant therapy, these drugs are now used primarily for refractory or atypical depressions. There has been a resurgence in their use in recent years, but they are still underutilized, particularly by psychiatrists trained within the past two decades. Their efficacy compared to TCAs has recently been reestablished, and is not limited to "atypical" depressions (White et al., 1984; Zisook, Braff, & Click, 1985). A review by Pare (1985) concluded that MAOI dosages are often too low and that psychiatrists may sometimes be unreasonably deterred from using them.

For the hydrazine group of MAOI, doses of up to 30 mg per day of isocarboxazid or up to 90 mg per day of phenelzine are commonly required. Tranylcypromine, the only nonhydrazine available in the U.S., is given orally at up to 50 mg per day. Dosage should begin at about half the maximum dose and should be increased slowly (over several weeks for phenelzine, one to two weeks for isocarboxazid or tranylcypromine).

The well-known dietary restrictions of MAOIs have probably contributed to their lessened popularity, since most other antidepressants are often prescribed without much medical attention. In fact, no antidepressant should be prescribed lightly; all require medical monitoring and follow-up. The dietary restrictions of MAOIs have probably led to more clinician worry than actual patient difficulty.

Nevertheless, in order to prevent a hypertensive crisis precipitated by histamine response, foods containing a great deal of tyramine should be avoided. The most important offenders, which should be eliminated from the diet, are aged cheeses, most red wines, beer, many kinds of sausage, fava beans, liver, smoked or pickled fish, and brewer's yeast. Other sources of alcohol, some overripe fruits such as banana or avocado, and some soured dairy products such as yogurt or sour cream should be avoided in large amounts. Caffeine, monosodium glutamate, and chocolate were formerly on the list of foods to avoid; however, they do not appear to cause many problems (McCabe & Tsuang, 1982).

Tranylcypromine is the most stimulating of the MAOIs and is considerably more so than any of the tricyclic antidepressants. Any of the MAOIs may cause insomnia, which should not be confused with depressive symptomatology.

Changing from one MAOI to another should be done by tapering the first, then adding the second after a week or two, unlike the TCA-to-TCA regimen. When changing from an MAOI to a TCA, two weeks off the former is recommended. Tapering is recommended when discontinuing MAOIs.

Combining tricyclic antidepressants with MAOIs has not been shown to increase antidepressant benefits to patients who already respond to one or the other; however, patients who do not respond to either class of drugs and/or for some reason either do not respond or cannot tolerate other forms of antidepressant therapy may benefit. The cautious addition of isocarboxazid or phenelzine to a TCA such as amytriptyline is now an established clinical regimen for certain nonresponders. The most conservative approach is to discontinue all antidepressants and then restart the MAOI and TCA at the same time.

One *should not* prescribe a TCA for patients already taking MAOIs. The tricyclic most likely to precipitate a serious hypertensive episode when given with MAOIs is probably clomipramine, which is not available in the U.S. Tranylcypromine may produce more problems than the other MAOIs in combination with TCAs.

Tetracyclics. The so-called "tetracyclic" antidepressants——amoxapine and maprotiline in the U.S.—were developed in an effort to find faster-acting antidepressant drugs, with fewer cardiac and anticholinergic side effects. Maprotiline has significant anticholinergic activity in some patients, but both the above drugs have fewer effects on cardiac conduction than the TCAs. Neither drug shows more antidepressant effect than the standard TCAs.

Amoxapine is marketed largely on the basis of its rapid action, frequently showing true antidepressant effects (as opposed to simply sedative effects) within the first week (McNair et al., 1984a). Evidence of dopaminergic activity can be seen in positron emission tomography (PET) data after only one or two days. The initial enthusiasm for amoxapine seen in the literature and clinical settings a few years ago has waned somewhat, largely because of common extrapyramidal side effects (EPS) and reports of seizures (apparently dose-related) (McNair et al., 1984b).

Maprotiline has not been shown to be as effective as amoxapine. It imparts a similar likelihood of EPS and lowered seizure threshold. Its relative lack of anticholinergic effects may make it useful for some elderly or medically ill patients.

Other Antidepressants. Most of the following should not be considered antidepressants of first choice for healthy patients, although they may be indicated for some patient groups, such as the elderly (Gerner, 1985). On the other hand, although the addition of new drugs, with more acceptable side-effects profiles is often hailed by pharmaceutical manufacturers as particularly relevant to treatment of the elderly and medically ill, most clinical studies indicate that the traditional tricyclics, particularly the secondary amines such as desipramine or nortriptyline, can be used safely for many such patients (Lazarus, Davis, & Dysken, 1985; Mahapatra et al., 1986). The psychiatrist should not disregard the pain, disability, and even lethality of severe depression when weighing the risks and benefits of various treatments.

Trazodone is useful in some medically compromised patients or those sensitive to anticholinergic side effects. It has no true anticholinergic activity, and little potential for cardiac conduction problems or orthostatic hypotension. (See later section for additional side effects and adverse effects.)

It is prescribed orally, up to about 450 mg per day. Although it is safe in higher doses, it is rather sedative. The patient should be started at lower levels, perhaps 100 mg per day, with the dose increasing over about two weeks. As with the TCAs, if response at high doses (300–600 mg per day) is insufficient, one should consider decreasing the dose and monitoring the patient. Unfortunately, blood levels are not yet either valid or reliable for the practicing clinician, and may not be well correlated with response.

Nomifensine maleate. Nomifensine is a second- or third-choice antidepressant, not currently available in the U.S., which may be useful for patients who do not respond to or are not appropriate for TCAs or electroconvulsive therapy. Its antidepressant action is significant, but monitoring for liver function, hemolytic anemia, hyperpyrexia, and allergic reactions is necessary. It is one of the few antidepressants which has a very high LD_{50}, making it a reasonable choice for some suicidal patients. The initial dose is 50 mg b.i.d., increasing to 200–300 mg/day. Kinney (1985) has recently reviewed this drug.

Mianserin. Mianserin has recently been successfully compared to nomifensine, flupenthixol, clomipramine, and indalpine (Dunbar, Naarala, & Hiltumen, 1985; Granier et al., 1985; Majid, 1986; Naylor & Martin, 1985). It is interesting that mianserin was felt to be superior to clomipramine, largely because of the side-effects profile, for patients with "mild depression." Mianserin may also have some anxiolytic activity.

Buproprion. Buproprion is well tolerated within its broad dosage range (150–450 mg per day). It has no significant anticholinergic action. It is chemically, and apparently neuropharmacologically, unrelated to other available antidepressants, and is at this writing being marketed largely because of its different side-effects profile. It is not available in the U.S.

Fluoxetine is a similarly new preparation, recently introduced to the U.S. market, with a convenient side-effects profile (little hypotension, anticholinergic effect, weight gain, or overdose danger). Both its safety and its efficacy remain to be proved in the clinical arena.

Other recently studied medications which show promise, but which cannot yet be recommended for general clinical use (or are not available in the U.S.) include *amineptine* (Scarzella et al., 1985), *valproic acid amide* (Puzynski & Klosiewicz, 1984), *zometapine* (Katz, 1984), and *diclofensine* (Capponi, Hormazabal, & Schmid-Burgk, 1985).

Alprazolam. Alprazolam is a benzodiazepine anxiolytic agent; however, it is largely prescribed as an antidepressant by clinicians apparently because of marketing recommending it for "anxious depression." When looking at common clinical indications for *antidepressant* prescription of alprazolam, one finds that it should be relied upon only after standard drugs and/or ECT have been unsuccessful. Its documented antidepressant effect is moderate at best.

Alprazolam is prescribed in divided doses beginning as low as 0.25 mg t.i.d., increasing to a manufacturer-recommended maximum of 4 mg per day. Some clinicians prescribe slightly larger amounts for depressed patients.

Alprazolam is well accepted by patients, perhaps because they begin to feel a "drug effect" almost immediately. This is probably not an antidepressive effect. It is habituating and requires tapering when moderate to high doses are discontinued. Alprazolam may be combined with tricyclic antidepressants.

Adjunctive Medications

Administration of serotonin, norepinephrine, and dopamine precursors, such as tyrosine, have been suggested and reviewed (Gelenberg & Gibson, 1984). One common precursor treatment in the U.S. is *L-tryptophan*, primarily for nondepressive syndromes. Up to 5 gm per day has occasionally been recommended as an adjunct to MAOIs (*International Drug Therapy Newsletter*, 1981). The sedative effect may cloud interpretation of the antidepressant augmentation. Phenylalanine and other amino acid precursor dietary supplements have been advocated by some (Kravitz, Sabelli, & Fawcett, 1984).

Although once a standard treatment for "involutional melancholia," there is little scientific evidence that *estrogen supplementation* adds to antidepressant effect (Shapira et al., 1985). Nevertheless, prescription of estrogen (or any of a number of other nonpsychiatric medications) may help certain individual patients, particularly those whose affective disorder accompanies a metabolic or endocrine disorder.

The addition of *lithium carbonate* to antidepressant drugs is probably helpful in some antidepressant-resistant patients (Louie & Meltzer, 1984). Lithium alone should not be a first choice in depressive disorders, even those associated with bipolar illness. In patients with recurrent depression or bipolar illness who are being maintained on lithium prophylaxis, there is some indication that the addition of folic acid decreases affective morbidity (see pp. 210–211) (Coppen, Chaudhry, & Swade, 1986).

The addition of *liothyronine (T_3, L-triiodothyronine)*, 25–50 mcg per day, to tricyclics is often helpful for TCA-resistant patients. It has also been used to increase the speed of action of the TCAs. There is no indication that it is helpful with MAOIs. Goodwin and colleagues (1982) and subsequent researchers have clarified the apparent clinical response, often seen within seven to 10 days. Although it suggests covert thyroid dysfunction as a source of depressive symptoms, it is not at all clear that this is the case, and most patients do not respond to endocrine treatment alone.

The use of true *stimulants* (e.g., methylphenidate, amphetamines) for depressive disorders is somewhat controversial. There are those who completely eschew their use, often citing the lack of neurochemical antidepressant activity. Other clinicians use them in small doses (e.g., 5–10 mg of methylphenidate in the morning) for elderly patients, usually already taking TCAs, who cannot tolerate therapeutic plasma levels of traditional antidepressants. Woods and colleagues (1986) found psychostimulants helpful in the treatment of depressive syndromes related to medical illness, and found that drug tolerance was unusual.

This author feels that such drugs as methylphenidate have a place in the short-term treatment of some depressive syndromes, particularly those in elderly or medically ill patients; however, there is no evidence to indicate their long-term usefulness. Clinicians should be familiar with the potential for toxic effects, abuse, and psychiatric symptoms (including psychosis), the last occasionally seen even at therapeutic doses.

Adding low doses of *antipsychotic medications*, especially phenothiazines, may help with patients who have psychotic (e.g., delusional) symptomatology associated with depression. This combination may also contribute to higher blood levels of the tricyclic (Spiker et al., 1981), but add anticholinergic concerns and the possibility of tardive dyskinesia if the neuroleptic is continued for more than a few weeks. Fixed-dose combinations (e.g., Triavil, Etrafon) should usually be avoided.

Benzodiazepine anxiolytics help with the anxiety and sleeplessness associated with serious depression; however, they do not apparently increase TCA blood levels. The anxiolytics do not contribute so much to anticholinergic side effects as do the phenothiazines. Fixed-dose combinations should be avoided.

Efforts to decrease the anticholinergic effects of the tricyclics in order to increase medication tolerance in patients who otherwise would not be able to reach therapeutic levels has been attempted with inconsistent results. Bethanechol, about 25 mg three or four times per day, may decrease constipation or problems with urination; however, it is not widely used.

Side Effects and Adverse Effects of Antidepressant Medications

Patient Information and Compliance. As is the case with other medications in other kinds of patients, the patient receiving antidepressants should receive a clear explanation of the reason for prescribing, the expected results, and the risks of side effects or adverse effects. Since depressed patients are sometimes not receptive to such facts and opinions from the physician because of unrealistic hopelessness, cognitive deficit, withdrawal from communication, and/or psychosis, the clinician should be prepared to discuss these matters with family, provide written information, and/or remind the patient of earlier discussions as needed. Compliance and development of side effects are not related solely to this kind of communication; however, a supportive, informative setting in which the patient can participate in his or her treatment is recommended (Myers & Calvert, 1984).

Tricyclic Antidepressants (TCAs). The most important adverse effect of the tricyclic antidepressants is lethal *overdose*. Cardiotoxic and anticholinergic actions are especially dangerous, when combined with patients who are sometimes at great risk for overdose. The pain of severe depression, its ability to give one an unrealistically hopeless outlook, and the impulsive characteristics of some patients make overdose a major consideration for many.

Serious toxic effects appear at two to three times the therapeutic blood level of tricyclics. At about four times the therapeutic level, cardiac arrhythmia and other medical complications can cause death.

Acute treatment for TCA overdose includes gastric lavage and physostigmine 2 mg IV every two to four hours to reverse anticholinergic delirium and coma. This must be accompanied by close monitoring, in part because physostigmine is metabolized rapidly and anticholinergia quickly returns. The accepted duration for cardiac-care monitoring is 24 hours after the electrocardiogram returns to normal. Seizures, when present, should be controlled with IV diazepam. Consultation regarding cardiac effects, electrolyte and acid-base balance, and hypoxia should be obtained. Dialysis has not been shown to be effective.

Elderly or medically compromised patients are more vulnerable to virtually all of the side effects or adverse effects enumerated below. Safe but effective treatment often includes lower doses, much lower starting doses, and divided doses rather than once-daily ingestion. Special attention must be paid to routes of absorption, possible impairment of plasma protein binding, and routes of degradation (especially the liver) if these may be impaired.

Organ systems in the elderly, such as the CNS or cardiovascular system, often have less reserve to handle even routine side effects, which means that ordinary doses can become toxic doses for some patients. Confusion, psychosis, or other toxic symptoms are often confused with worsening of the depression itself, leading to increased dosage or polypharmacy. The most prudent course when new symptoms arise, even apparently psychological ones, is usually to decrease or discontinue the medication for a time. This is particularly true of any effect that might arise from the anticholinergic properties of these drugs.

The interaction, chemically or additively, of antidepressants with the variety of other medications often taken by elderly or medically ill patients is a topic too broad to treat in this text. The physician must always be aware of the patient's other prescriptions and treatments, and of the known interactions among them. (See **Appendix A**.)

Induction of mania or hypomania is a potential effect of virtually all of the antidepressants, and may appear in patients not previously known to have bipolar illness. This possibility has long been observed for the TCAs, and has now been recorded for the "second generation" and "third generation" antidepressants as well (de la Fuente, Verlanga, & Leon-Andrade, 1986; Knobler et al., 1986). In some cases, manic symptoms have occurred with abrupt changes in antidepressants, probably because of increased clinical action of the new drug rather than any specific manic properties (Haggerty & Jackson, 1985). ECT and T_3 (L-triiodothyronine, liothyronine) have also been associated with switch to mania in patients prone to rapid cycling (Evans et al., 1986; Lewis & Nasrallah, 1986).

Cardiovascular and cardiac conductance effects of the tricyclics are often the physician's greatest worry. These effects have been somewhat exaggerated in the past, and many patients who are probably not at risk have been denied potential benefits of TCAs and related antidepressants. Healthy young patients (under about 40) do not require any medical workup beyond a thorough medical history and physical examination. Rare supraventricular ectopic beats may be seen in some patients at therapeutic levels (Mahapatra et al., 1986). For patients over 45, or those with a history of cardiovascular disease, a physical examination and electrocardiogram before beginning polycyclic drugs are indicated.

Postural hypotension is a far more common complaint, and does not appear to be correlated with blood levels of medication. For most middle-aged or older patients, the vascular system does not accommodate and the symptom remains unless the drug is changed or discontinued. It is usually an inconvenience rather than a serious problem, provided the patient remembers to rise slowly and there is no particular danger of serious falls or, in elderly patients, a history of compromised CNS perfusion. Nortriptyline may be the TCA of choice if postural hypotension is a serious problem (Blackwell, 1984).

Lowered seizure threshold has been documented in the literature; however, actual seizures related to tricyclics are unusual.

Anticholinergic side effects are significant for all of the tricyclics and many other antidepressants. Such effects have been described elsewhere in the text, and include dry mouth, sedation, and occasionally more serious effects such as gastric slowing or urinary hesitancy (especially in older male patients, for whom prostate enlargement may create an emergency). Anticholinergic delirium is a significant risk for elderly or CNS-compromised patients. When discontinuing TCAs, they should be tapered rather than stopped abruptly, to avoid cholinergic rebound.

Metabolic or endocrine effects include occasional inappropriate ADH secretion and weight gain. Fatty necrosis of the liver, probably idiosyncratic, has been reported. Other changes in liver function tests are generally benign and resolve without changes in the medication. Sexual changes, especially erectile impotence, has been recorded with almost all tricyclics and many other antidepressants (Mitchell & Poplin, 1983).

Ophthalmic symptoms are generally related to anticholinergic effects. The most common is blurred vision, often accompanied by problems with visual accommodation. Narrow-angle glaucoma has been cited as a potential adverse effect; however, it is now known to be rare, and most cases reported are probably not related to the antidepressant itself (Reid et al., 1976).

Since all the polycyclic antidepressants readily cross the placenta, they should be avoided in *pregnancy*, at least during the first trimester. It is prudent to discontinue the drug well before childbirth in those patients for whom treatment through pregnancy has been necessary. For many pregnant patients, ECT is a better choice of treatment for severe depression. *Nursing* should be discouraged.

TCAs are distantly related to the antipsychotic medications described elsewhere. They are capable of producing dyskinetic syndromes, although this is quite unusual.

Monoamine Oxidase Inhibitors (MAOIs). *Overdose* of MAOIs is not as dangerous as that of tricyclic antidepressants, provided the overdose does not involve complicating medications or tyramine reaction. Nevertheless, it is potentially lethal. Medical support for multiple organ failure, including defects in temperature regulation, is imperative.

Dietary considerations and avoidance of tyramine-containing foods and medications are important to prevent untoward histamine response and possible hypertensive crisis (see p. 223). Patients unable or unwilling to understand and follow dietary instructions should not be given MAOIs in unmonitored settings.

Insomnia is one of the most common complaints of patients taking an MAOI. Tranylcypromine is the most frequent offender, and should be taken early in the day. *Anticholinergic* (or anticholinergic-like) side effects have been seen with most MAOIs, particularly phenelzine (Evans et al., 1982). *Peripheral nerve symptoms,* including carpal tunnel syndrome, may result from pyridoxine deficiency, most often reported with phenelzine. This is ordinarily not serious, and can be reversed with oral vitamin supplements (Stewart et al., 1984). *Sexual disturbance* is fairly common with the MAOIs, and occurs in both men and women. It sometimes responds to decreases in dose; however, change of medication may be necessary to maintain antidepressant response.

Cardiac and liver effects are considerably fewer than those found in the polycyclic drugs. If *hypotension* occurs, it tends to be persistent, not orthostatic. *Inappropriate ADH secretion* occasionally occurs. *Weight gain* for other reasons is fairly common as well.

The MAOIs can *induce mania,* even when bipolar illness has not been diagnosed. They may rarely precipitate other psychoses, particularly in patients prone to thought disorder.

Although not considered "addictive," *discontinuing MAOIs* abruptly may result in a withdrawal syndrome virtually indistinguishable from relapse of depression. Tapering is recommended.

Amoxapine. Amoxapine is closely related to the phenothiazines, increases prolactin levels, often produces *extrapyramidal symptoms* (including dystonia) and other *neuroleptic-like side effects,* and carries some risk of *dyskinesia.* Dose-related *seizures* have been reported.

Trazodone. Trazodone has significant *anticholinergic* side effects. It is often *sedative* and sometimes seems to cause a distressing feeling of *disorientation* or mood change. It is probably not as likely as the TCAs to decrease seizure threshold and has few direct cardiotoxic effects. *Postural hypotension* does occur, however.

Clinically significant *priapism* is now a well-known, if unusual, adverse effect, which sometimes leads to serious penile problems. As several years have passed since its introduction as one of the first non-TCA antidepressants, several of the TCA-associated side effects that were once thought not to be part of its side-effects profile have been reported (including *delirium, hepatotoxicity, induction of mania*).

One significant advantage of trazodone is its decreased lethality, compared with MAOIs or TCAs, in *overdose*. Although it may cause death in combination with other drugs or alcohol, it is difficult to find cases in which trazodone was the probable cause of death.

Maprotiline. Maprotiline has a number of *anticholinergic* and *sedative* side effects. Although it is marketed as having less *cardiotoxicity* than the TCAs, there is some doubt about this claim (Coccaro & Siever, 1985). Maprotiline lowers the *seizure threshold*, probably more than the TCAs, and is sometimes associated with a benign *rash*. It is dangerous in *overdose*, with frequent cardiac and seizure-related complications. It clears from the body less rapidly than other antidepressants, a fact that may be helpful in some dosage regimens, but makes management of side effects or overdose more complex.

Nomifensine. Although this antidepressant was recently taken off the U.S. market, it is useful to point out that nomifensine is *stimulating or agitating* for some patients. It has not been found to lower seizure threshold, and is considerably safer in overdose than are MAOIs or TCAs. A *flu-like syndrome*, probably an allergic reaction, develops in 5%–10% of patients. *Liver function* tests may become abnormal. Rare *hemolytic anemia* has been associated with deaths; monitoring of liver function and blood count is recommended.

Mianserin. Mianserin, currently not available in the U.S., has significant *sedative* effects which may be related to its anxiolytic effects. Other side effects appear to be common. There has been little clinical experience with mianserin overdose.

Buproprion. Buproprion is not yet available in the U.S. and is undergoing further testing of *seizure-producing potential*. Its antidepressant activity has not been well established; however, the side-effects profile does not include weight gain, appetite stimulation, or orthostatic hypotension, which may make it a choice for some patients. Plasma levels vary broadly, as does recommended daily dosage (see p. 226). There is little experience with overdose; however, significant lethality has not been established (Preskorn & Othmer, 1984).

234 The Treatment of Psychiatric Disorders

Fluoxetine. Fluoxetine's side effects may be less troublesome than those of the TCAs, particularly with respect to anticholinergic or orthostatic symptoms. Future clinical experience may or may not change this impression. It probably does not lower seizure threshold significantly, and appears safer than TCAs or MAOIs in overdose.

Alprazolam. Although not an antidepressant *per se*, alprazolam is often prescribed for depressed patients, with or without established antidepressant medications. Its side effects are generally those of the benzodiazepine anxiolytics. It is safer than any known antidepressant in overdose, unless taken with alcohol or other drugs. Habituation can be a problem.

Electroconvulsive Therapy (ECT)

ECT has established safety and efficacy for the treatment of severe depression, depression and some mania in bipolar disorders, and some schizophrenic patients compromised by or refractory to traditional medications. Numerous studies have established its effectiveness and general superiority over antidepressant drugs with respect to mortality and morbidity (American Psychiatric Association, 1979; Tanney, 1986; Weiner, 1983).

The clinician should at least consider ECT if the patient does not respond to the first one or two choices of antidepressant. For older patients, those with cardiac disease or other medical contraindications to standard antidepressants, acutely suicidal patients, or those with histories of good response to ECT, it should be considered earlier.

The following summary of ECT procedures, side effects, and possible adverse effects should not be considered a complete guide. The reader is referred to Martin (1986), the American Psychiatric Association Task Force Report (1979), or any of several excellent papers or book chapters in the recent literature for more detailed information.

Contraindications (mostly relative rather than absolute) include intracranial hemorrhage or known aneurism, recent myocardial infarction, and known posterior fossa mass or other sensitivity to transient increases in intracranial pressure. MAOIs should be discontinued two weeks prior to ECT, because of possible interference with anesthetics or emergency medications. Cardiac pacemakers are not significant contraindications, nor is normal pregnancy.

Consent. Consent should be obtained as for a surgical procedure, since anesthesia will be involved. Complete written informed consent is necessary, with assurances that the patient (and family if applicable) understand all potential procedures, benefits, and risks. This is sometimes accomplished via a videotape which actually shows a treatment. Such videotapes often allay patients' and families' anxieties about ECT, since the actual procedure is far less distressing than most people's fantasies and movie portrayals.

The *pre-ECT workup* should include:

Complete history and physical exam
Complete blood count
Serum chemistries and electrolytes
Sickle cell screening for Black patients
Urinalysis

Patients over 40 should receive an electrocardiogram. Spinal radiographs are usually not necessary, but should be obtained in older patients and those with histories of arthritis, osteoporosis, or other orthopedic problems. Lithium should be discontinued in most patients taking it. Patients in whom lithium is continued during ECT should have a level drawn before treatment and twice a week during treatment. Baseline memory and intelligence testing is a defensive measure, but sometimes clinically useful some time later. Routine laboratory determination of plasma pseudocholinesterase activity is recommended by some, but most anesthesiologists suggest such measurements be limited to patients with certain risk factors: personal or family history of abnormal response to succinylcholine, current use of anticholinesterase medication (e.g., for glaucoma or myasthenia gravis), exposure to chemicals with anticholinesterase actions (e.g., some insecticides), or severe respiratory illness. Abnormalities are not absolute contraindications, but mandate anesthesiology consultation.

The *procedure before each treatment* includes:

The patient has been NPO for six to eight hours.
Empty bladder if possible.
Remove dentures and dental appliances.
Check routine and emergency drugs and equipment. A special emergency/life-support cart, with resuscitation equipment, should be in the room, if not permanently installed. A defibrillator should be nearby.
See that bed or treatment table is insulated.
Assemble loaded syringes (anticholinergic agent, muscle relaxant, anesthetic).
Establish and secure venous pathway.

No pretreatment anxiolytic or sedative drugs are recommended, as these increase seizure threshold. The specific agents used for anticholinergia, muscle relaxation, and anesthetic may vary (and the anticholinergic is often omitted). The anesthetic should be short-acting and should not increase seizure threshold (e.g., methohexital, thiopental). Although some anesthesiologists suggest a venous catheter, the venous pathway is often merely a taped "butterfly" in a hand vein, since the patient will require the procedure six to 15 times over several weeks.

Anesthesia may be provided by the psychiatrist, an anesthetist, or an anesthesiologist. Medically complicated patients require anesthesiologic consultation. In any event, the person responsible for anesthesia and recovery must (1) be competent to handle anesthesia-related emergencies and life support, and (2) understand the special anesthetic needs of ECT as differentiated from those of surgical procedures.

Treatment itself begins with mask breathing of 100% oxygen for several minutes, followed by the anticholinergic (if used, to block cardiac cholinergic block) and the anesthetic. Mask ventilation with 100% oxygen is continued until stimulus (and reinstituted after stimulus). The muscle relaxant (usually succinylcholine) can now be administered. Tourniquets or cuffs used to prevent muscle relaxation for test purposes should already be in place.

Once maximum paralysis has occurred, the gag or bite block is inserted (if not placed earlier) and electrodes placed unilaterally or bilaterally. Nondominant unilateral placement is used by many North American clinicians (Squire & Slater, 1983), but evidence of advantage over bilateral placement is controversial.

The electrical stimulus should be just enough to produce an adequate seizure. The necessary stimulus setting will increase with age, and (slightly) with each treatment. Presence of seizure is ascertained in a number of ways, such as EEG monitoring or movement of a limb protected from the muscle relaxant. Although significant patient movement is unlikely, care should be taken to prevent injury or falling. The seizure is necessary to treatment. If it does not occur, the stimulus should be increased and repeated after one to two minutes. Glissando is not recommended.

After the seizure, the bite block or gag should be removed, any tourniquet or cuff loosened, and the oropharynx checked for blockage and secretions. Ventilation is continued until breathing is clearly re-established and continuous. The patient is closely observed for vomiting or regurgitation. Monitoring should continue in a recovery area until vital signs are stable and the patient has been reoriented.

Many patients remain somewhat confused for several hours, with the period of disorientation lengthening as the number of treatments increases. The patient and family should be reassured that this is expected (and temporary). Staff must supervise and protect the patient during this period.

Outpatient ECT must be done with the understanding that the patient will be in the company of a responsible adult for several hours after recovery. Cautions against driving, operating machinery, cooking, and so forth should be clear to all concerned.

Treatments should be given every two to three days, for a total of eight to 15 sessions, although improvement may occur within the first few days. More may be indicated in ECT treatment of schizophrenia. Seizure duration, and probably total time in seizure, is important to treatment success and prevention of relapse (Maletsky, 1981). Multiple seizures in one anesthetic session or treatments scheduled more often than every two days have not been shown superior to traditional scheduling (Tanney, 1986), and may cause unnecessary confusion. Degree of amnesia, usually none-to-slight after six to nine months, appears correlated more with number of treatments than total seizure time, however (Weiner et al., 1982).

Tolerance to ECT is virtually unknown. Remission is usually lasting. Relapse, such as that associated with cyclic depressions, can often be prevented with lithium, carbamazepine, or antidepressants.

Side Effects and Adverse Effects of ECT. The common myth of lasting, significant memory deficit associated with modern ECT has been disproved many times (Martin, 1986; Weiner et al., 1982). *Transient anterograde and retrograde amnesias* occur during the course of treatment, but permanent deficit of either type is very rare. Other cognitive impairment is quite unusual as well. It should be noted that the impairments associated with severe depression are significant themselves. "Holes" in the patient's memory appear related to the depressed periods, not to ECT, except for the time immediately following treatment sessions.

Although *confusion and headache* are common after treatment sessions, permanent EEG changes apparently do not occur with modern ECT. Epilepsy following ECT is very rare. Prolonged (greater than three to four minutes) seizures during sessions must be treated immediately, and are uniformly stopped by IV diazepam or barbiturates. Continuous oxygenation is essential. Most serious morbidity or mortality in ECT is related to anesthetic complications; the rate is probably lower than that for inpatient dental surgery (Martin, 1986).

Treatment of Depression in the Elderly

Affective disorder in the elderly should not be viewed solely as a consequence of environment, physical or social loss, or anticipation of aging or death (Talley, 1987). On the other hand, the elderly patient must usually be seen as one in whom there are physical (e.g., pain, fatigue, accompanying medical illness), emotional (e.g., loss, grief, despair), and social (e.g., environmental change, loss of prior living settings or social skills) complications for the disorder and its treatment.

Several of the biological considerations for elderly patients, such as changes in dosage requirements, vulnerability to side effects, and special attention to polypharmacy (Ban, Guy, & Wilson, 1984) have already been discussed. Careful evaluation and diagnosis of medical disorders will offer many elderly patients presenting with depression additional avenues for help, through treatment of medical illness related to the psychiatric presentation.

Although it is clear that appropriately diagnosed major depression in the elderly should be treated with the same general approaches and vigor as depression in any other age group (Murphy, 1985), older patients offer an excellent example of the usefulness of nonbiological psychosocial treatments as well. They should not be excluded from psychotherapy, whether in a residential environment such as a nursing home, an acute inpatient setting, or an outpatient office. For some, reminiscing in a guided, therapeutic way is helpful (Parsons, 1986). Counseling for "life enhancement," which takes into consideration ethnic and cultural variations, has also been recommended (Szapocznik et al., 1982). Structure, respect, gentleness, and sensory enhancement such as touch and music are all important to the prevention of serious depression in living facilities for the elderly (Kartman, 1984; Rowlands, 1984).

Sleep and the Treatment of Depression

The most common sleep-related concerns have to do with the treatment of sleeplessness or *depression-related sleep disorders*. Helping the patient to sleep almost always helps him or her to feel better, and often restores optimism with respect to the somewhat slower antidepressant therapy. It is common to see sedative antidepressants prescribed in the evening; however, the psychiatrist should be aware that the actual sleep generated by antidepressants is not particularly restful.

Modern approaches suggest short-acting sedative benzodiazepines, such as temazepam or triazolam. These drugs help normalize sleep cycles, increase REM content, do not mask symptoms of either depression or therapeutic response, and rarely interfere with antidepressant medications. They should be given in doses that allow complete clearing before morning; if the patient is sleepy or disoriented the following day, the dose is probably too high.

Therapeutic sleep deprivation is a seemingly paradoxical approach to the treatment of depression. At this time, it must still be considered experimental, although studies have for several years tried to reconcile anecdotal reports with knowledge of biological rhythms and neurotransmitter function (Joffe & Brown, 1984; Wehr et al., 1985). Chronobiological effects either of bright light or of additional hours of sunlight imply that there is at least a subgroup of patients who develop symptoms of major affective disorder on a seasonal (usually winter) basis. Some of these regularly-cycling depressive patients improve significantly after as little as one week of exposure to bright light in the morning (but not in the evening) (Lewy, Sack, & Singer, 1985; Lewy et al., 1987). A number of other symptom-relieving effects of "biologically active" bright light under specifically controlled conditions are described by Dietzel and colleagues (1986).

Maintenance Drug Treatment of Depression

Since many depressive episodes remit of their own accord, it is reasonable to consider stopping the antidepressant medication at some point during remission. Many—perhaps most—serious depressive disorders follow a natural course of relapses and remissions throughout one's life, however, with the periods of remission often becoming shorter and shorter as the patient grows older.

Formulas used until a few years ago suggested keeping the patient on medication for at least several months, or at least half of the duration of pretreatment depressive symptoms, whichever is longer. The medication would then be slowly tapered, with monitoring for the return of symptoms.

Rush (1986) suggests that a rough estimate of the time for which medication will be needed can be made by means of a careful history of the recurrences of the depressive episodes. This may be particularly useful for elderly patients or patients who do not tolerate medication well, and who should be free of it during those periods in which the natural course of the episodes would leave them free of symptoms in any event. This presupposes that antidepressant medications are solely symptomatic and do not "cure" or even alter the natural course of relapsing and remitting depressive disease.

Course. The several possible courses of depression make simplistic comments about outcome impossible. Those patients whose cycling of symptoms allows return to baseline functioning between episodes have a generally good prognosis. Those with "double depression," that is, dysthymic disorder or character accompanied by occasional episodes of major affective disorder, are more difficult to treat, since biological treatment for the major affective episodes often merely brings the patient back to his dysphoric, dysthymic "baseline" (Rush, 1986).

Prognosis. In general, the prognosis for major depressive episodes, either simple depressive or bipolar, is quite good. Patients whose depressive disorders resemble Schizoaffective Disorder, tend to have a long-term course more consistent with schizophrenia, however (Coryell et al., 1984).

Psychotherapy of Major Depression

As mentioned many times in this text, biological treatment should almost never be given in psychosocial vacuum. Whether one sees patients in a purely psychiatric setting, or in consultation-liaison settings in which the psychiatrist works within the medical or surgical specialties, the "biopsychosocial" approach provides for broader response of the patient to treatment efforts of all kinds (Vasile et al., 1987).

Various forms of psychotherapy have been attempted as primary treatments for severely depressed patients. Studies with outpatients, in which the depressive illness was mild enough to allow outpatient treatment, indicate that *cognitive* therapy is useful alone, and can add considerably to the effectiveness of antidepressant medication (Rush et al., 1982). *Psychodynamically oriented* psychotherapy or psychoanalysis has been successful for some patients; however, studies of its efficacy are lacking. In either case (cognitive or psychodynamic), the therapist must be experienced and must understand the depressive illness clearly.

Behavior modification is useful for decreasing nonproductive thoughts and activities. Those who use it extensively hope that changing behavior will result in concomitant change in the patient's depressive outlook.

Psychotherapy is particularly helpful for reintegrating the patient into normal interpersonal and social settings. Patients who have been depressed for some time may literally have lost the skills necessary to participate in their families, work, and so forth. Individual or group therapy to support their efforts, bolster confidence, increase interpersonal skills, and fight inevitable fears of relapse can be very important. *Self-help groups* (e.g., local chapters of the National Alliance for the Mentally Ill and local Depressive and Manic Depressive associations), particularly when guided by psychiatric consultation, can provide a great deal of support.

Group or individual psychotherapy may also address situations of substance abuse or illegal activity which has been related to the patient's depression. Many patients will have developed problems with, for example, alcohol abuse, either as self-medication or as self-destructive behavior. It is sometimes difficult to know which is the "primary" disorder, substance abuse or depression; indeed, the treatment of combined or "dual diagnosis" disorders is a large part of the work of most clinicians. Finally, a psychotherapeutic relationship with patients, whether by the psychiatrist or by a nonphysician who understands the importance of psychiatric treatment, can help the patient understand biological treatment, comply with treatment regimens, and develop a realistic concept of his illness.

Physical Activity. For years, physicians have prescribed activity for the treatment of depression and other illnesses. There are now a number of accepted papers, including a few controlled studies, which note the benefits of regular, usually aerobic, exercise of patients, ranging from simple feelings of well-being and mastery (Mellion, 1985), to specific antidepressant activity (McCann & Holmes, 1984).

Psychotherapy Alone. A few studies indicate that psychotherapy, particularly behavior or cognitive therapy, is sometimes adequate treatment for major depression (Beck et al., 1985; Murphy et al., 1984). Others sometimes show an advantage—usually of specific cognitive therapies—over medication (Rush et al., 1977). Most of the latter studies were done prior to 1983, and some (e.g., Simons et al., 1984) indicate that some of the comparatively good results of psychotherapy may be related to the higher dropout rate for medication-alone treatment.

300.40 Dysthymia (Depressive Neurosis)
In spite of the implications that Dysthymia or "Depressive Neurosis" is by definition a less serious condition than the "major" or bipolar affective disorders, it is in many ways more difficult to treat and can

lead to more cumulative discomfort for the patient. Uncomplicated dysthymia is not generally associated with suicide risk, serious social or interpersonal deterioration, or hospitalization. Nevertheless, these patients are in pain, and deserve vigorous clinical attention.

Some psychotherapists, and many laypersons, suggest environmental approaches to treatment. They expect, or wish, the patient to "snap out of it" as a result of a job change, vacation, geographic move, or the like. Since Dysthymic Disorder is not, however, a reactive disorder or sign of "maladjustment," these approaches rarely produce lasting results.

Psychotherapy is the treatment of choice for most patients, given qualifications that make it emotionally and realistically available. In today's cost-cutting mental health arena, the majority of patients referred for "therapy" or "counseling" are seen by individuals with master's-level training or less, who, because of training, experience, or time and financial constraints, offer superficial or supportive counseling. Treatment is often done in groups which, although they can be sophisticated and carry specific psychotherapeutic value, are sometimes created more for their low per-patient cost, increased total therapist revenue, and scheduling efficiency than for solid therapeutic process and content. It should be said, however, that many patients can benefit from supportive work.

Suitable, motivated patients who receive intensive therapy from competent therapists of any clinical orientation have a fairly good prognosis, with cognitive therapy often showing the best results (Covi et al., in press; Wilson, Goldin, & Charbonneau-Powis, 1983). Psychoanalytic psychotherapy or psychoanalysis remains a treatment of choice for those patients with neurotic conflict and other criteria for this form of treatment. An excellent discussion of psychotherapeutic approaches for depression is found in Jarrett and Rush (1986).

No matter what the form of psychotherapy, supportive measures are important. These may range from simple reassurance and education of the patient, to unqualified acceptance of the patient (who may at times appear hostile or draining to the therapist), to working with significant others in the patient's life. Successful therapy usually involves warmth and availability on the part of the psychiatrist, not the classically "neutral" stance which the patient easily misperceives as noncaring.

The treatment of depressed patients, particularly in individual or group psychotherapy, is a draining experience, fraught with countertransference and simple exhaustion. Therapists who treat many such patients should be aware that although not infectious, depression can be "catching." The patients may be hostile; may trigger feelings of anger, frustration, or rescue needs in the therapist; and at times will be so demanding as to appear extremely dependent. The clinician can defend himself and his patient against these personal reactions in three ways: by being aware that they are likely to surface in the therapist, by having some understanding of his or her own emotional makeup (perhaps through personal psychotherapy), and by having sufficient outlets and gratifications in his or her personal life that the unique stresses of psychotherapy of depression can be dissipated.

Medication. If the patient presents with evidence of agitative signs, serious emotional dysfunction, or episodes of deep "double depression" between which the symptoms are depressive but less severe, one may consider a course of antidepressant medication. Trazodone may be useful in moderate-to-severe neurotic depression (Goldberg, Rickels, & Finnerty, 1981). In most instances, however, antidepressants are ineffective. There is, incidentally, no clinical rationale for giving "a little" antidepressant to treat "a little" depression; low doses of these drugs are homeopathic. Pharmacologic intervention should generally be limited to symptom relief, such as temporary treatment for insomnia.

The patient often will have read or heard from others, perhaps from his or her family physician, about the "chemical imbalance" kinds of mood disorders for which medication can lead to a striking improvement. The clinician should carefully explain to the patient the reasons for not choosing antidepressant drugs, while conveying an understanding of the depth of the patient's pain, assessment of self-destructive potential, and optimism for the future.

Outcome. The outcome of most forms of psychotherapy is positive to some extent, given appropriate patients and a competent therapist. However, complete alleviation of symptoms, or prevention of relapse, is less common. Psychoanalytically oriented treatment is probably the most likely to bring lasting relief. For other treatments, relapse rates of 35%, given initial success, are not uncommon.

The prognosis for Dysthymic Disorder ordinarily does not include deterioration into more serious affective disorder. There are some exceptions to this; dysthymia does not provide immunity from other psychiatric disorders. In the absence of family history, however, the patient is unlikely to develop major affective disorder or bipolar illness.

311.00 Depressive Disorder Not Otherwise Specified

One form of "not otherwise specified" Depressive Disorder is depression superimposed on another mental or physical illness. Since several of the established treatments for depression are generic (e.g., cognitive therapy), one should consider both pharmacologic and nonpharmacologic treatments based upon the severity and course of the symptoms, using the concepts discussed earlier in this section. It is important to determine the extent to which the depression is linked to the primary disorder. For some, such as schizophrenia, remission of the primary disorder often eliminates the need for continued antidepressant treatment.

The high frequency of organically associated depressions (symptoms of general medical illness or adverse effects of any of a wide variety of medications) makes continuing monitoring of diagnosis an important part of treatment. The number of patients who improve after discontinuing or decreasing even apparently benign medications is striking.

For those depressions not associated with other illness or treatment, but still not represented in the *DSM-III-R*, the symptoms, course, and family history of both depression and response to treatment should be the clinical guide. Although it is tempting to try one of the medication regimens already described, the psychiatrist should understand that in the absence of "endogenous" symptoms, the number of positive responders is probably only slightly greater than that for placebo.

Chapter 18

Anxiety Disorders (Anxiety and Phobic Neuroses)

For most patients, treatment of the anxiety disorders can be aimed at alleviating uncomfortable or disabling symptoms. For some others—for example, many patients with post-traumatic stress disorders—in-depth treatment may be required or advisable. Since the last edition of the *DSM-III*, the chronic treatment of anxiety disorders has made considerable strides, as has our understanding of their neurochemistry.

Although most new strategies are pharmacologic or behavioral (with support and education), insight-oriented psychotherapy (including psychoanalytic psychotherapy when appropriate and available) continues to be recommended for patients whose symptoms stem from identifiable neurotic conflict, whose anxieties or compulsions are readily identified by the patient as going beyond specific symptoms, whose chronic anxiety has not responded to the more straightforward treatments described below, or who develop additional complaints when the presenting symptoms are removed.

As a number of specific treatment techniques, ranging from the behavioral to the psychoanalytic, are mentioned in the following pages, it is important to reiterate that the clinician must be familiar with both the indications for and the technical aspects of a given therapeutic approach before expecting it to be effective. This is true for any treatment modality, whether it outwardly appears simple, or obviously requires extensive training.

300.xx Panic Disorder
with Agoraphobia (300.21)
without Agoraphobia (300.01)

Acute Treatment. The primary acute treatment of Panic Disorder, once other problems (particularly organic sources of the panic, such as caffeinism) have been ruled out, is blocking of the panic attacks, coupled with brief psychotherapy and reassurance that, although extremely uncomfortable, the disorder does not lead to severe mental illness. Telling the patient that the symptoms *can* be managed and are very probably transient is quite reassuring. Acute treatment is similar for Panic Disorder alone, or Panic Disorder with Agoraphobia.

A number of different medication* classes have been shown effective, some of which are primarily anxiolytic, others antidepressant (although probably not acting in the same way as they do when combatting depression), and still others related to the physiologic indices of anxiety and panic (e.g., cardiovascular signs).

Imipramine is the standard treatment for blockade and prevention of panic attacks (Liebowitz, 1985; Rifkin & Siris, 1985). Other tricyclics have also been shown effective, particularly desipramine and clomipramine, the latter being available only outside the U.S. Doses are often lower than those required for treating depression. As little as 10-25 mg per day of imipramine, increasing in 25 mg increments every few days, often leads to rapid blockade while the clinician monitors for side effects or hypersensitivity. Patients with anxiety disorders sometimes experience different side effects than those with affective disorders (e.g., agitation and insomnia). The eventual daily dose occasionally reaches 200 mg or 300 mg of imipramine or its equivalent.

The *monoamine oxidase inhibitors (MAOIs)* (especially *phenelzine*) and *alprazolam* compare favorably with imipramine (Alexander & Alexander, 1986; Charney et al., 1986; Buigues & Vallejo, 1987; Hollister, 1986). Up to 90 mg per day of phenelzine may be required. It has been noted in one study (Buigues & Vallejo, 1987) to block panic attacks virtually 100% of the time.

Alprazolam is often effective even in low doses (1-2 mg twice a day). Although patient acceptance of alprazolam is high, and it has fewer serious side effects than either the tricyclics or the MAOIs, there is a potential for overuse of this medication. Many psychiatrists and other physicians report that it is difficult to get patients to discontinue

---
*The reader is referred to **Appendix B** for generic and trade names of medications.

alprazolam once it is no longer needed. Alprazolam has been associated with induction of manic episodes in at least two patients with Panic Disorder, although they had some biological markers of underlying affective disorder as well (Pecknold & Fleury, 1986).

Another benzodiazepine derivative which has been successfully used in the treatment of recurrent panic attacks is *clonazepam*. This long-half-life drug appears to block panic attacks independently of its anxiolytic properties. It has been favorably compared with the TCAs, MAOIs, and alprazolam (Pollack, et al., 1986; Tesar & Rosenbaum, 1986), particularly for treatment-resistant patients. Other benzodiazepines also have panic-blocking ability, although they do not appear as specific in their actions.

Propranolol and other *beta-adrenergic blockers, clonidine,* and several other drugs have been used in atypical patients, and are sometimes useful in other anxiety disorders; however, they have not outperformed the more effective (and sometimes safer) medications already mentioned.

As pharmacologic control is being established, the psychiatrist, with or without an additional therapist, should be establishing rapport with the patient and preparing him or her for further treatment. Drugs that block panic attacks do not necessarily address other kinds of anxiety. The patient almost always anticipates, with some dread, the return of these often-terrifying episodes. Benzodiazepines may be helpful for this anticipatory anxiety. Reassurance from the clinician, who should repeatedly point out the patient's ability to control and prevent panic attacks either with medication or with one of the behavioral treatments described in the sections to follow, helps prepare the patient for gradual tapering of the drug.

At this point, treatment becomes similar to that for Generalized Anxiety Disorder (300.02) (see pp. 255–258). Once the panic-blocking medication has been discontinued after several months, many patients will not require it again.

300.22 Agoraphobia without History of Panic Disorder

Pharmacologic Treatments. The treatment of panic attacks associated with agoraphobia is discussed in the preceding section. This section assumes either that panic attacks were absent, or they are being treated as already described.

Although there is evidence for the specific effectiveness of some medications, pharmacologic intervention alone is not the optimal treatment for agoraphobic patients. Long-term treatment with imipramine or alprazolam favorably affects noradrenergic function and is probably safe (Charney & Heninger, 1985), but may deprive the patient of additional gains from psychotherapeutic or behavioral treatments. Clonazepam has also been found safe and effective (Pollack et al., 1986).

Nonpharmacologic Treatments. Several behavioral treatments, either alone or with medication, can be applied. Success depends largely upon one's expertise and experience with the treatment (and sometimes on one's confidence in it).

In vivo desensitization, exposure, or *flooding* implies a situation in which the patient is placed in the phobic setting—in this case an environment related to agoraphobia—and allowed to become emotionally and physiologically adapted to it. Sometimes this occurs in a gradual stepwise fashion (gradual desensitization), in which the patient becomes comfortable with one level of phobic stimulus before moving to a more stressful one. In "flooding," on the other hand, the patient is rapidly exposed to situations of great anxiety.

In each kind of exposure, and variations of both, the therapist supports the patient, sometimes by actually participating or modeling the desired behavior. Flooding can be quite stressful, and should not be undertaken by inexperienced therapists, nor with patients who may be physically or emotionally vulnerable to the significant physiologic and psychological reactions that are likely to occur.

There are a number of "imaginal"—as opposed to in vivo—versions of desensitization and flooding. All use some form of relaxation or hypnosis, in which the patient creates an anxiety-producing image and then either holds it in his or her mind until the anxiety has dissipated or "escapes" to a pleasant thought or image when anxiety arises.

The literature generally recommends in vivo exposure, although there are individual differences in response. Some studies report improvements in up to 75% of patients. More realistic estimates, from unselected populations, suggest about one-third "total improvement" for in vivo treatment, with 50%–65% "significant improvement" (Jansson, Jerremalm, & Ost, 1986). Imaginal exposure is effective for a significant number of patients, although fewer than for in vivo treatment. The reasons for this are not clear. Imaginal treatment may be more practical, or better accepted for certain patients. Self-exposure assignments, in which the therapist is not present, usually fall between these two methods in effectiveness; a therapist is necessary to guide the patient's treatment course.

It is unrealistic to ask the patient to "promise" that he or she will succeed at the therapy (e.g., never avoid a crowded concert). Indeed, such broad promises of "giant steps" in treatment are countertherapeutic and may represent neurotic resistance. That is, one sure way for the unconscious to guarantee failure of the treatment, and thus perpetuate the defensive symptom or habit, is to make a nonkeepable promise. The therapist should refuse to accept such broad promises and instead have the patient focus on small steps in treatment, and in life: e.g., "I feel confident after our first three sessions, doctor, and I will try out my progress on my next business trip." It is particularly important to let the patient know that each step in the treatment process represents real gains, which are not erased by temporary setbacks or return of symptoms.

Combined treatments offer a more comprehensive approach to the patient. They provide an opportunity to give the patient personal control over his symptoms, address anticipatory anxiety, and help him deal with the desire to avoid situations that previously caused phobic anxiety. This last concern is often overlooked by physicians, whose patients report that medication alleviates discomfort, but may not discuss the fact that they are continuing to avoid certain settings or situations. This can be addressed with simple suggestion or exhortation by the psychiatrist that the patient test his or her improvement.

Combining imipramine and in vivo flooding has been thought to greatly increase the number of patients who respond positively to treatment (Mavissakalian & Michelson, 1982). Later studies (Mavissakalian & Michelson, 1986a) and follow-up after several years (Mavissakalian & Michelson, 1986b) note less response variance related to combining the treatments, but considerable correlation between clinical outcome and chronicity or severity of the agoraphobia. Patients who responded best initially tended to have more favorable long-term treatment outcomes.

300.23 Social Phobia

The social phobias often respond to the same kinds of psychotherapy or behavioral therapy (especially in vivo) used for Agoraphobia Without History of Panic Disorder (p. 247). The lack of studies specifically addressing this syndrome makes specific treatment recommendations or predictions difficult, however. Some suggest training or education focusing upon social skills, with a combination of role-playing, exposure, and practice provided in a group setting. For specific descriptions see the section on Agoraphobia Without History of Panic Disorder or Simple Phobia.

Performance Anxiety. It is now well-known that beta-adrenergic blockers, particularly propranolol, can alleviate performance anxiety ("stage fright") in patients without additional anxiety symptoms or syndromes. Assuming no medical contraindications, 20–40 mg of propranolol taken an hour or so before, say, public speaking or a musical performance often alleviates the anxiety without affecting mental or physical dexterity. The medication should not be taken just before the performance, but at least an hour beforehand, so that peripheral symptoms do not have a chance to develop. The dosage should ordinarily be acute, as needed; however, the author has treated several patients chronically exposed to anxiety-producing social settings involving performance anxiety (i.e., regular sales presentations) with regularly scheduled doses. One should expect to taper the medication after several months since, at this writing, the safety and effectiveness of this medication regimen for this indication have not been formally established.

300.29 Simple Phobia
The phrase "simple phobia" implies little significant underlying psychopathology or neurotic conflict. That is, removal of the phobic symptoms can be accomplished with behavioral treatment, with little or no symptom substitution or emotional decompensation by the patient. Most authors and clinicians report success for most patients using some form of *exposure*, such as systematic desensitization (in vivo or imaginal), or *paradoxical intention*. The various forms of exposure have already been described in the section on Agoraphobia Without History of Panic Disorder.

Paradoxical intention is a method by which the patient can enter into the treatment process with less anxiety and more control than is the case with, for example, flooding. Several different paradoxical techniques are reviewed and compared with other behavioral and exposure methods by Dowd and Swoboda (1984) and Michelson and Ascher (1984). Marks (1985) provides a concise discussion of several rapid, effective behavioral treatment strategies for phobias and other anxiety disorders.

Alleviation of the phobia can change the patient's life considerably. This is particularly important in the treatment of medically ill patients whose phobias prevent, for example, necessary injections or other treatments. Hypnosis, relaxation training, and/or desensitization can easily be performed in the hospital or physician's office, even for patients with considerable pain.

Self-administered computer programs, videotaped sessions, or audiotapes have all been used with some success (Chandler, Burck, & Sampson, 1986; Horne et al., 1986), although the support and guidance of an experienced therapist is recommended.

Traditional psychotherapy for phobias has not by any means been abandoned. Phobic patients often recognize that their symptoms are not "simple," and that their fears have meaning beyond the anxiety that they cause. Psychotherapy is particularly helpful for "phobias" that are not very specific, such as academic anxiety in college students (Sifneos, 1985).

Drug Therapy. As is the case for other anxiety disorders, the tricyclic antidepressants and MAOIs have been reported effective for treating Simple Phobia. The doses of antidepressant medication approximate those used for depression. Some patients respond quickly; however, others take six to eight weeks for maximum improvement. The incidence of side effects and the tendency for relapse limit their usefulness for some patients, particularly when behavioral therapy is often effective (Noyes, Chaudry, & Domingo, 1986). Adjunctive use of the benzodiazepines, preferably those with short half-lives, is recommended by many (Hollister, 1986). The tricyclic clomipramine continues to enjoy favor in the treatment of anxiety disorders outside the U.S. (see the following section on Obsessive Compulsive Disorder) (Allsopp et al., 1985).

300.30 Obsessive Compulsive Disorder (Obsessive Compulsive Neurosis)

Drug Treatments. The discovery that Obsessive Compulsive Disorder and severe obsessive symptoms often respond to a variety of medications, particularly antidepressants, has been welcome news for both clinicians and patients, since traditional psychotherapy is quite difficult. The tricyclics, MAOIs, trazodone, and fluoxetine have all been reported effective in at least a few studies. This disorder is the only one for which clinical research indicates a relationship between the antidepressant activity of these drugs and an anxiety disorder, with dexamethasone suppression, sleep electroencephalography, plasma growth hormone response, and platelet 3H-imipramine binding indicating some relationship between endogenous depression and obsessive-compulsive disease (Cottraux et al., 1984; Insel et al., 1984).

The medication most associated with relief is clomipramine, a tricyclic not readily available in the U.S. (Ananth, 1986; Insel et al., 1985; Volavka, Meziroglu, & Yaryura-Tobias, 1985). Nevertheless, the other tricyclics should be tried when clomipramine is not available. Murray (1986) found that compulsive rituals respond more often than obsessive actions to both behavioral and pharmacologic therapy; most other authors agree.

The MAOI phenelzine (Mahgoub, 1987), trazodone (Lybiard, 1986; Prasad, 1986), and the benzodiazepine alprazolam (Tollefson, 1985) have all shown some effectiveness with obsessive-compulsive patients, the most consistent being with trazodone. Fluoxetine, in doses between 40 mg and 80 mg per day, was reported successful in open-label trials (Fontaine & Chouinard, 1986).

Low doses of neuroleptic drugs, commonly prescribed in years past, are no longer the treatment of choice. Similarly, most benzodiazepines, although they have good patient acceptance and relieve anxiety, appear to have little or no effect on the core symptoms of Obsessive Compulsive Disorder (Lelliott & Monteiro, 1986).

Biological approaches to treatment-resistant patients include addition of lithium or tryptophan to tricyclics (Rasmussen, 1984) and antiandrogens (Casas et al., 1986). For severely disabled patients, for whom pharmacologic and behavioral therapy are ineffective, cingulotractotomy has been prescribed.

Behavioral Treatments. Although a variety of behavioral therapy methods have been tried for Obsessive Compulsive Disorder, two—exposure and response prevention—have been more useful than the others (Murray, 1986). Exposure therapy has included in vivo techniques, systematic desensitization, and the use of either tapes or fantasies to simulate in vivo exposure (Taylor, 1985; Thyer, 1985). The imaginal techniques are often carried out under hypnosis. Compulsive behavior (rituals, checking) is generally more responsive to treatment than is intrusive obsessional thinking.

Psychotherapy. Psychoanalytic psychotherapy, commonly used in the past, is probably an excellent choice for patients who are acceptable candidates, and who see their obsessive-compulsive symptoms as related to neurotic conflict which requires more than superficial treatment.

Salzman (1985) and Sifneos (1985) suggest psychodynamic approaches within a short-term therapeutic context.

309.89 Post-traumatic Stress Disorder (PTSD) (Acute or Delayed)

Acute Treatment. The backbone of successful treatment of Post-traumatic Stress Disorder (PTSD) lies in recognition and prompt treatment. Recognizing the potential for emotional or adjustment problems after a significant trauma, and then providing support and opportunities for ventilation, can prevent the post-traumatic syndrome from fully establishing itself or becoming chronic. Treatment is primarily psychotherapeutic, with different kinds of interventions and goals for different kinds of trauma: violent crime, automobile accident, combat, and so forth.

The immediate approach should be gentle and nonconfrontive, acknowledging the patient's loss and the fact that certain symptoms and strong feelings are normal under the circumstances. The patient may have to be protected from or counseled about countertherapeutic responses, either in himself or herself (e.g., acting on vengeful impulses) or from others (e.g., pressures associated with "debriefing" after the event, criminal investigations, or litigation). For the most part, this kind of support allows the patient to experience the natural process of the "stress response," leading to a return to baseline functioning or even emotional growth.

If the patient suffers from deficits in attention, alertness, or social or vocational functioning, one may advise against immediately returning to everyday life; however, overprotection or *expecting* that the trauma will have a permanent effect is usually countertherapeutic.

Subacute Treatment. For those patients who do not return to baseline functioning within several days or a few weeks, depending upon the trauma, brief psychotherapy should begin without delay (in order to prevent the chronic syndrome). Treatment should include discussion of the original trauma and open examination of psychodynamic concepts such as survivor's guilt to help the patient view his or her experience realistically. Encouraging normal and higher-order neurotic mechanisms for resolving the trauma support the patient's progress. Conversely, giving subtle permission for the patient to continue to be disabled often delays improvement and encourages unconscious secondary gain. The patient's responsibility for his or her own life should be gently communicated to prevent unnecessary sequelae.

Post-traumatic psychotherapy should be brief. This is a poor time to suggest that the patient consider additional psychotherapy for deeper conflicts or vulnerabilities, although these may be discussed. Emotional progress and insight, once consolidated, should be used in the termination of therapy. Termination, in turn, becomes a reexperienced loss, this time able to be handled and integrated with optimism instead of anxiety alone.

Delayed PTSD. If symptom onset is at least six months following the trauma but the presentation is acute, then treatment principles are similar to those described above. The psychological characteristics which led to the delay of symptoms may portend a less optimistic course (although not necessarily). The patient may feel even less control over his symptoms, since they do not appear directly related to the traumatic event. Nevertheless, serious, even psychotic symptoms often respond to supportive and psychodynamic psychotherapy which includes the reexperiencing and reintegration of the event.

Chronic PTSD. Many clinicians feel that the treatment of chronic PTSD is more difficult, and more pessimistic, than intervention during the acute phase. While this is probably statistically true, two related patient characteristics suggest that a poorer response to treatment may not be related simply to the chronicity of the disorder.

First, patients whose post-traumatic symptoms have been present for a long time may have avoided meaningful psychotherapeutic intervention. Such avoidance is sometimes a personal issue, sometimes related to secondary gain, and often related to the consciously motivated rewards of pending litigation or worker's compensation. Second, patients who have had their symptoms for many months or years often represent a subgroup for whom treatment response was poor when the disorder was acute, and continues to be poor by virtue of the disorder and/or patient, not just chronicity.

Tricyclic antidepressants (Falcon et al., 1985) and lithium carbonate (Kitchner & Greenstein, 1985) have been suggested for some patients; however, most studies and reviews attest the superiority of psychotherapeutic or psychosocial interventions (Grigsby, 1987; Lindberg & Distad, 1985; The Quality Assurance Project, 1985). Behavioral techniques such as exposure are sometimes helpful (Kuch, Swinson, & Kirby, 1985), as are temporary uses of benzodiazepines or other anxiolytics.

Related Psychosocial Disorders. The treatment of psychiatric or psychosocial problems that may accompany post-traumatic syndromes is an important part of total care. Two of the most common are depression and substance abuse.

Depression frequently remits with psychotherapy of PTSD, but should be vigorously treated if it remains behind when other symptoms remit. Substance abuse disorders are considerably more complex, and should usually be treated as if they were primary. That is, the clinician should not expect the substance abuse to disappear with psychotherapy for the Post-traumatic Stress Disorder (and, conversely, the substance abuse treatment program should specifically address PTSD). Increasing self-image, decreasing guilt, and reexperiencing and reintegrating the trauma are common parts of combined substance abuse/PTSD treatment programs for, for example, Vietnam veterans (Jelinek & Williams, 1984; Schnitt & Nocks, 1984).

Finally, many PTSD patients, particularly combat veterans or victims of mass disasters, benefit from lay support groups. Where possible, these groups should have the benefit of psychiatric consultation or participation.

300.02 Generalized Anxiety Disorder

A recent controlled trial of treatments for generalized anxiety (Lindsay et al., 1987) found that although anxiolytic drugs (benzodiazepines) were rapidly and significantly effective at reducing anxiety early in treatment, groups receiving drugs alone tended quickly to relapse. The most significant and consistent improvements were seen in groups receiving cognitive-behavioral therapy or anxiety management training. Nevertheless, most patients who reach the physician's (including the psychiatrist's) office receive anxiolytic medication, and perhaps brief psychotherapy. Choice of drug and dosage schedule should be clearly separated from medication for panic attacks or relief of acute anxiety.

Drug Treatment. Benzodiazepines are the anxiolytics of choice. Treatment may take two forms. First, the medication may be prescribed with the understanding that it will be available for only a short time, while psychotherapy, behavioral treatment, or merely the passage of time remove the source of generalized anxiety. Because of development of tolerance, medication abuse, potential physical dependence, and the long half-life of several of these drugs (e.g., diazepam), the short-half-life benzodiazepines (e.g., oxazepam) are preferred. In spite of many cautions, particularly in the lay literature, benzodiazepines are very effective, quite safe in both therapeutic regimen and overdose, have excellent patient acceptance, and cause few side effects. Except for side-effects profile and half-life, all of the common benzodiazepines, including alprazolam, are similarly effective (Cordingley, Dean, & Hallett, 1985; Dunner et al., 1986; Fontaine et al., 1986).

Reid (1983) suggests a second approach, in which the benzodiazepine need not actually be ingested in order for it to contribute to the patient's improvement. Formation of a therapeutic relationship with a patient often allows therapeutic reassurance and the mere carrying of the medication (perhaps as symbolic representations of the therapist) to supplant the chronic taking of drugs. In this plan, the medication is prescribed on a per-day or per-week basis (e.g., two tablets per day, or 10 tablets per week, no matter when they are taken) rather than in a fixed schedule. This is a logical way to prescribe for Panic Disorder (see p. 246), if one is using benzodiazepines, as well.

Some of the benzodiazepines, notably clorazepate (Zung, 1987) and alprazolam, are said to be effective for depressed mood in patients who are anxious. Careful evaluation of the patient should allow one to separate primary affective disorder with anxiety from primary anxiety disorder with concomitant depression.

Buspirone. The first nonbenzodiazepine anxiolytic to be introduced for many years, buspirone has been heavily studied, but has had insufficient clinical exposure to conclusively establish its usefulness in the U.S. The primary indication for buspirone is chronic or generalized anxiety without panic attacks. It acts quite slowly, often taking two to three weeks for complete effect.

One should begin with small doses, around 5 mg twice a day, increasing to 20–30 mg per day within the first week to 10 days. It has little or no immediate effect, and thus should not be used for acute relief or as-needed anxiolytic treatment. Patients notice little or no medication effect, and should not expect to feel better immediately. Interestingly, patients who have been taking benzodiazepines usually respond poorly to buspirone. Whether this is a pharmacologic effect or is related to buspirone's not providing any immediate feeling of well-being is not clear.

Buspirone provides some advantages, and a couple of disadvantages, in comparison to other anxiolytics (including meprobamate or barbiturates). It apparently has little or no interaction with or potentiation of alcohol or other CNS depressants. It is thus far not known to have a potential for tolerance or physical dependence, and is unlikely to encourage emotional dependence. It is apparently fairly safe in overdose. It does not block the withdrawal effects of alcohol, benzodiazepines, meprobamate, or sedatives/hypnotics, and has little or no anticonvulsant activity. Side effects are occasional and generally benign, including dizziness, headache, nervousness, and lightheadedness (*International Drug Therapy Newsletter*, 1984; Newton et al., 1986).

Other Nonbenzodiazepines. Hydroxyzine is a useful anxiolytic but is somewhat sedative and anticholinergic. Meprobamate, once commonly prescribed for anxiety, is a poor choice because of its limited effectiveness, high addictive potential, and serious withdrawal syndrome.

Some experimental medications, as well as some drugs currently experimental for generalized anxiety, should be briefly mentioned. The tricyclic and MAOI antidepressants have both been prescribed, although they are probably more indicated for primary blockade of panic disorder than for chronic anxiety. Atenolol has been studied outside the U.S. (Saul et al., 1985), as have the benzodiazepine methylclonazepam (Ansseau et al., 1985) and a buspirone relative, gepirone (Csanalosi et al., 1987), all with some success.

Psychotherapy. It is often effective for the therapist to inform the patient that although this condition is quite uncomfortable, it has predictable patterns (and is thus potentially understandable) and is quite separate from more serious, "psychotic" mental illness. The possibility of frequent relapse should be frankly addressed as part of reassurance that the course of the disorder is fairly predictable and is likely to improve with time. As with Panic Disorder (p. 246) intensive or psychoanalytic psychotherapy may be helpful for a few patients; however, it is usually not cost-effective unless there are clear underlying conflicts which the patient is motivated to address, and for which the patient can tolerate psychodynamic exploration.

Many patients with Generalized Anxiety Disorder have personality characteristics or coping styles that must be considered as one shapes the psychotherapeutic plan. Some have anxiety accompanied by considerable dependency or clinging to the clinician. Specific rules for when and how the therapist will be available may alleviate some of the therapist's discomfort and provide an atmosphere of consistency for the patient. It is unreasonable, and usually countertherapeutic, to be so "available" to the patient that he or she is encouraged to call whenever symptoms arise.

Cognitive and Behavioral Treatments. Relaxation training, desensitization, biofeedback, and "stress inoculation" have all been used successfully, with and without medication, for the short-term treatment of anxiety disorders. Relaxation therapy (often including training the patient to carry out the therapy himself or herself) and other, behavioral methods for giving the patient control over his or her anxiety tend to be associated with continued improvement months or years later (Holcomb, 1986; Spencer, 1986; Tarrier & Main, 1986).

Other Treatments. Inhalation of carbon dioxide (diluted with air but in concentrations well above normal expiration) has long been known to alleviate anxiety and "hyperventilation." There is now at least behavioral evidence that carbon dioxide inhalation may provide anxiety reduction which lasts up to several weeks, perhaps because of an operant conditioning effect: weakening of the anxiety response by competitive response to carbon dioxide (Wolpe, 1987). Anecdotal evidence for its effectiveness is frequently reported, with occasional controlled studies (Lanza, 1986). An ancient Chinese remedy, suanzaorentang, was recently studied in a double-blind clinical trial and found to possess anxiolytic effects comparable to diazepam, in doses of 750 mg per day (Chen, Hsie, & Shibuya, 1986).

300.00 Anxiety Disorder Not Otherwise Specified
The treatment of other anxiety disorders should be predicated upon the symptoms presented and the underlying situational and psychodynamic issues elicited during evaluation. Many of the principles mentioned in this chapter may apply. Practical counseling, in an atmosphere of support and reassurance, is a good adjunct to any treatment program. An understanding of the patient's personality or character style, as well as careful evaluation for medical or environmental correlates, increases the opportunity for treatment success.

Chapter 19

Somatoform Disorders

300.70 Body Dysmorphic Disorder (Dysmorphophobia)
300.70 Hypochondriasis (Hypochondriacal Neurosis)
In this section we will discuss the two above disorders together, since there are many similarities and insufficient differentiation in the modern treatment literature to separate them. Similarities in treatment concept with the several other somatoform disorders are apparent as well; the reader is encouraged to examine this entire Somatoform Disorders section for suggestions related to treatment of individual patients with any of these diagnoses.

Two issues that must be addressed before treating a patient for primary hypochondria are the adequate exclusion of medical illness (including brain disease which manifests as delusions of bodily symptoms or dysmorphia) (Takeda et al., 1985) and treatment of accompanying psychiatric disorders which may be giving rise to the anxieties, obsessions, or delusions of bodily disease. The symptomatic treatments below are unlikely to be helpful for patients in whom the source of the illness behavior is, for example, a guilt-ridden depression or a paranoid psychosis.

A practical means for the primary physician to treat hypochondriasis and several other somatoform disorders is described by Kellner (1982a). Patients are given accurate information about the interaction between their emotions and possible physical symptoms; the benign nature of the somatoform disorder is emphasized; and the fact that there is a good medical prognosis is celebrated by the physician. Good physical examinations are performed and the patient is allowed to have regular, brief physician visits. The patient is not allowed to expand his illness behavior into frequent, "as-needed" medical calls, but is strongly encouraged and reassured that he has a consistent place in the physician's appointment schedule.

In hypochondriasis, and to some extent in the other somatoform disorders, concern over loss of the physician (and the object that the physician symbolizes) can be a significant impediment to lasting improvement. Thus, the physician who tells the patient "I have good news. Your tests are all negative. You don't need to come back and see me" may well precipitate further symptoms or complaints which are designed to recover the lost physician or object.

Individual psychotherapy that focuses on the here-and-now complaints, fears, and beliefs of the patient is frequently successful, with good long-term outcome associated with fairly brief symptom duration and the absence of a personality disorder diagnosis. Outcome is not particularly associated with age, sex, severity of symptoms, or severity of anxiety (Kellner, 1983). Psychotropic drugs are effective in reducing anxiety, and for treating patients with mixed psychiatric disorders (Kellner, 1985).

Although patients with somatoform disorders are often felt to be difficult to treat with psychotherapy, when both the primary physician and the psychotherapist can communicate their understanding of the patient's distress, he or she can be engaged in treatment (Galatzer-Levy, 1982). The presence of the psychiatrist as part of a medical team emphasizes the integration of psychiatric issues with medical fears and symptoms.

Traditional insight-oriented psychotherapy can be helpful for patients whose hypochondriasis is symptomatic of neurotic conflict, and who are willing to engage in it. Once the patient has entered treatment, it may be useful to discourage talk about the hypochondriacal symptoms during certain phases of therapy, with the idea that this topic is a resistance and prevents the surfacing of other important material.

Group therapy is a cost-effective alternative to individual psychotherapy or visits to the primary physician, and can provide ventilation, interpersonal relationships, and help with dependency needs.

The source of the illness behavior can be a form of manipulating others or responding to stress, for example, in a patient who wishes to generate guilt in others or bring them closer to him or her. These reasons can be used to develop a psychosocial treatment program which may include the patient, the family, and training in other ways to accomplish the needed aggression, attention, or caring from others. A few behavioral protocols have been described for treating hypochondriasis, disordered body image, or disease phobia. The most common is exposure, which treats the disorder as a phobia (Tearnan et al., 1985).

Monosymptomatic Hypochondriasis. The obsession with a particular serious physical disorder or symptom, such as a delusionally aberrant body image, body smell, internal parasite, or malformation, is frequently associated with a severe personality disorder, psychosis, or organic central nervous system deficit. Evaluation should be vigorous, particularly if one of the senses (e.g., smell, taste, touch) is involved. Treatment often requires antipsychotic medication, even if a brain lesion is present. The high-potency drugs, such as haloperidol (Andrews, Bellard, & Walter-Ryan, 1986) or (outside the U.S.) pimozide, may be helpful.

When talking of disorders of body image or obsessions with bodily defects, it is important that a differentiation be made between patients with a somatoform disorder and those with eating disorders (Anorexia Nervosa, Bulimia Nervosa) or Transsexualism, all of which are addressed elsewhere in this text.

300.11 Conversion Disorder (Hysterical Neurosis, Conversion Type)

Conversion reactions often disappear of their own accord in hours or days—sometimes in response to lost opportunities for secondary gain. In some cases the rapid loss of symptoms is misunderstood as always connoting "malingering."

Response to symptomatic treatment is usually quite good. If symptom removal is the only goal of treatment, then hypnosis or behavior therapy should be considered. Simple suggestion or "magical" symptom removal through amytal interview or other clinical trickery should usually be avoided, and treatment provided in a broader context. Particular attention should be given to making improvement permanent, generalizing it to other maladaptive ways of handling the underlying conflicts that gave rise to the physical symptom.

Suggestion or amytal interview may be used for diagnostic purposes, although mere disappearance of symptoms is not conclusive evidence of their functional origin. The psychiatrist may thus assist when conversion patients present in a general hospital setting, by helping to differentiate conversion from organic symptoms or malingering, and by educating the hospital staff in methods of humane management and approaches to the patient (e.g., discouraging direct confrontation or accusations by staff) (Cohen et al., 1985; Lazara, 1981).

The clinician should establish himself as someone who has genuine respect for the patient and his or her difficulties. He should have a medical background, since up to 25% of patients originally diagnosed by nonpsychiatric physicians to have conversion disorders are eventually found to have organic disease, often of a degenerative type (Watson & Buranen, 1979).

Involvement of the spouse and/or other important family members in the patient's care, with an understanding of the social and psychodynamic issues that may be involved, can promote better communication and decrease the need for future conversion symptoms.

If the patient has a true hysterical neurosis, intensive or psychoanalytic psychotherapy is indicated. Unfortunately, conversion symptoms are nonspecific, and patients with more severe underlying pathology (e.g., personality disorders) may appear clinically similar to those with hysterical neurosis before treatment is begun (Shalev & Munitz, 1986). For those patients, dynamic psychotherapy may help with symptoms but is usually not the best approach in the long run.

Patients with good premorbid adjustment, absence of major psychiatric syndromes, and the presence of a stressful event associated with acute onset of the conversion symptoms are associated with good prognosis. Most patients without severe underlying psychopathology continue to be significantly improved several years after treatment, although for some the conversion reaction is an indicator of ongoing emotional problems or, as mentioned above, developing physical disease.

300.81 Somatization Disorder
(See also Somatoform Pain Disorder—307.80.)

The first tenet of treatment is understanding that patients with Somatization Disorder (or Briquet's syndrome) are not immune from physical illness. It is a serious mistake for any physician, much less a psychiatrist, to underestimate the patient's symptoms and the discomfort that they are causing, or to label them using discriminatory terms (e.g., "crock"). Excellent diagnostic procedures are usually possible without invasive techniques. Excessive medical care is expensive, however, sometimes dangerous, and can usually be avoided (Ries et al., 1981; Zoccolillo & Cloninger, 1986).

There are a number of clinical approaches to the somatizing patient (including those represented among the other somatoform disorders). The primary physician can manage many, if not most, of these patients by developing a good physician–patient relationship, applying rudimentary techniques of behavior modification, expanding the patient's care to include attention to life stresses, treating symptoms conservatively, watching for depression, and understanding the importance of ongoing contact with the patient (Smith, 1985).

The psychiatrist in a consultation-liaison setting can help the nonpsychiatric treatment team both understand the patient's complaints and, perhaps more importantly, understand the concept that because these patients cling to their symptoms for emotional reasons, "care" rather than "cure" is the cornerstone of management (Lichstein, 1986).

Symptomatic outpatient follow-up is recommended for those patients who are willing to engage in psychotherapy. A number of techniques are helpful, including short-term, anxiety-provoking psychotherapy (Sifneos, 1984), relaxation therapy (Johnson, Shenoy, & Langer, 1981), combination approaches such as the coping-rest model (Moss & Garb, 1986), and reality- and insight-oriented group psychotherapies (Schreter, 1980). Each should provide support and mild, tolerable confrontation. In both group and individual therapy, the clinician should be alert for nonsomatic symptoms of underlying conflict (e.g., depression), and be prepared to recognize and treat them accordingly.

Definitive treatment of Somatization Disorder involves the removal of the emotional precursors of multiple medical complaints and/or the channeling of coping mechanisms for those precursors into behaviors or emotions that are more effective for the patient than are the symptoms of Somatization Disorder. Unfortunately, most clinicians report only limited success for traditional psychodynamic intervention (Karasu, 1979; Kellner, 1975).

Karasu (1979) recommends that the psychotherapist relate to the patient as a physician to a medically ill individual, well informed about the patient's illness. Once this empathy and understanding have been established, a "life alliance" promotes friendly and educational interactions. After several weeks, the patient may eventually be able to explore feelings toward the therapist, feelings toward the symptoms, and the possibility that these are related. Once the patient has meaningful insight into the relationships among affect, behavior, and somatization, symptoms of anxiety or physical distress should lessen. Nevertheless, patients who have expressed feelings in terms of bodily sensation may, by definition, be those who are reluctant to accept a psychotherapeutic approach.

In the absence of serious underlying psychiatric illness, the use of medications to treat this and similar somatoform disorders is not recommended. On the other hand, the psychiatrist should remain aware that somatic symptoms can be atypical presentations of, for example, depression.

307.80 Somatoform Pain Disorder

This disorder, called Psychogenic Pain Disorder in *DSM-III*, should be viewed multidimensionally (Getto & Ochitill, 1982). This places the psychiatrist treating a somatoform disorder into the multidisciplinary group of physicians and others who have a common goal of alleviating and preventing the patient's pain. One important aspect of this approach is that it may allow the patient to accept psychiatric intervention more readily in a situation that the patient perceives as nonpsychiatric.

Another important part of treatment is the clinician's belief that the patient actually feels pain and requires treatment. This—and the corollary belief that the patient is being honest with the physician—may be lacking in many of the patient's previous interactions with physicians. This does not preclude the psychiatrist's expressing his or her belief that even very considerable pain can begin in, and be mediated by, the human mind.

The psychiatrist should be a person who works well within medical settings and is comfortable discussing and evaluating medical illness in his or her patients (Murphy & Davis, 1981). The dual orientations of medicine and psychology offer reassurance that the patient continues to be medically monitored.

One view of Somatoform Pain Disorder compares it to other forms of chronic pain, and recommends treatment along similar lines. Pain clinics, usually found in larger medical institutions, use clear guidelines for evaluation, treatment goals, and attaining those goals. This structuring activity, often in an inpatient setting, transforms a confusing and overwhelming pain experience into one with manageable parts. The patient participates in the program to a great extent, and thereby gains some measure of mastery over feelings and sensations toward which he or she was formerly passive.

The programs are primarily behavioral, with reinforcement for decreasing "pain behavior" as well as for the more obvious goals of decreased use of medication and lessened perception of pain. Biofeedback and group therapy are often used. Since the chronic pain takes place in, and is part of, the patient's family and social life, attention must be paid to education and counseling for the family and preparation for activities of daily living. Such programs generally last for several weeks or months, and frequently have high success rates among patients who have not done well with previous (usually drug-oriented) regimens.

Treatment is sometimes criticized for its emphasis on simply decreasing hospital visits and demands on the physician's time. Such goals should, however, be seen as being attained because the pain behavior is no longer necessary from the patient's viewpoint, and not merely as the result of "punishment" for visiting the clinic. Indeed, reassurance that the doctor and other means of alleviating pain are available is a large part of showing the patient that he or she does not need to *use* the medical facilities to prove that they are there.

Many forms of chronic pain are treated with tricyclic antidepressants and some other psychotropic medications. In some reports, psychogenic pain responds as well. The best patient response often occurs at doses consistent with antidepressant activity; however, it has not been shown that effectiveness of the medication is due to its antidepressant qualities. Some recommend the tricyclics as an early choice, before resorting to inpatient pain control programs.

It is virtually impossible to change severe, often personality-related pain behavior, usually associated with secondary gain, in an outpatient setting. Insight-oriented psychodynamic psychotherapy is not often a treatment of choice, and when applied should carefully isolate the pain symptom from the bulk of the verbal therapy. Supportive therapy may seem helpful, and may serve to keep the patient functioning in his or her social environment, but generally has little more than superficial value.

300.70 Undifferentiated Somatoform Disorder
300.70 Somatoform Disorder Not Otherwise Specified

The treatment of Undifferentiated Somatoform Disorder or Somatoform Disorder Not Otherwise Specified should be based upon the principles already outlined in this section, the presenting symptoms, and the clinician's understanding of the underlying medical and psychological disorders.

Chapter 20

Dissociative Disorders (Hysterical Neuroses, Dissociative Type)

300.14 Multiple Personality Disorder
The treatment of this rare disorder is far more complex and lengthy than that of any of the other, relatively encapsulated dissociative disorders. The condition should not be considered synonymous with schizophreniform disorders, and should not be treated with antipsychotic medication unless indicated by the symptoms presented. The traditional approach, popularized by Thigpen and Cleckley (1957), is intensely psychodynamic or psychoanalytic, often aided by hypnosis. The hypnotic portion of treatment may be used to uncover material for therapeutic exploration outside the trance or, if the clinician is trained in the psychoanalytic use of trance, may be an aid to restructuring the patient's character in such a way as to integrate the various separated parts, each of which is incomplete without the others.

The psychotherapeutic treatment of multiple personality requires sufficient subspecialization that the clinician should either be experienced in this area or seek supervision. The patient, with his or her various, often uncooperative parts, will tend to be demanding and frustrating. Nevertheless, many clinicians feel that when understood as a chronic dissociative Post-traumatic Stress Disorder—that is, arising out of in-

Dissociative Disorders 267

tolerable childhood traumata—Multiple Personality Disorder has an excellent prognosis if treated by an experienced clinician using intensive, prolonged psychotherapy (Kluft, 1987).

The recent marked increase in reported cases of multiple personality patients is difficult to explain. This author believes that much of the increase is related to the "popularity" of the disorder, and particularly its popularity among certain therapists who "specialize" in its treatment. Considerable caution with respect to diagnosis and treatment is indicated for at least the following reasons.

1. Focus on the "multiple personality" aspects of the patient as his or her most interesting characteristics and as sources of extra attention from the therapist creates a setting in which the often highly suggestible patient unconsciously creates (or worsens, by adding additional parts) the very disease being treated. This is especially likely with hypnotic treatments in relatively inexperienced hands (see below).
2. The therapist may be seduced by the notoriety—among other professionals, patients, or the public—of treating these exotic individuals.
3. Individual, especially legal, responsibility for one's actions may be questioned or avoided altogether. Whether or not the patient has Multiple Personality Disorder, to exonerate him from responsibility for his actions is often inappropriate and almost always countertherapeutic.
4. Serious countertransference reactions, including anger, exasperation, exhaustion, and even sexual seduction or violence are not uncommon (Coons, 1986a; Watkins & Watkins, 1984).

Because Multiple Personality Disorder is commonly felt to represent a chronic, global reaction to childhood trauma, some authors suggest early, even childhood diagnosis and treatment (Coons, 1986b).

Hypnotic Treatments. It has long been recognized that patients with dissociative disorders are easily hypnotizable. Spiegel (1984) notes multiple personality patients' spontaneous dissociation to protect themselves from emotional and physical pain. Bliss (1980) even suggests that the core of multiple personality is in unrecognized self-hypnosis, by which the patient has created a number of personalities and allowed experiences or functions to be delegated to alter egos.

Using hypnosis as a means for communicating with and eventually integrating the parts of the patient's personality (which should be clearly understood as *parts*, and not separate personalities) raises the danger that either the therapist or the patient will actually create new parts or "personalities" in response to the highly suggestible emotional milieu. The danger is exacerbated by trance and by the strong implication that the therapist expects, and will be gratified by, the uncovering of additional "personalities."

The process of uncovering, appearing to uncover, or communicating with parts of the personality in trance and then suggesting that they will be remembered by, and integrated with, the dominant personality is simplistic and incomplete. The patient must see his or her parts as parts of an already existing "whole." It is probably countertherapeutic even to refer to each part by a separate name. If this seems unavoidable, one should make it clear that the names are merely labels, and do not connote any acceptance by the therapist that the patient actually contains more than one "person."

No matter what the psychotherapeutic treatment choice, resistances related to repression, denial, secrecy, and crises that threaten to disintegrate the treatment process must be addressed (Coons, 1986a). The anxiety-ridden perceptions, memories, and screened memories that have given rise to dissociative and depressive symptoms must be dealt with, and more adaptive resolutions found. In particular, depression and loss may need to be addressed with either psychotherapy or biological approaches as treatment progresses.

Restraint. A word should be added about the therapeutic use of physical restraint suggested by a few authors (Young, 1986). This technique suggests voluntary, intermittent use of restraints to work through "dangerous" situations of the bringing out and treatment of angry or aggressive parts of the personality, with the aim of providing a physically and emotionally safe environment for both patient and therapist.

This author would suggest great caution in this and other abreactive techniques, and recommends experienced supervision if it is attempted. There is considerable danger of (1) creating a "special" setting for this "special" and potentially gratifying symptom, (2) creating considerable potential for patient abuse and sensationalism, and (3) creating a seductive, "secret" affect-laden experience with the therapist.

300.13 Psychogenic Fugue

Psychogenic Fugue may be considered similar in purpose to amnesia but as involving a necessity for more dissociation from an affect-laden event and/or from the self. Many of the treatment techniques described in the next section on Psychogenic Amnesia are useful for fugue. The clinician should expect treatment to be more lengthy, consistent with the more massive defensive mechanism (or with a premorbid character structure which was predisposed to it). Since Psychogenic Fugue may last longer than amnesia, therapeutic strategies that include more intense psychodynamic therapy are often suggested. At the least, a continuing supportive relationship with a psychotherapist is recommended for preventing future dissociative episodes.

Many treatment techniques, particularly hypnosis and amytal interview, are aimed at recovering the patient's memory for things that happened during the fugue state. As was implied in the previous section on multiple personality, caution should be used when hypnotic techniques are used to "reconstruct" memory, since what may appear to be restitution of old memory is often actually construction of new "memory" (Orne, 1979). In some patients, this is not a significant problem; however, when the recovering of a specific memory is important (e.g., for legal reasons), hypnosis should be used only with the greatest of care in order to assure that the "memory" is not actually an iatrogenic confabulation which becomes permanently imbedded in the patient's past.

Symptom-oriented approaches such as hypnosis, amytal interview, or even brief psychotherapy sometimes imply that the patient's symptoms are interesting and worth keeping because of the attention they generate. When possible, psychotherapeutic approaches should try to uncover the stressful and conflictual sources of the fugue, and provide alternative needs for dealing with the painful affects against which fugue is a defense.

300.12 Psychogenic Amnesia

The most common clinical presentation of Psychogenic Amnesia is in an emergency room or military clinic, often following severe emotional trauma (which may be accompanied by physical injury). In spite of the fact that Psychogenic Amnesia frequently clears without treatment, early intervention to prevent stabilization of the amnesia and its incorporation into the patient's emotional structure is recommended.

Both active and passive treatment methods have been advocated. Since amnesia produces anxiety in family and friends, there is usually pressure to alleviate it quickly. Barbiturate interviews and hypnotic techniques often give access to the suppressed memories.

One may suggest that the patient will recall the events upon arousal; however, most clinicians prefer to allow the *patient* to make this decision, saying something like: "When you become alert, you will be able to remember as much of our interview as you like; the rest will come to you in time, when you are ready to recall it." This allows the mind to use the amnesia for its intended, defensive purpose while eliminating as much of the symptom as is practical.

The fact that patients almost always have access to their memories under hypnosis or during barbiturate interview is reassuring to patients and families, and helps establish the diagnosis (MacHovec, 1981; Ruedrich, Chu, & Wadle, 1985). Small amounts of IV amphetamine during barbiturate procedures, to titrate the level of consciousness and allow more verbal interchange, is helpful for some patients.

Conservative Treatment. Another approach, which may be used alone or in combination with the above methods, is that of providing a supportive environment in which the psyche may allow its barriers to be lowered. In some such settings, long, supportive interviews with the patient allow him or her to discuss at length the memories, associations, and feelings that come to mind. In others, the memory returns over a period of days or weeks of support and gentle reminders. Dependency should not be encouraged; brief psychotherapy may be aimed at helping the patient find defenses other than amnesia by which he or she can cope with the emotions and stressful event that precipitated the symptoms.

No matter what method is used, the conflict that precipitated the amnesia should be explored if the patient can tolerate such investigation. One should recall that in this, as well as other neurotic behaviors, the precipitating event is *idiosyncratically* associated with inner conflict, and may not appear particularly stressful to persons other than the patient.

300.60 Depersonalization Disorder (Depersonalization Neurosis)
Nemiah (1980) provides an elegant description of the clinical features of Depersonalization Disorder which are relevant to its treatment and prognosis. He notes that the disorder tends to be chronic, but that many patients experience long periods without symptoms of depersonalization. The association of acute anxiety with onset (or reemergence) of symptoms suggests that many of the treatment approaches for acute

and chronic anxiety (q.v.) may be helpful in the management of symptomatic periods.

Muller (1982) describes successful treatment of acute, severe depersonalization with benzodiazepines. Blue (1979) suggests psychotherapy in which the therapist is quite directive, gaining control of the therapeutic relationship with positive expectations for rapid behavioral change, requiring the patient to think about his or her feelings of depersonalization, and even using paradoxical intention, in which the patient is asked to try to recreate the symptoms.

Barbiturate interviews or hypnosis may provide access to the source of depersonalization symptoms for diagnostic purposes or to provide material for psychotherapy; these acute techniques do not appear to have lasting therapeutic value by themselves.

The patient is usually aware of the dissociative episodes. In those situations in which some *belle indifférence* is present, many clinicians would speak of Briquet's syndrome and apply treatment measures related to those for hysteria (q.v.). In most patients, however, the symptoms are quite frightening.

The depth of psychopathology in persons with severe depersonalization is seen by some as a contraindication to psychoanalytic psychotherapy; however, progress in the analysis of character disorders and disorders of the self should cause the clinician to consider consultation with, or referral to, a qualified psychoanalyst.

Although feelings of "unreality" may sound psychotic, this condition appears clinically and biochemically unrelated to the thought disorders, an observation that is consistent with the lack of success of neuroleptic medication or ECT. Depersonalization sometimes protects against the painful affects of depression. Antidepressant medication may be helpful, but occasionally induces manic psychosis.

300.15 Dissociative Disorder Not Otherwise Specified

Treatment of patients with dissociative symptoms which do not fit any of the above *DSM-III-R* categories should focus upon the symptoms and syndromes as they present, and upon the apparent underlying psychopathology. As implied in the preceding pages, the presence of dissociation suggests a massive defensive effort in the patient. This, in turn, suggests a relatively acute trauma which has rekindled earlier conflicts by virtue of either the strength of the conflicts or the strength of the trauma.

For those patients with relatively good premorbid functioning and/or well-encapsulated symptoms, a symptomatic approach is likely to be helpful. One example is the treatment of some forms of sleepwalking (somnambulism). Many such patients, after sleepwalking as children, are free of the symptom until some external stress appears in an otherwise uneventful life (e.g., an important loss). Treatment approaches described by Reid (1975; Reid, Ahmed, & Levie, 1981) indicate that symptom removal can occur without psychodynamic complications.

For most dissociative disorders, however, it is important to address both the symptoms and their sources. Dissociative syndromes usually do not lead to serious disability, but return of symptoms at some future time is common.

Chapter 21

Sexual Disorders

21A: PARAPHILIAS

General Treatment Principles

There are a number of general treatment considerations common to many of the paraphilias. Although treatment is commonly seen as quite difficult because of the apparent lack of dysphoria, great physical gratification, and frequently associated personality disorders, patients often come to psychiatric attention in one way or another. The psychiatrist should be prepared to treat the patient, or at least to talk with him or her about treatment before referral to a subspecialist. Before talking specifically about the sexual symptoms, it should be pointed out that patients with paraphilias are prone to other kinds of problems, including marital and family difficulty, social crises that may give rise to adjustment disorders and depression, and anxiety or depression during times at which the paraphilic behavior produces guilt or shame.

The clinician who treats these patients must have a therapeutic orientation rather than a punitive one, and must be comfortable with his or her own feelings regarding these sometimes criminal patients. This is particularly important when the patient's behavior is exploitive, aggressive, or pedophilic. Serious manifestations of countertransference will almost certainly arise, and must be understood and managed.

It is practical, although not always psychodynamically accurate, to draw distinctions among those paraphilias that do not intrude upon the wishes of others (e.g., Fetishism, Transvestic Fetishism), those that intrude but are nonviolent (e.g., Exhibitionism, Voyeurism), and those that are not only intrusive but physically aggressive and potentially injurious to others (e.g., Sexual Sadism, Pedophilia). Patients with primarily aggressive disorders sometimes manifested in sexual terms (e.g., rapists) are addressed to some extent in this section; however, their conditions are more properly seen as disorders of impulse control, antisocial behavior, and the like.

The patient may come to treatment in a variety of ways. One should be suspicious of the individual who requests treatment simply because he "wants to change." Far more often, some sort of family, social, or legal crisis is the motivating factor. One must take great pains to clarify this before deciding whether to accept the patient for treatment. Patients anticipating trial on criminal charges or otherwise being coerced into treatment are not in a position to make long-term treatment decisions. Once the case has been settled in some way, however, patients who seek (or remain in) treatment often have a good prognosis.

It is not always necessary for the patient to be completely committed to treatment at the outset. If, for example, a marital crisis or a condition of probation brings the patient to the psychiatrist for a few visits, there is an opportunity to discuss treatment motivation and coercion, and to work to motivate the patient further (e.g., "I know you don't want to be here, but perhaps we can use this time to explore some ways to make your life go more smoothly"). There are also certain situations in which treatment may be forced upon the patient. These usually occur in correctional settings, although courts can order outpatient medication in some jurisdictions, especially outside the U.S.

Paraphilic behavior is often associated—by patients or clinicians—with some transient stress. If a disorder is clearly chronic, the therapist should not allow the patient to rationalize or devalue the symptom with statements such as "The job pressures were too great" or "I understand now that the whole thing happened because my wife was pregnant." On the other hand, patients in insight-oriented psychotherapy should view the paraphilic behavior as a symptom of conflict (and thus as worthy of exploration by clinician and patient), rather than as a heinous and irreversible part of the personality. Even though many of these conditions are refractory to therapy, punitive attitudes for punishment's sake have no place in the treatment program.

There are three primary kinds of treatment for many paraphilic disorders and a fourth, combination approach. *Psychoanalytically oriented psychotherapy* is helpful for many patients who meet the usual criteria of motivation, ego strength, intelligence, and so forth. There are many anecdotal reports of success with patients, but no controlled outcome studies.

Behavioral paradigms vary considerably in effectiveness. Masturbatory satiation and covert sensitization have shown considerable success. Aversion therapy has been successful for some conditions, but not for others. These are described in more detail in the sections that follow.

Antiandrogenic medication shows great clinical promise but its use is fraught with social and political difficulties. It is described in more detail in the section on Pedophilia.

Finally, *combinations* of behavioral, psychotherapeutic, and psychosocial approaches, such as that developed by Abel et al. (1984) and described in the section on Pedophilia, are probably the best overall approach for many patients.

No matter what form of treatment is chosen, many authors recommend some level of participation by the patient's family. Kentsmith and Eaton (1979) particularly recommend counseling for spouses, conjoint therapy, and/or participation of the spouse as a co-therapist in various treatment programs. This not only helps the patient, but allays family anxiety and increases the spouse's acceptance of the patient and the treatment.

Spouses (or patients) who loudly complain that the fetishistic behavior is intractable or ruining their relationship can often be found to be scapegoating the paraphilia. In such cases, complete treatment must include a serious attempt by all involved to uncover other, often nonsexual issues which may be contributing to family difficulties.

302.40 Exhibitionism

Exhibitionism is among the most common paraphilias presenting to the psychiatrist's office. The patient's resistance to change, either with treatment or with time, approaches that of pedophilia, although it is far less intrusive or exploitive for victims. A number of treatment methods have been tried, including those discussed under General Treatment Principles.

Both antiandrogenic medications and the behavioral/psychosocial combination described in the section on Pedophilia are effective, although antiandrogenic medication is rarely the treatment of choice. Case reports of success with hypnotherapy (Mutter, 1981) and cognitive-behavioral approaches (Snaith & Collins, 1981) imply success; however, there is no general acceptance of these methods. Simple hypnotic suggestion alone is useless. Lamontagne and Lesage (1986) describe a case of covert sensitization with success at two-year follow-up.

Individual psychotherapy can be useful for those patients who fill the usual criteria, provided motivation continues and denial is not allowed to exert too great a resistive influence. Group psychotherapy has been a common approach, with a number of anecdotal reports of success. Participation or co-treatment of spouses of exhibitionists is advocated by many (Bastani & Kentsmith, 1980). Treatment approaches that focus on the situational components of exhibitionism and other impulsive paraphiliac behaviors, which often appear strikingly obsessive and anxiety-related, may be helpful (Smaith & Collins, 1981).

302.81 Fetishism

The treatment of fetishism rarely involves concerns about criminality or danger to others. Presenting complaints generally focus on guilt or difficulty with one's sexual partner. If the complaint is mild, education about the condition and its benign course may alleviate the patient's anxiety about, for example, whether his or her symptom indicates deep-seated mental illness. It is necessary that the therapist be comfortable with this sort of "permission" for the patient to practice his sexual preference. In situations in which the guilt is more significant, the patient recognizes the fetishistic symptom as only one of a constellation of neurotic symptoms, and/or the fetishism interferes with desired or necessary activities in other spheres, more intensive treatment is needed.

There is disagreement in the literature about the usefulness of the various psychotherapeutic, behavioral, biological, and hypnotherapeutic treatments. This author prefers psychodynamically oriented treatment aimed either at resolution of underlying conflicts or at development of more efficient ego defenses. Once this approach to treatment is undertaken, it is important that the therapist not ally himself or herself with the symptom-producing portion of the patient's ego. Thus, although the symptom should be seen as neither good nor bad, it must be confronted as something that is undesirable. This is particularly true if the fetishism has led to some sort of mild criminal activity such as stealing women's underclothing.

Wise (1985) and others have noted the potential usefulness of behavioral paradigms such as aversive conditioning (electrical shock, apomorphine injections), covert sensitization (see below), snapping rubber bands attached to the wrist (see below), and so forth. Masturbatory satiation, useful in many paraphilias, can be helpful in fetishism as well (see section on Pedophilia).

Involving the patient's sexual partner in treatment is imperative if marital difficulty is part of the presentation, or if the spouse has rejected the sexual behavior. Sex education is important, and should take place in a conjoint setting if possible.

302.89 Frotteurism
The general understanding and treatment of Frotteurism is often seen as similar to those of Exhibitionism and Voyeurism. There are no controlled studies of treatments for Frotteurism in the literature. The fact that Frotteurism (or *toucherism*) involves physical contact with a victim, unlike Voyeurism or Exhibitionism, implies more inappropriate intrusion, and perhaps a greater potential for escalation to the more aggressive disorders. Freund describes patients whose symptoms overlap among Frotteurism, Exhibitionism, Voyeurism, and obscene telephone calls, and suggests that these may be seen as distorted counterparts of normal human courtship behavior (Freund & Blanchard, 1986; Freund, Scher, & Hucker, 1984).

In cases that appear intractable or particularly aggressive, antiandrogenic medication may be considered (see next section).

302.20 Pedophilia
A famous philosopher, upon his second arrest and lengthy sentence for Pedophilia, was asked why he returned so quickly to the behavior when he knew his punishment would be severe. He replied, in effect, "Because it is worth it." This statement seems to reflect the intractability of Pedophilia, an intractability that is sometimes common to the other paraphilias but which, for a variety of reasons, seems more prominent in those who molest children.

It is not possible in this text to differentiate in detail groups of pedophilic offenders. The importance of baseline testing and categorization will be pointed out, however. Careful initial evaluation, with penile plethysmography if possible, is imperative to clarify treatment objectives and—as a beginning for treatment—breach the denial almost always seen in the patient. This assumes that most patients are male; treatment of the female pedophilic (usually incestuous) will be only briefly addressed.

Pedophilics almost uniformly describe their behavior as limited to one form of offense (the one for which they were caught), a posture also held by other paraphilics. Thus, the patient discovered in incest may say (and indeed believe) that he has no interest in other children, or the person caught with an adolescent boy may deny any interest in prepubescent children. In a large number of cases, however, standardized penile plethysmography produces graphic evidence of arousal to several ages and sexes of children. The results can then be shown to the patient and used as a foundation for therapy.

Treatment of Pedophilia is often complicated, or constrained, by legal conditions such as probation, incarceration, or loss of custody of one's children. In some cases, these are used to advantage, for example as motivating factors and barriers to denial. In others, society's legitimate need to protect its children interferes with treatment voluntariness and confidentiality.

Ethical and legal decisions regarding breach of confidentiality to protect potential victims must sometimes be made. Most states, for example, have reporting criteria which are so strict that should an actively pedophilic patient come voluntarily for treatment, the psychiatrist (or other mental health professional) must report him to a law enforcement or child protective agency.

The possibility of suicide after discovery of pedophilic activity is significant, particularly in the professional person or one who is highly visible in the community. This is true as well, but to a lesser extent, for public discovery of any of the other paraphilias.

Psychotherapy. The principles of psychotherapeutic treatment are similar to those for the other paraphilias. There is a psychodynamic assumption of immature or improperly fixated choice of sexual objects, whether because of basic defects in development per se or because of regression based upon underlying depression, organic impairment, or other significant psychopathology. The insight-oriented psychotherapies are not well accepted for this disorder, however. Once the patient has become visible, society demands more rapid, observable modes of treatment, which can be given under at least a semblance of social control. The social magnitude of the pedophilic activity being greater than that for any of the other paraphilias, the opportunity for denial, guilt, self-castigation, marital problems, and the like is also greater. Conjoint marital therapy, or cotherapy of one's spouse, should be accomplished whenever possible.

Biological Reduction of Sexual Drive. Biological treatments are often recommended for Pedophilia, particularly aggressive forms, as well as other disorders in which sexual and aggressive drives combine to give rise to socially intractable behavior. Surgical approaches, including castration and stereotaxic surgery, are carried out in some parts of the world, but only very rarely in North America. There is considerable doubt about the specificity of orchiectomy in paraphilic disorders, since a great deal of the neurochemical and hormonal activity involved arises outside the testes.

Antiandrogenic Medications. These are a more palatable method of sex-drive reduction. The most common agents currently in use are medroxyprogesterone acetate (MPA) and cyproterone acetate (CPA). The former is available throughout North America, although not generally approved for sex-drive reduction in the U.S. The latter is available only outside the U.S. Both are effective in controlling deviant hypersexuality and paraphilia by reducing libido and overt sexual behavior.

There are now a large number of controlled and uncontrolled studies that attest to the safety and effectiveness of both drugs (Berlin & Mienecke, 1981; Bradford & Tawlak, 1987; Freund, 1980; Gagne, 1981; Herrmann & Beach, 1980; Micheroli & Battegay, 1985; Wincze, Bansai, & Malamud, 1986). Nevertheless, and in spite of society's great need for treatment and control of pedophilic and/or aggressive sex offenders, these medications are inaccessible to most patients.

One reason for their nonavailability is the perception of a "coercive" setting, in which the patient may have to choose between consenting to the medication or being incarcerated. Another has to do with a misperception, in this author's opinion, of the dangers of adverse medication effects. These are indeed complex and must be understood by any physician who prescribes MPA or CPA; however, the disorders for which they are indicated are so devastating for the patient and those around him that the risk-benefit ratio would appear favorable in many cases. Finally, it is clear that society itself, while complaining about our lack of treatment modalities for these patients, is angry and fearful, and does not want them to be treated as "sick" if this means avoiding incarceration.

Some of the advantages of pharmacologic treatment include a therapeutic posture that is medical rather than punitive, effects that are reversible in most cases, the ability to preserve some secondary sex characteristics and appropriate sexual behavior in some patients, and the ability to provide the medication on an infrequent, depot basis.

MPA, CPA, and related drugs must not be given in a therapeutic vacuum. Psychotherapy to address changes in the patient's symptoms is imperative. Treatment dropout is common, particularly when one tries to give the medication without appropriate psychosocial support. Some of the reasons for noncompliance are denial of the chronicity of the disorder, a wish to return to the highly gratifying paraphilic behavior, lowered self-image and the need to punish oneself, and specific stresses or crises (e.g., marital problems, job loss, substance abuse).

Behavioral Approaches. Conditioning programs, primarily aversive ones, are perhaps the most widely used treatment approach. Various success rates are reported, usually with optimistic results for the first few months (especially while the patient is either in active treatment or under legal scrutiny). Some of the techniques are similar to those used for the other paraphilias, and include negative reinforcers such as electric shock, apomorphine injections, and so forth. Conditioning to milder shocks or the use of the "rubber band" technique (in which the therapist or patient snaps a rubber band against the patient's skin as a reminder) have largely replaced the more severe reinforcers.

During the past decade, emphasis has moved from passive aversion therapy to self-management programs (including self-administration of aversion) and sexual skills training (Marks, 1981a, b). These treatments are often similar to those for phobic and obsessive-compulsive symptoms; however, several highly specific techniques have shown particular promise:

> *Fading,* in which fantasies are gradually shifted from deviant to conventional sexual contact during periods of sexual arousal. The patient may focus on visual stimuli (such as photographic slides which automatically fade from one kind of scene to another) or fantasy while masturbating (Laws, 1985).
> *Masturbatory satiation* involves carefully designed instructions to masturbate to orgasm with conventional fantasy or stimuli, and then to continue masturbation for up to an hour while visualizing the deviant object(s).
> *Covert sensitization* pairs fantasies of deviant arousal (or, more effectively, pre-arousal scenes) with immediate "switching" of the fantasy to terrible consequences (e.g., getting caught, being sent to prison, hurting an innocent child).

Combination Treatments. Abel and colleagues (1984) have developed a treatment system which provides intensive use of covert sensitization, masturbatory satiation, sex education, social skills training, and other psychosocial concepts in a group setting. The program, which is available from the address given in the reference list, provides roughly 40 hours of therapist and group contact and another 40 to 50 hours of "homework." The patient receives instructions for specific masturbatory and covert sensitization techniques, records his practice sessions, and discusses them with the therapist and group.

Outcome for patients who complete this program, most of whom remain in follow-up care, is good, given the specific patients for whom it is recommended. There is some overlap with patients who are candidates for antiandrogenic medication, and some controversy about which may be more effective; however, the Abel et al. program can be set up with little social or legal interference, does not require exclusively psychiatric therapists, and, particularly when provided in a group setting, is extremely cost-effective.

Incest. Pedophilic incest involves all of the above treatment considerations, with greater attention to the family dynamics involved. Although many pedophilics categorically deny that they are attracted to their own children, the possibility (or probability) cannot be ignored. Conversely, the incestuous offender is virtually always aroused by other children as well, his or her own children being more readily available and less likely to tell other adults.

There are a number of programs for families involved in incestuous relationships; it is likely that each member requires treatment. Unfortunately, reporting laws which may be necessary for the protection of victims have a chilling effect on some families who might otherwise seek treatment. There are apparently no studies that differentiate treatment of incestuous pedophiles from other pedophilic offenders.

302.83 Sexual Masochism

The treatment of Sexual Masochism per se, which is now known to be less a disorder of women than was once thought, is (like that of the other paraphilias) actually the treatment of only those masochistic persons who come to clinical attention. There is little in the literature about treatment, although much discussion and many case reports exist on the topic of masochism in general. The clinical cases described in those publications often do not approximate the *DSM-III-R* diagnosis.

Superficial symptomatic treatment with such methods as assertiveness training, bolstering of self-image and self-worth, and the like, may be helpful for some patients (e.g., those who have in the past accepted a "victim" role but are no longer satisfied with it). If evaluation reveals roots of the masochism in depression, *ennui*, or existential apathy, then specific treatment for these (psychotherapeutic and/or pharmacologic) may be helpful.

More intensive psychotherapy, aimed at discovering and resolving causative conflicts and or developing more efficient, less destructive defense mechanisms, is indicated for those patients who can utilize and tolerate this treatment approach. This sexual behavior, like the other paraphilias, will retain its gratifying value for a long time and will probably be used during periods of regression.

302.84 Sexual Sadism
Once this disorder has been differentiated from primarily violent, quasi-sexual behaviors, decisions about treatment may be divided into two approaches, neither of which is well addressed in the literature.

For those patients who inflict physical or emotional suffering on nonconsenting others, especially when the disorder is not marked by dysphoria, the social and legal issues discussed earlier in the sections on Pedophilia and on General Treatment Principles become important. Society may dictate control, prescribe certain treatments, or constrain other treatment approaches, as already discussed.

Antiandrogenic medication may be necessary and should be considered when the protection of others is an issue. In the absence of dysphoria, however (or at least discomfort induced by threat of arrest, unemployment, or divorce), adequate consent may be impossible to obtain.

For those patients who practice Sexual Sadism with a consenting partner, the presence of dysphoria during some phase (e.g., between sexual activities) or threat of family loss may bring the patient to treatment. Behavioral approaches similar to those already discussed are worthy of consideration (e.g., fading, masturbatory satiation, combination approaches).

Sometimes a cooperating partner is severely injured. Such cases usually indicate severe psychopathology in both partners, and necessitate protection of the victim even if his or her participation seems "consenting." It goes without saying that this issue is all the more important when it involves persons unable to consent (e.g., minors, elderly or incompetent individuals). In such situations, control of the sadist, with appropriate legal constraints, must be part of the treatment.

302.30 Transvestic Fetishism (Transvestism)
One of the most important treatment considerations in Transvestic Fetishism (Transvestism) is that its resemblance to transsexualism or homosexuality is only superficial. Treatment principles are related to those for Fetishism. Issues of anxiety, guilt, social difficulty, and family

dissatisfaction are usually more prominent than in other paraphilias, since the symptoms are more visible, are probably less common, and require more effort to carry out. Unlike simple Fetishism, the clinician usually should not give "permission" for the activity.

Treatment is frequently sought because of discovery by a spouse or age-related changes. In this regard, both Transvestism and Fetishism are much more erotic in adolescence and early adulthood than later in life. Mature and older transvestites associate their cross-dressing with feelings of relaxation and reassurance more than with sexual activity (Croughan et al., 1981; Frances & Wise, 1987).

Psychotherapy is the treatment of choice. Wise (1979) described some of the psychodynamic underpinnings and tasks of therapy, including identification of important losses, reassurance of gender identity, and recognition of the hostility and aggression often implied by transvestic behaviors (Frances & Wise, 1987). Wise also recommends that the therapist never encourage the spouse to tolerate or participate in the patient's fetishistic activities, but rather ally herself with parts of the patient (and of the family) that are working toward change.

As implied above, the clinician should not confuse treatment for Transvestism with that for transsexualism. Feminizing hormones and surgery have no place in the management of this disorder. Brantley and Wise (1985) describe the use of diethylstilbestrol to reduce cross-dressing impulses in a gender-dysphoric, 65-year-old patient, and suggest that antiandrogenic drugs may be of use in some patients.

302.82 Voyeurism

The symptoms of the true voyeur are often as resistant as those of the exhibitionist, although the former's dangerousness to society and intrusiveness upon those around him may be less. Treatment approaches are similar to those for paraphilias such as Exhibitionism. Family, social, and legally related considerations are likewise important. This author does not recommend antiandrogenic treatment for patients whose primary disorder is Voyeurism in the absence of accompanying chronic symptoms of violence, exploiting of children, or intractable hypersexuality.

302.90 Paraphilia Not Otherwise Specified

The treatment of individuals who fall into this residual category should be predicated upon their presenting symptoms and underlying psychopathology. The extent of which treatment should be vigorously pursued by the clinician, and the extent to which the more invasive therapies (e.g., antiandrogenic drugs) should be used, depends in large measure upon how intrusive or injurious the paraphilia is for persons other than the patient, upon the depth of dysphoria attached to the symptoms, and upon the magnitude of the social and legal implications of the repeated paraphilic behavior.

21B: SEXUAL DYSFUNCTIONS

General Treatment Principles

The treatment of psychosexual dysfunction has been extensively discussed by a number of authors, from a variety of clinical points of view. The well-known and often highly successful Masters and Johnson techniques will be briefly touched upon, but are described in more detail elsewhere (Masters & Johnson, 1970). It should be noted that superficial knowledge of these and other treatment modalities is insufficient for their successful use.

Graber (1981) suggests that most physicians and psychotherapists with legitimate clinical interest can assume a role in the treatment of specific sexual dysfunctions. Marmor (1982), however, notes that psychiatrists tend to see patients who have already been to other therapists, and who thus may have deeper problems or be more difficult to treat. It is now clear that the treatment of sexual dysfunctions is much more likely to be successful when carried out by professionals with specific training and experience, and that the dangers of countertransference or inappropriate behavior by the therapist are reduced by training, experience, and clinical consultation.

Several of the *DSM-III-R* sexual dysfunctions fall under the rubric of *desire, arousal,* or *orgasm*. Patients with disorders of sexual desire tend to have deeper psychopathological reasons for their conditions, and may benefit most from psychodynamic or psychoanalytic treatment (although situational factors, particularly in those patients in whom symptoms are of recent onset, may be more important). Disorders of orgasm, on the other hand, are more likely to be successfully treated behaviorally or with other short-term approaches, in spite of psychodynamic factors.

Limited treatment objectives, often aimed at a single dysfunction or symptom, may eliminate the complaint. Removal of the sexual dysfunction may be a catalyst for growth in other areas of one's self and the relationships involved; however, more comprehensive approaches, often involving the sexual partner as well, are usually indicated.

In spite of the financial and practical temptations to treat individuals and couples on an outpatient basis within the traditional once-a-week context, the original Masters and Johnsons recommendation for two or more weeks of daily, intensive work has stood the test of time. This approach tests the motivation of the couple, weeds out many patients for whom treatment may be unsuccessful, establishes the dedication of both partners to the importance of their sexual relationship and their marriage, fosters an intensive immersion in the treatment method that would otherwise be diluted by the days between treatment sessions, and allows more rapid improvement than would occur with weekly outpatient scheduling.

Heiman and LoPiccolo (1983), however, found little difference in eventual outcome between daily and weekly treatment (15 sessions of each). The same group found no differences in effectiveness of therapy for erectile failure, premature ejaculation, or female orgasmic function between single therapists (whether sex-matched or not) and traditional male-and-female cotherapist treatment (LoPiccolo et al., 1985).

Methods of sex therapy have changed somewhat since Masters and Johnson's early publications. However, the therapist still must understand the basic tenets of treatment modules such as "sensate focus" exercises, help with attitudinal change, therapeutic "permission," correcting misinformation or faulty learning, and removal of emotional and social roadblocks that impede sexual expression (Rosenbaum, 1985).

Prognosis in sex therapy is generally associated with quality of the relationship between the partners, motivation of the couple, accurate assessment of the sexual relationship, and to some extent the presence of improvement early in treatment (Hawton & Catalan, 1986). Many writers feel that the motivation must include motivation or insight into one's conflicts and interpersonal communications, and not just "cookbook" methods (Cole, 1985).

Psychotropic Medication. Although no specific psychotropic medications are indicated in sexual dysfunction, and authors sometimes disagree about their place in its treatment, the use of drugs for underlying disorders such as depression or disorganized thinking is generally accepted. Alleviation of an accompanying disorder may by itself improve sexual function, particularly when the sexual symptoms are related to depression.

The more common situation is that in which the sexual dysfunction is caused (or appears to be caused) by the medication. The neuroleptics and antidepressants are particularly likely to cause problems. Most of these are reversible or can be balanced with other clinical needs (Harrison et al., 1986). Trazodone raises additional concerns because of the possibility of painful priapism.

Nonpsychiatric Medications. Many other medications, as well as surgical treatments and irradiation, affect sexual functioning. Oral contraceptives have been reported to both impair and enhance sexual performance and desire in women (Bancroft et al., 1980). Many antihypertensives have been implicated as well. The complete list is too long to address in this text. The emotional and psychosocial importance of sexual functioning makes sexual symptoms a common focus for psychosomatic responses to virtually any drug, particularly in men. When such complaints arise, the physician should review the known side effects of the medication involved, consider the probability that the patient's complaint is a physiologic one, change or adjust the medication if possible, and bear in mind the likelihood of emotional overlay.

Sexual Dysfunction After Surgery or Irradiation. The issues above should be considered when counseling the patient who has had surgery or radiotherapy, particularly that which may be disfiguring or related to cancer. Many such complaints are treated by the primary physician, surgeon, or oncologist. Surgical treatments for disorders such as prostatic cancer or carcinoma of the cervix appear in some studies to be less sexually damaging than irradiation (Bergman et al., 1984; Siebel, Freeman, & Graves, 1980). Frank and caring explanations of the treatment, with discussions, for example, of myths about pelvic cancer and its treatment, markedly increase chances for good return of sexual functioning and—not coincidentally—preservation of intimacy between the patient and his or her partner.

There are a number of medical/sexual disorders that may initially be treated by the nonpsychiatric physician, usually because of relationship to a known organic cause. Sexual dysfunction in diabetics, for example, is well studied, and indeed may be the presenting symptom. The dysfunction, in both males and females, is generally related to peripheral neuropathy, and not to treatment with insulin as was once thought (Jensen, 1985).

Successful treatment depends upon discovering the condition (since many patients do not raise the complaint), differentiating the organic from psychogenic factors (el-Bayoumi, el-Sherbini, & Mostafa, 1984), and working with the patient and his or her partner in an understanding, educational manner. Referral for more specialized consultation is often helpful. The therapist, if not a physician, should remain in close contact with the doctor. Treatment usually is incorporated into the overall care program (Schover et al., 1984; Szasz, Paty, & Maurice, 1984). Medical interventions for specific complaints are discussed in the subsections below.

Homosexual Patients. Treatment of specific sexual dysfunction in gay or lesbian patients has not been well addressed in the literature, and no controlled studies could be located for this text. Psychodynamic and psychosocial issues probably take a more prominent role than in heterosexual couples. Brown (1986) examines the relationship of dysfunction among lesbians to cultural homophobia and misogyny and presents a theoretical framework for intervention.

Presenting complaints of homosexual dysfunction should not always be accepted at face value any more than the psychiatrist should accept heterosexual dysfunction as the "only" problem without thorough psychiatric (including medical) investigation. Concerns about AIDS, whether voiced or not, should be carefully addressed. Once this has been carried out and a decision made that sex therapy is indicated, the therapist should evaluate his or her skills and feelings about treating homosexual dysfunction. As in the treatment of other specialized disorders, referral may be indicated.

Psychotherapy vs. Directive Therapy vs. Behavioral Treatments. Kaplan (1986) notes that the basic treatment strategy for all sexual dysfunctions is to modify sexual performance and address immediate defenses through behavioral or directive interventions, and to address resistance with psychotherapy. She points out the commonly recognized problems of "performance anxiety," self-observation to the point of loss of arousal or pleasure, and negative thoughts or "anti-fantasies."

The structured behavioral approaches to treatment of sexual dysfunctions outlined below are quite powerful, particularly for temporary relief, but usually do not address unconscious conflicts and processes, often critical to lasting success. Simply changing sexual behavior and response can sometimes set the stage for emotional change without much additional therapy, however. The reader is referred to Kaplan's more comprehensive work as well (Kaplan, 1979).

SEXUAL DESIRE DISORDERS

302.71 Hypoactive Sexual Desire Disorder
302.79 Sexual Aversion Disorder

Disorders of this phase of sexual activity require greater consideration for psychodynamic psychotherapy than do the other dysfunctions. Nevertheless, ascertaining that the patient has accurate and relevant *information* about sexuality, his or her personal sexual activity, and (often overlooked) reproductive issues is an important first step. This and the nonthreatening but matter-of-fact taking of the complete sexual history, with attention to feelings and activities that are avoided or suppressed in the interview, represent the beginning of the therapeutic relationship and desensitization of the patient.

The most successful behavioral technique involves the prescribing of highly structured tasks, in an authoritative manner, using techniques similar to those recommended by Kaplan (1979) and/or Masters and Johnson (1970). The tasks explore the giving and receiving of pleasure, development of the ability to fantasize, comfort with the sharing of sexual experiences with one's partner, and the broader issue of the relationship between the partners. Treatment should be provided in an atmosphere that can offer consistent and multifaceted attention not only to symptoms, but also to accompanying and peripheral feelings and behaviors.

"Desensitizing" with audiovisual materials, including that which would be called pornography by some readers, is not as universally recommended as in the past. Giving permission to examine such materials ad lib may be helpful; however, indiscriminate use may produce counterproductive increases in anxiety and resistance to therapy (Neidigh & Kinder, 1987).

Decreased sexual interest is occasionally a sign of underlying medical illness (although physical signs, such as erectile failure, are more common). Bancroft and colleagues (1984) report, for example, a man in whom hyperprolactinemia presented in this way and who was successfully treated with bromocriptine. The authors point out the usefulness of sexual counseling for the patient and his wife, even in such a "medical" disorder.

Physiologic assessment of sexual response, including focus on pubococcygeal control, lacks the clinical value it was felt to have a few years ago. Hoon (1984) questions the need for assessment of sexual arousal, particularly in women, in the sterile, artificial context of the laboratory.

A 1986 survey of the American Association of Sexual Educators, Counselors, and Therapists (AASECT) (Kilmann et al., 1986) indicated that discrepancies of sexual desire between partners was the most common problem seen. Success rates for treatment among this experienced group of professionals were reported to be about 53%. The most commonly used methods stressed communication skills, sex education, homework assignments, sensate focus, and discussion of nonsexual individual and/or relationship issues.

Fichten et al. (1983) reported that in females, sensate focus exercises in combination with a temporary ban on intercourse led to significant increases in enjoyment of noncoital sexual activity. Snyder and Berg (1983), in a small study, suggested that marital dissatisfaction was correlated with lack of treatment success (and with marital distress) after sex therapy. This study agrees in part with one by Hartman (1983a,b), who found that in couples complaining of sexual difficulties who received both sex therapy and marital therapy in a balanced, crossover design, women showed greater improvement as a result of the sex therapy, whereas men showed a trend favoring greater improvement from the marital therapy.

SEXUAL AROUSAL DISORDERS

Although more physically visible and anxiety-producing in males, the increasing ability of women to recognize inhibitions in sexual arousal as something that interferes with pleasure leads individuals of both sexes to seek treatment. In addition, a large segment of the public now knows that there are many treatment techniques available.

302.72 Female Sexual Arousal Disorder

Many treatment characteristics are similar to those just discussed under Hypoactive Sexual Desire Disorder and Sexual Aversion Disorder, including "pleasuring" prescribed by the therapist but taking place in privacy. A female therapist is recommended in most cases. Initially, there is a proscription against genital stimulation; later it is allowed, but orgasm is avoided. Most techniques are similar to the behavioral concept of desensitization (not the same as desensitizing with erotic literature), with each step designed to create little or no opportunity for "failure" (e.g., making initial physical contact brief). The threat of "failure" is more important in Male Erectile Disorder.

This symptomatic treatment should not be carried out without considering educational, psychotherapeutic, and sometimes religious needs. Outcome is generally optimistic (Fichten, Libman, & Brender, 1983), although few outcome studies exist. This is further discussed in the section on Inhibited Female Orgasm.

302.72 Male Erectile Disorder

Non-*DSM-III-R* causes of erectile dysfunction should be ruled out, most of which are best treated by nonpsychiatric physicians. Erectile dysfunction is still considered "impotence" by many. Urologists and endocrinologists are sometimes unaware of the psychiatric differential diagnosis and accede to patients' requests for testosterone injections or penile prostheses. These have their place in a few cases, as do some newer treatments with dopamine agonists, intracorporeal injections, and alpha-2-adrenergic receptor blockers (Baum, 1987).

Endocrine and other systemic causes should be ruled out. Restoration of libido and erectile ability is usually possible when endocrine causes can be found (except for those related to diabetes) (Braunstein, 1983). The effect of drugs (prescribed or abused) on sexual functioning has already been discussed; withdrawing or adjusting medications may be sufficient.

Several authors discuss the occasional advisability of penile prostheses in patients for whom the erectile disorder is psychological (Watters, 1986). This should only be done with full investigation of the individual, the sexual partner, and other forms of treatment. In any case in which a penile prosthesis is used, regardless of the reason, professional sexual counseling should follow (Schover & von Eschenbach, 1985).

Sex therapy for Erectile Disorder and Inhibited Orgasm must incorporate the concept of "performance anxiety" and prescribe settings in which sexual stimulation is present but demands (or perceived demands) for performance are minimized. The "pleasuring" and "sensate focus" techniques described in the past few pages are recommended by most therapists.

Unfortunately, outcome for erectile problems is among the poorest of sexual dysfunctions treated with traditional sex therapy (Heiman & LoPiccolo, 1983). The AASECT survey already reported (Kilmann et al., 1986) indicated that primary erectile dysfunction made up about

2% of referrals to this group of treatment professionals, and that the success rate was about 25%.

LoPiccolo and colleagues (1985) indicated better satisfaction with traditional sex therapy. Everaerd and Dekker (1985) compared systematic desensitization to a modified Masters and Johnson treatment approach. Both led to improvement in sexual functioning over that of a waiting list control, but little improvement in marital satisfaction. Rational emotive therapy also appeared to provide some sexual improvement and was successful in changing couples' relationships in some cases.

ORGASM DISORDERS

302.73 Inhibited Female Orgasm

Both psychodynamic and behavioral approaches to the treatment of Inhibited Female Orgasm stress the lowering of barriers to the releasing aspect of sexual climax. Traditional psychotherapeutic methods of addressing excessive control (or fear of being out of control) have generally been unsatisfactory. Education and specific training regarding clitoral stimulation or pubococcygeal control (Graber, 1982), for example, are often useful.

A single therapist, usually a woman, is recommended. Group therapy has been advocated, in which discussions of masturbatory techniques and further "permission" are fostered. Kaplan (1974) discusses the importance of "distracting" the patient and the use of erotic paraphernalia. The judicious use of manual masturbation, vibrators, or other objects between therapy sessions carries few or no dangers, despite occasional comments in the literature about dependence upon mechanical aids.

Libman and colleagues (1984) compared three therapeutic formats: standard couples therapy, group therapy, and "minimal contact bibliotherapy" (self-help) in 23 couples. A cognitive-behavioral sex therapy program was effective, with the standard couple condition being favored. Cotten-Huston and Wheeler (1983) found that women in preorgasmic group treatment developed more frequent orgasms, better feelings about themselves, and better communication with their partners than a control group. Fichten, Libman, and Brender (1983) noted that with sensate focus and intercourse-ban techniques alone, orgasmic responsiveness was not affected (although arousal was; see Sexual Arousal Disorders). Orgasmic dysfunction is among the most successfully treated disorders reported by AASECT providers (Kilmann et al., 1986).

302.74 Inhibited Male Orgasm

Inhibited Male Orgasm or ejaculatory inhibition, without medical cause, is among the least common reported sexual disorders. Many characteristics of the disorder are similar to those of Inhibited Female Orgasm, just discussed. Since orgasm is an extremely common experience for most males in most cultures, and since reproduction is closely associated with male orgasm, educational or simple counseling approaches are less likely to be effective. Nevertheless, education, "permission," and behavioral approaches should be tried, particularly if the sexual history indicates aberrant psychosexual development or strong cultural taboos. Psychogenic inhibition of male orgasm is likely to reflect a condition for which exploration of psychodynamic issues is indicated.

Relative inhibition of male orgasms, such as that found in individuals who require extraordinarily long periods of stimulation or intercourse before ejaculation, may be of concern to the patient and/or the partner. Exercises that employ manual stimulation prior to intromission are generally useful, often combined with additional stimulation during intercourse. The latter may come from fantasy, from erotic paraphernalia, or from the partner in the form of stroking, anal stimulation, particular kinds of thrusting, or sexual conversation. "Distraction" techniques may also be used.

So-called "anesthetic ejaculation" is a somewhat uncommon symptom. Williams (1985) reviewed seven cases in which no physical cause could be found. The men shared problems in recognition and expression of emotions, and an orientation toward performance. Traditional sex therapy was not effective.

302.75 Premature Ejaculation

Premature Ejaculation is the sexual dysfunction most associated with complete, successful treatment by behavioral means. The "squeeze" technique, in which the female partner stimulates the penis almost to orgasm and then prevents orgasm and ejaculation with firm pressure below the ventral glans, is an effective, hierarchical desensitization method. It is now widely accepted that the squeezing itself is not always necessary. The male partner can merely tell the woman when he is near orgasm, at which point she stops stimulating him, the sexual feelings are allowed to dissipate, and the process is repeated.

After several repetitions, the couple moves a step closer to intercourse, perhaps by using a lubricant. Later the start-and-stop activity is done with the penis inside the vagina, with the woman controlling the movements and stopping when ejaculation is near. As the hierarchy progresses, male thrusting is allowed until a sensation of loss of control is felt. Later, other positions are used.

The similarity to other desensitization techniques, in which "failure" is not allowed to occur, is obvious and is extremely important to treatment success. Premature ejaculation had the highest recorded success rate (62%) in the Kilmann survey of AASECT providers (1986).

SEXUAL PAIN DISORDERS

302.76 Dyspareunia
Sexual pain, particularly Dyspareunia, should be medically evaluated before a diagnosis of functional disorder is accepted and treatment begun. Functional Dyspareunia may be approached in a manner similar to that of Somatization Disorder (300.81) and some other somatoform disorders, in that it is a physiologic manifestation of emotional conflict. As with the somatoform disorders, the pain is—for the patient—a means of dealing with an unacceptable fear or impulse. With this in mind, approaches to treatment should consider psychodynamic issues and may include insight-oriented psychotherapy. The possibility of secondary gain associated with avoidance of intercourse or manipulation of the sexual or marital relationship should be addressed.

Behavioral approaches that employ gentle, nonpressured, perhaps graduated attempts at arousal and intercourse are recommended; however, informal attempts at this have probably already been tried by the couple. It is thus important that behavioral methods take place in a professional, structured context, accompanied by individual or conjoint psychotherapy.

306.51 Vaginismus
As in the case of functional Dyspareunia, functional Vaginismus is likely to reflect emotional characteristics similar to those found among the somatoform disorders. Psychodynamic exploration and understanding of potential manipulation and secondary gain are highly recommended, with either conjoint or concomitant counseling of the male partner, since this condition involves and threatens the couple's relationship.

Physical deconditioning of the vaginal musculature using graduated dilation is an effective treatment but should not be undertaken without psychotherapeutic involvement, at least to the extent of supportive counseling. Most behavioral approaches are similar to desensitization of phobias, beginning with visual inspection and touching and proceeding through insertion of one, then more, fingers (or lubricated graduated dilators), first by the patient herself and then by her partner. When the penis is finally used, initial control of the speed and depth of penetration, as well as of coital position, should rest with the patient.

As with all of the experiential techniques described herein, the exercises are described in detail and in writing by the clinician, but carried out in privacy by the patient.

302.70 Sexual Dysfunction Not Otherwise Specified

Disorders similar to those described earlier, but placed in this residual diagnostic category, can usually be treated using principles already outlined. Desensitization techniques are useful, but should be undertaken by trained and experienced therapists in appropriate surroundings, with attention to the interpersonal and psychological dynamics involved. Understanding underlying pathology is especially important when the atypical dysfunction appears to involve thought disorder, major affective disorder, personality disorder, or other significant mental or medical illness.

Medical aspects of sexual dysfunction should never be overlooked. Disorders that resemble "functional" *DSM-III-R* diagnoses but do not completely fit *DSM-III-R* criteria often involve physical illness or are iatrogenic (e.g., from medications or surgical trauma).

OTHER SEXUAL DISORDERS

302.90 Sexual Disorder Not Otherwise Specified

Patients whose sexual disorders are felt to be primarily psychiatric, but do not fit the above categories, should be treated using the principles described above when it appears appropriate to do so (i.e., when symptoms are similar to those for the disorders already discussed).

Ego-dystonic homosexuality no longer appears in the official APA nomenclature, but is a relatively common focus for treatment. Although many such patients come to treatment because of overt family, social, or legal problems, a significant number appear for alleviation of painful affects and inner conflicts with family or cultural mores.

For those who have been mislabeled homosexual or who painfully see themselves as homosexual because of a few impulses or experiences, education and brief counseling may bring significant relief. The patient may then continue his or her sexual behavior with less conflict, may experience a relief and strengthening of self-image which will allow entry into psychotherapy, or may stop feeling so badly about past "homosexual" events which are no longer taking place.

For those patients accurately "diagnosed" homosexual, and for whom this state is ego-dystonic, the treatment is far more complex and less likely to result in global alleviation of symptoms. Marks (1981b) speaks of "increasing heterosexuality" in these and in paraphilic patients, citing aversive techniques such as covert sensitization, which requires no external equipment and little participation by the therapist except for training and monitoring of progress. Marks and others also discuss "fading" in this regard. For details of these methods, see the section on Paraphilias.

Socarides (1979) has written extensively on the psychoanalytic treatment of the homosexual male, including patients with symptoms not identified as related to sexual preference and patients in whom the homosexuality was largely latent. Positive predictors are similar to those sought in other psychotherapy patients (good premorbid adaptation, circumscribed symptoms, good ego strength, ability to tolerate anxiety and the transference relationship, etc.). As with other patients in analytically oriented treatment, attention must be paid to secondary gratifications (e.g., the "neurotic equilibrium"), which become practical barriers to lasting change.

An alternative view of the treatment of ego-dystonic homosexuality would address the dysphoria rather than the homosexual orientation of the patient. For many therapists and patients it seems advisable to address those matters that make the patient feel badly, and to leave established homosexuality alone, at least for the time being.

Chapter 22

Sleep Disorders

by

Jerry J. Tomasovic

VARIATIONS OF NORMAL SLEEP
Longitudinal studies indicate a normal reduction in total nightly sleep time from birth until age 20, after which there is a plateau until age 35. After that, the total time asleep gradually declines further (yet the total time in bed begins to climb again). Thus, older patients may lie in bed, unable to sleep, as they approach their seventies and eighties. There is a gradual decline in total delta sleep (stages III and IV) from birth until it reaches less than an hour by the ages of 50–70 years.

One also notes that insomnia is manifested differently in the young than in the old. The young insomniac has difficulty initiating but not necessarily maintaining sleep, whereas the older patient can neither initiate nor maintain sleep through the entire night (Hauri, 1982; Williams, Karacan, & Hursch, 1974). Parasomnias vary with age, with sleepwalking and night terrors appearing more frequently in children, narcolepsy beginning in the second decade, and sleep apnea becoming more common with increasing age.

It is important to recognize the wide variation in total time required for sleep from person to person. Identification of a sleep disorder is therefore largely predicated on the patient's daytime behavior and drowsiness.

SLEEP HYGIENE

All of us have experienced disturbances of the balance between the state of wakefulness and sleep induction systems. Rules for improving the quality of sleep have evolved which can be quite useful to those with transient and milder forms of insomnia. They will not, however, eliminate the more severe forms of sleep disturbance (particularly insomnia). Table 4 provides guidelines for patients who experience minor sleep disturbances.

22A: DYSSOMNIAS

Treatment considerations are predominantly addressed for the chronic or recurring symptom complex. Although the diagnosis often becomes apparent through a detailed history, differentiation of primary vs. secondary insomnia frequently requires polysomnography. Medical consultation may be necessary. Complaints about inadequate sleep are much more significant when the patient also complains of tiredness when awake. To become significant, inadequate sleep should appear at

TABLE 4
Sleep Hygiene

1. Maintain a regular sleep and arousal time.
2. Don't remain in bed after awakening, particularly if you feel rested. Regular morning or afternoon exercise can improve the efficiency of sleep.
3. Avoid warm rooms, which interfere with sleep.
4. Consider a light bedtime snack.
5. Avoid evening caffeine, other stimulants, or alcohol. Nicotine is problematic for many.
6. Mask loud or disturbing noises with an air conditioner, fan, or other source of "white noise." Ear plugs may be helpful.
7. When unable to fall asleep, do not struggle but simply turn on the light, read, write, or even have a light snack until sleepy.

least three times a week for at least one month and remain significant enough to cause daytime fatigue or drowsiness.

INSOMNIA DISORDERS

307.42 Insomnia Disorder Related to Another Mental Disorder (Nonorganic)

This is the most common condition presenting with chronic insomnia. Axis I disorders include depression or other affective disorders, anxiety, and/or adjustment or reactive disorders with anxiety. Many Axis II personality disorders are associated with secondary insomnia. Treatment is directed toward the primary disorder.

In nonpharmacologic management, one must begin with the general sleep hygiene regimen just presented. Kales and Kales (1984) and Coleman and colleagues (1982) have presented excellent recommendations for adjustments in the sleep environment, and in daytime and nighttime activities. Success has been described with behavioral treatments such as biofeedback, stimulus control, relaxation therapy, and the previously mentioned "sleep hygiene."

Spielman, Saskin, and Thorpy (1987) reported sustained improvement in all sleep parameters for up to 36 weeks after a sleep restriction therapy. Extension of an initial marked restriction of time for sleep was based upon improved sleep efficiency. Compliance with this schedule was difficult, but selected patients did achieve satisfactory goals.

At times conjoint marital therapy, particularly when sexual issues are involved, can compliment behavior management. Exercise may be useful, as long as significant exercise activities are avoided near bedtime.

Transient insomnia lends itself quite favorably to pharmacologic management. Inappropriate pharmacologic management can lead to drug abuse. Behavior management is usually more effective in the long run. This is particularly true for the elderly; hypnotic agents should be considered adjuncts to multifaceted treatment. Over-the-counter medications are of no significant assistance in pharmacologic management.

Among the hypnotics, the benzodiazepines have emerged as the primary class of drugs. Roth and colleagues (1982) have demonstrated their effectiveness in reduction of sleep latency, total wake time, and extension of the total sleep time. Benzodiazepines are preferred over barbiturates, antidepressants, antihistamines, and nonbarbiturate sedative-hypnotics. (See Table 5 for a list of benzodiazepines often used to treat insomnia.)

Drug therapy is complicated by side effects such as psychological dependence, drug tolerance, withdrawal symptoms, and daytime hangover. Intermittent use minimizes rebound insomnia, which is particularly common with abrupt discontinuation of the medication. Rebound sleep disorder can be reduced by tapering of the drug (Greenblatt et al., 1987).

In the elderly, diminished metabolism and elimination of all central nervous system depressant drugs prompt one to begin with a minimal dose and to monitor the patient carefully. Many clinicians select compounds with intermediate absorption and elimination rates in order to reach a compromise among daytime sedation, tolerance, and rebound symptoms. Several new benzodiazepines are being studied in this regard (Clark et al., 1986; Dominguez et al., 1986; Rickels et al., 1986).

Chlormethiazole is a rapidly metabolized sedative hypnotic derived from vitamin B1. It has proved to be a popular choice in Europe for treatment of insomnia in elderly patients. In several double-blind studies, published by Bayer and his group, chlormethiazole was as effective as triazolam or temazepam (Bayer et al., 1986; Pathy, Bayer, & Stoker, 1986). Interest in the delta-sleep-inducing peptide (DSIP) remains in experimental stage at this time (Schneider-Helmert, 1986).

L-tryptophan, a precursor of serotonin, is quite popular for the treatment of insomnia. The effective dose is 1–2 gm at bedtime. A recent review suggested that L-tryptophan is effective in both situational

TABLE 5
Benzodiazepines Frequently Used in the Treatment of Insomnia

Drug	Hypnotic Dose (mg)	Absorption Rate	Elimination Rate
Diazepam	5–10	Rapid	Slow
Flurazepam*	15–30	Intermediate	Slow
Triazolam*	0.125–0.5	Intermediate	Rapid
Lorazepam	2–4	Intermediate	Intermediate
Alprazolam	0.25–0.5	Intermediate	Intermediate
Prazepam	10–50	Slow	Slow
Oxazepam	15–30	Slow	Intermediate
Temazepam*	15–30	Slow	Intermediate
Halazepam	20–40	Slow	Slow

* marketed as a hypnotic

and chronic psychophysiologic types of insomnia. Absence of serious side effects and lack of tolerance in long-term trials make it an attractive first-choice prescription (Schneider-Helmert & Spinweber, 1986).

780.50 Insomnia Disorder Related to a Known Organic Factor

This condition addresses 15%-20% of patients with chronic insomnia, and includes conditions that occur only during sleep (e.g., nocturnal myoclonus, restless leg syndrome, sleep apnea, childhood onset insomnia, sleep-related seizure disorders, and nonrestorative sleep).

Among the somatic disorders that commonly lead to insomnia, infectious diseases with high fever, heart disease, hypertension, pulmonary disorders, and gastrointestinal diseases lead the list. Chronic renal insufficiency, endocrine disorders such as hypothyroidism and diabetes, and both acute and chronic states of pain may be associated with insomnia or hyposomnia.

Insomnia secondary to drug use may be the result of bronchodilators, energizing antidepressants, central nervous system stimulants, steroids, and central adrenergic blockers. Adjustments in medication or treatment side effects can prevent most symptoms, without resorting to inappropriate use of hypnotics to counteract these side effects. Benzodiazepine hypnotics with short half-lives can induce insomnia in the latter portion of the night. Caffeinated beverages and cigarette smoking may impair the initiation of sleep. Alcohol will interrupt sleep, inducing difficulty maintaining sleep.

Sleep-related seizure disorders may prove quite difficult to identify but produce symptoms of nocturnal awakening, reducing sleep efficiency. Appropriate diagnostic studies, which include overnight EEG monitoring, may lead to anticonvulsant therapy. Standard polysomnography may not provide adequate EEG channels for proper diagnosis.

Childhood-onset insomnia suggests a developmental, neurochemical imbalance which persists into adulthood and may be accompanied by secondary behavior such as fear of sleep. This condition is frequently associated with learning disabilities and attention deficit disorders. Treatment for those conditions may also alter sleep efficiency. These patients are often quite sensitive to environmental stimulants such as caffeinated beverages. In addition to the standard general recommendations for activity and sleep hygiene adjustments, low doses of amitriptyline (10-50 mg) at bedtime often reduces sleep latency in these patients.

Nonrestorative sleep suggests a difference in the distribution of sleep staging, implying an altered arousal threshold. These patients appear to have adequate total sleep time but continue to complain of daytime malaise and joint aches and pains. L-tryptophan does not appear to be useful; low doses of amitriptyline may relieve the symptoms. Moldofsky and Lue (1980) demonstrated reduction of sleep disturbance and alpha intrusions and improvement in the patient's daytime well-being with chlorpromazine, 100 mg at bedtime.

307.42 Primary Insomnia

After one has eliminated insomnias secondary to psychiatric and medical disorders, 15%–30% of patients (in whom poor sleep patterns represent the only complaint) remain. Total sleep time appears to be within normal limits, but the patient complains of lack of satisfaction with his night's sleep. This group may include naturally short sleepers, subtle sleep-phase syndromes, and individuals with abnormal expectations about sleep. Some are labeled hypochondriacal in spite of psychophysiologic sleep disturbance.

The resolve to obtain a satisfactory night's rest following prolonged stress leads to increased effort which often leads to greater difficulty yet. Such patients often have difficulty returning to efficient sleep after the stress has resolved. This group might benefit from the sleep restriction therapy discussed previously.

Additional therapies which have proved useful include stimulus-control behavior therapy, described by Bootzin and Nicassio (1978). Many can benefit from relaxation therapy and intermittent judicious use of hypnotics. Stress reduction, which must be closely monitored and controlled, is tied to the success of the behavioral techniques.

HYPERSOMNIA DISORDERS

Patients with these disorders experience excessive daytime sleepiness or somnolence despite an adequate night's rest: individuals with one-to-two-hour daytime sleep attacks, excessively prolonged nocturnal sleep, or prolonged transition from the sleeping to fully awake state. Those patients who have a disturbed night's sleep from anxiety, insomnia, or poor health are excluded. The consequences of these symptoms may be devastating to the individual with regard to social impact, employment, underachievement, and impaired school performance.

While studies of excessive daytime somnolence would suggest a prevalence of 0.3%–4% of the adult population (Bixler et al., 1976; Karacan et al., 1976), the percentage of patients presenting to a sleep laboratory is considerably greater. The incidence of treatable medical problems is much higher than in patients complaining of insomnia.

Besides the patient's complaint, the standard approach to measurement of the daytime drowsiness is the Multiple Sleep Latency Test (MSLT) developed by Richardson and colleagues (1978). Sleep latency following the command to fall asleep on five successive occasions is measured every other hour from 10 a.m. A consistent latency of less than 5-10 minutes is abnormal.

307.44 Hypersomnia Disorder Related to Another Mental Disorder (Nonorganic)

This disorder affects about 15% of hypersomnic patients. It is particularly common in the depressive phase of bipolar illness, as well as in dysthymic disorders. It is also common in younger patients with symptoms of depression, schizophrenia, and borderline mental disorders. It is to be distinguished from amnesias and fugue states. One important feature is that the patient awakens unrefreshed even after prolonged sleep. Such individuals may also manifest weight loss, reduced concentration, appetite disturbance and fatigue.

Treatment for this condition is directed toward the primary nonorganic mental disorder. Hypersomnia will often respond to tricyclic antidepressants and monoamine oxidase inhibitors (O'Regan, 1974).

780.50 Hypersomnia Disorder Related to a Known Organic Factor

This disorder affects over 85% of hypersomnic patients, including those with physical conditions, substance abuse, or medication use. Medications that induce these symptoms include hypnotics, tranquilizers, stimulants (rebound from their use), and alcohol. Treatment is dosage adjustment or withdrawal. Withdrawal from caffeine and other stimulants can also be complicated by hypersomnolence.

A second type of hypersomnia is apparent only during sleep: sleep apnea, restless leg syndrome, and narcolepsy. In one series of 283 consecutive patients with daytime drowsiness, 180 were diagnosed with narcolepsy and cataplexy, while only 10 patients were found to have sleep apnea (Parkes, 1981). In the majority of sleep disorders centers, sleep apnea is the most common diagnosis. These primary disorders must be distinguished from hypersomnolence due to medical disorders such as uremia, liver failure, diabetes, hypothyroidism, brain tumors, and anoxic encephalopathies.

Narcolepsy. Treatment of narcolepsy (and frequently accompanying cataplexy or hypnagogic phenomena) must consider its psychosocial and economic impact. The patient may mistakenly be considered psychotic or lazy (Kales et al., 1982). The narcoleptic must adjust his daily activities to his sleep attacks. A nap of 30-60 minutes should be scheduled as needed, after which the narcoleptic symptoms will abate for several hours. These individuals should avoid shift work and occupations involving frequent travel or driving. Their symptoms are exacerbated by drugs with sedative side effects.

Central nervous system stimulant therapy will be required in most cases, most commonly methylphenidate or dextroamphetamine. Guilleminault, Carskadon, and Dement (1974) noted that in a series of 31 patients, dosages greater than 100 mg of dextroamphetamine daily were no more effective than lower doses. In some patients higher doses actually increased daytime drowsiness. Higher doses and long-term therapy are associated with headache, irritability, palpitations, and insomnia. One should try to limit dextroamphetamine to 10-30 mg per day and methylphenidate to 10-40 mg per day. When tolerance appears, the drug should be withdrawn for several weeks or an alternative drug instituted. The danger of medication abuse is obvious.

Pemoline, 40-120 mg per day, is often favored for its longer half-life and once-daily administration. Pemoline has been used for hyperactivity in children with reasonable safety. Phenmetrazine, 25-75 mg daily in up to three divided doses, may be used as an alternative therapy. Since it was introduced in the 1950s for its anorectic affect, phenmetrazine has been noted also to induce mood changes and has a high incidence of misuse (Martin et al., 1971).

The monoamine oxidase inhibitors have not routinely been utilized for this condition, although a recent British report by Roselaar and colleagues (1987) suggests improvement with selegiline, a specific monoamine-oxidase-B inhibitor, in 21 patients. Its effectiveness may be related to its internal conversion to amphetamine. Twenty mg induced subjective improvement in the alert state for four to eight hours. Propranolol in doses of 40-360 mg per day has provided subjective improvement in selected patients (Kales et al., 1979). Finally, gamma-hydroxybutyrate has been demonstrated by several investigators to show promise in the reduction of narcoleptic symptoms (Mamelak & Webster, 1981).

At times, symptoms of cataplexy persist despite the successful treatment of narcolepsy. Tricyclic antidepressants such as clomipramine, 10-100 mg per day, have been described as effective. Some patients develop tolerance (Shapiro, 1975). Clonazepam, 1-4 mg per day, is an alternative.

Menstruation-Associated Hypersomnia. A long-cycle hypersomnia with intervals of sleep prolonged for more than a day has been described with several disorders, including the Kleine-Levine syndrome and a menstruation-linked periodic hypersomnia. Menstruation-associated hypersomnia occurs with a regular and temporal relationship to the menstrual period and is occasionally accompanied by megaphagia. Sleep study often reveals normal nocturnal sleep, but several patients demonstrate paroxysmal EEG discharges (Sachs, Persson, & Hagenfeldt, 1982). Billiard, Guilleminault, and Dement (1975) found that a combination of ethinylestradiol and lynestrenol (oral contraceptives) was successful for many patients.

Kleine-Levine Syndrome. This uncommon disorder involves males with periodic hypersomnia of up to 18–20 hours of sleep per day (recurring monthly to yearly), affective symptoms, and hypothalamic dysfunction. On recovery, the patient may experience total or partial amnesia for his symptoms. Patients appear normal between attacks (Critchley, 1962). Although the condition is considered self-limiting, with recovery occurring in most cases by age 40, Billiard (1981) and others have noted persistence of symptoms for 56 of 96 cases followed for five to nine years. Amphetamines have been reported to reduce both the frequency and severity of the attacks. Lithium carbonate may be an alternative treatment (Goldberg, 1983).

Restless Leg Syndrome. Patients with this condition complain, particularly as they are entering sleep, of an unpleasant, creeping dysesthesia which produces discomfort, weakness and an irresistible need to move the legs (Coleman, 1982). The symptoms have been associated with motor neuron disease, amphetamine use, caffeinism, iron deficiency, anemia, and other metabolic or neoplastic disorders. Patients with restless leg syndrome usually also experience sleep-related myoclonus. When significant arousal occurs during the night, the patient may present with daytime somnolence (Montplaisir et al., 1985).

Treatment is initially directed toward associated medical disorders and deficiencies. Clonidine, up to 0.3mg hs, may bring symptomatic relief (Handwerker & Palmer, 1985). Hening and colleagues (1986) reported relief of restlessness, dysesthesias, dyskinesias while awake, and sleep disturbance following administration of opioids, including propoxyphene, codeine, and methadone.

Sleep Myoclonus. Nocturnal arrhythmic, repetitive twitching is more common than the restless leg syndrome; approximately one-third of patients also have restless legs. Sleep-related myoclonus appears in 12% of insomniacs and 3% of patients with excessive daytime somnolence (Coleman, 1982). The patient is often unaware of the movements yet complains of nonrefreshing sleep. Duration varies from five minutes to several hours during non-REM sleep. Medications, including levodopa, tricyclic antidepressants and anticonvulsants, and withdrawal of hypnotic drugs have been associated with the symptoms.

Clonazepam and temazepam have provided symptomatic relief in some patients (Mitler et al., 1986). Guilleminault and Flagg (1984) reported that baclofen decreased the amplitude of the leg movements but not their frequency.

Sleep Apnea. Sleep apnea is found in approximately half of those patients presenting with hypersomnia related to an organic factor. The condition is pathological when more than 30 episodes of 10 seconds or more occur during a single night's sleep, specifically when associated with symptoms of excessive daytime somnolence.

Several types of apnea (central, obstructive, others) can be identified through polysomnography. A number of psychiatric symptoms may develop or be associated with the syndrome, including deterioration in both memory and judgment (particularly during early morning), personality changes, anxiety, and depression. Adults very often have related medical problems, often associated with poor oxygenation of the blood. The diagnosis is confirmed by referral to a sleep laboratory for polysomnographic studies.

Treatment depends upon the severity of the patient's symptoms, oxygen desaturation, and medical status. Milder cases need only avoidance of aggravating medication or substances and/or weight reduction. Avoidance of the supine position for sleep may be effective. In patients with frightening medical sequelae, more aggressive management, beginning with milder surgical procedures, may be necessary.

Treatment should include avoidance of hypnotics, antihistamines, and CNS depressants (including alcohol) before sleep, and may involve a behavior management program. High altitude trips may aggravate problems. Shift work may induce sleep deprivation and aggravate mild sleep apnea. Many patients with chronic obstructive pulmonary disease, appearing as a consequence of sleep apnea and/or contributing to its severity, are made worse by smoking. Steroids may induce obesity and soft tissue hypertrophy, thereby aggravating the obstructive component.

Significant obesity requires the combined approach of diet, stress reduction, and behavior modification. Surgical procedures for weight reduction may be necessary.

In severe conditions, low-flow oxygen therapy (Smith, Haponik, & Bleeker, 1984), nasal CPAP (continuous positive airway pressure) (Guilleminault et al., 1986, 1987), mechanical devices for positioning the jaw or tongue, and various forms of surgery may be indicated.

Drug therapy is often ineffective. Protriptyline has been suggested for increase in the muscle tone of the upper airway and reduction of REM sleep (Brownell et al., 1982; Smith et al., 1983). The effectiveness of this approach remains unclear. The data are inconclusive concerning the effectiveness of medroxyprogesterone acetate (Rajagopal et al., 1986), naloxone, theophylline, acetazolamide, and L-tryptophan.

780.54 Primary Hypersomnia

This condition has no obvious organic cause or relationship to any other disorder. Van den Hoed and colleagues (1981) suggest that this idiopathic disorder represents a neurochemical imbalance. For some patients, there is prolonged nocturnal sleep (12–20 hours) with sleep drunkenness upon awakening, but little refreshed feeling. Symptoms, including sleeping through alarms, often begin in adolescence. This is a non-REM sleep disorder in which approximately one-third of patients have an affected first-degree relative.

Morning doses of stimulants (e.g., dextroamphetamine 10 mg, methylphenidate 20 mg, pemoline 37.5 mg) may be effective. In those patients with almost a 24-hour hypersomnia cycle, a late evening dose may prove useful. Wyler, Wilkins, and Trupin (1975) suggested a trial of methysergide, 2–6 mg per day.

307.45 Sleep-Wake Schedule Disorder

The sleep-wake cycle is directed by a biological, circadian rhythm of approximately 24–28 hours which persists even in a time-free environment. Disorders of sleep schedule can be produced by damage to the suprachiasmic nuclei of the hypothalamus from trauma, infection, degeneration, and/or other disorders (Hauri, 1977). Synchronization or resetting of the biological clock is accomplished through "zeitgebers" which represent time indicators, the most powerful of which is the regular wake-up time. Others include clocks, positions of the sun, work periods, mealtimes, and even low-frequency electromagnetic fields. Medications may lengthen or shorten the circadian rhythms cycle.

There are three types of sleep-wake cycle disorders: the delayed and advanced sleep-phase syndrome, disorganized sleep or irregular sleep-wake patterns, and symptoms that accompany frequently changing sleep-wake times (e.g., from shift work or "jet lag").

Advanced or Delayed Type. Individuals with this disorder experience a shift in their entire sleep process, for example, falling asleep at 3:00 a.m. and awakening seven to eight hours later. The most popular treatment approach is to progressively delay onset of sleep for two to three hours each night until the cycle has been shifted to a more appropriate setting (Weitzman et al., 1981). Following this shift, the individual must strictly adhere to his or her new schedule. There have been several reports of successful treatment of the advanced sleep-phase syndrome by phase-advance chronotherapy moving in the opposite direction (Moldofsky, Musisi, & Phillipson, 1986).

Brief trials of short-acting benzodiazepines have been attempted. Seidel and colleagues found that triazolam, 0.5 mg, modified both the nocturnal insomnia and daytime drowsiness in five patients. Recent studies indicate that exposure to bright light (2,000–2,500 lux) between 8:00 and 10:00 p.m. may be quite effective in treating the advanced sleep-phase syndrome. The delayed sleep-phase syndrome has been shown to respond to bright light exposure in the morning (Lawy, Sack, & Singer, 1985; Lawy et al., 1983).

Disorganized Type. This problem occurs throughout adulthood, more commonly in the older patient who has no set work schedule. It is often self-perpetuating, and requires a gradual reestablishment of the regular day/night cycle, perhaps with mild exercise when the patient becomes drowsy. Daytime naps should be abolished and time in bed should be restricted to those hours designated for sleep. An in-house trainer or even hospitalization may be needed to reestablish a regular cycle. Weekends are particularly dangerous for return to old habits.

Symptoms Due to Frequent Changes in Sleep/Wake Times. Occasionally, individuals (for example, "on-call" workers, international travellers) will attempt to alter these symptoms with stimulants or sedative-forced sleep. Individuals with a permanent night shift have difficulty establishing a consolidated sleep period. Previously efficient sleepers fare better with work shifts and night shift responsibilities than do persons with histories of sleep problems. Transient use of bedtime short-acting benzodiazepines can be tried, if the patient's schedule change is permanent, to establish the new sleep/wake cycle. In severe cases, the patient may have to change jobs (Afchoff, Hoffman, & Pohl, 1975).

307.40 Dyssomnia Not Otherwise Specified
Complete discussion of all other dyssomnias is not possible. The clinician may consider the principles just outlined, and should make use of referral resources in other specialties as appropriate.

22B: PARASOMNIAS

307.47 Dream Anxiety Disorder (Nightmare Disorder)
Nightmares or dream anxiety episodes frequently do not contain the screams nor the excessive autonomic symptoms noted in night terrors. Instead, the patient manifests a motor component with rolling or thrashing about in the bed, but upon awakening is able to recall the dream and present a clear sensorium. These events occur predominantly out of REM sleep in the middle and latter parts of the night. Patients experiencing a Post-traumatic Stress Disorder may manifest a striking imagery during the drowsy state between wakefulness and sleep.

These symptoms are frequently transient, particularly in the younger age groups, and require only temporary psychiatric support or benzodiazepine hypnotic. It is important to recall that nightmares may be associated with drug treatment withdrawal.

307.46 Sleep Terror Disorder
Among the parasomnias, night terrors evoke the most concern from the patient. These episodes are characterized by extreme terror and panic, often punctuated by a piercing cry. They are associated with autonomic discharges such as tachycardia, sweating, mydriasis, and hypertension. These events are distinguished from nightmares because they are not followed by a full degree of alertness with clear sensorium. Sleep terrors occur 60–90 minutes after sleep onset.

They are relatively more common in children; adult presentation is often associated with psychopathology. Many patients demonstrate inhibition of aggression. Obsessive-compulsive tendencies and phobias accompanied by both anxiety and depression are common accompanying features which should be thoroughly investigated by the clinician.

Psychotherapy may be appropriate following the diagnostic evaluation. Suppression of Stage III/IV sleep with benzodiazepines or other carefully chosen hypnotics may prove useful, although many hypnotics increase Stage III/IV sleep time and thus may worsen symptoms.

Imipramine has also been used. Medication is rarely required for this condition in children.

307.46 Sleepwalking Disorder

Somnambulism or sleepwalking manifests as an automatism which varies from sitting up in bed to leaving one's bed and walking about in a confused part-waking, part-sleeping state. Most episodes last only a few seconds or minutes, with occasional recall of the events upon awakening. The risk of injury mandates adjustments in the patient's environment similar to those mentioned above for sleep terrors.

In children, sleepwalking is generally benign and rarely requires therapy. There is very often a family history of similar symptoms. In adults, the appearance of symptoms is often associated with unusual tension or stress in a person with a childhood history of sleepwalking. The clinician must identify any psychopathology or neurologic disease and initiate appropriate measures. There is frequently no diagnosable mental or physical illness.

The management of patients with sleepwalking requires stringent safety measures to prevent the patient from accidental injury. This may mean special locks for the doors and windows as well as sleeping on the ground floor. The old adage about precipitating violent behavior if one interrupts sleepwalking is largely myth, although awakening should be gentle and confusion should be expected.

Reid (1975) demonstrated sustained effect of six hypnotherapy sessions in young adults with uncomplicated, intractable sleepwalking, using specialized conditioning to tactile cues. Low doses of diazepam (5–10 mg at bedtime) have worked for similar patients (Reid, Ahmed, and Levie, 1981). Tolerance is not a problem, as the effect appears to be related to regulation of sleep cycles rather than alleviation of anxiety. Imipramine, 10–50 mg at bedtime, has also been reported to be of use, particularly in children with intractable symptoms and/or combinations of parasomnias.

In the elderly, one should consider low doses of neuroleptics (e.g., haloperidol 0.5 mg) rather than the benzodiazepines. Geriatric symptoms are often associated with an organic brain syndrome.

307.40 Parasomnia Not Otherwise Specified

The motor parasomnias include restless leg syndrome or periodic repetitive myoclonic-like leg movements (particularly occurring as the patient enters sleep). The benzodiazepines—particularly clonazepam 1–3 mg hs or hypnotic doses of temazepam—remain the accepted treatment for such disorders. Clonidine may also be effective (cf., its use in Tourette's Disorder).

Nocturnal head-banging or body-rocking, sometimes seen in adolescents or adults following head injury, may respond to imipramine.

Other parasomnias should be carefully evaluated and treated according to their symptoms and the principles already discussed. Referral to a neurologist or other sleep disorders subspecialist is often indicated.

Chapter 23

Factitious Disorders

301.51 Factitious Disorder with Physical Symptoms
The treatment of patients with Factitious Disorder is clouded by the lack of established approaches to which the disorder will respond, the absence of controlled studies of its treatment, and the assumption, sometimes well-founded, that the patient will leave medical care soon after the disorder is discovered. Such measures as blacklisting of patients and denial of hospitalization are repugnant to most physicians and could have disastrous consequences (Hyler & Sussman, 1981). Hyler and Sussman have suggested that extensive behavior modification programs may be helpful; however, these are almost never feasible.

Consultative Role. Since most patients present as inpatients or in emergency rooms, the psychiatrist is usually called as a consultant. He or she is often given the job of confronting the patient. Although confrontation is recommended, the psychiatrist should suggest that the primary or attending physician carry it out. The psychiatrist may be with the other physician, in order to establish a nonambivalent setting and ensure that the confrontation, while firm, will be as kind and therapeutic as possible.

The best treatment is sometimes merely a coordinated discharge of the patient and defusing of the staff's anger and other feelings. A number of cases are reported in which patients with no incentive for emotional change responded to humane behavioral approaches while in the general hospital, leading to at least temporary reversing of deceptive, self-destructive behavior (Myall et al., 1984; Simmons et al., 1987).

The psychiatrist may also help by communicating with medical and nursing staff about the nature of the disorder and the inadvisability of punitive approaches. The psychiatrist's input may particularly assist in decisions regarding whether or not to perform potentially hazardous procedures for diagnosis or treatment.

Although some feel that patients with factitious disorders are usually unsophisticated, most clinical experience indicates intelligence and professional background consistent with at least exploring therapeutic options. Folks and Freeman (1985) suggest the best treatment may simply be rapport, with continuation of necessary medical treatment and limits on illness behavior. Personality-disordered patients have a worse prognosis than those with obvious depression. Antidepressant medication may clear the way for psychotherapy in the latter (Earle & Folks, 1986).

Apparent factitious illness in children may in fact be related to parental abuse, sometimes as a result of mental illness in the parent. Meadow (1984) found that fictitious epilepsy in children was sometimes related to anoxic episodes caused by a parent. Recognition and protective action are imperative.

For those occasional patients who are successfully encouraged to pursue psychotherapy, the uncovering, in a supportive surrounding, of reasons for masochistic or substitutive behavior may bring marked improvement. Psychotherapy may also address the patient's need for attention and caring, and his anger against objects who withhold this from him. A dynamic issue which has been discussed in this context, as well as in other self-mutilating patients, has to do with an apparent need to sacrifice one part of the body (e.g., through surgery) in order to protect the whole from suicide or decompensation into psychosis. Behavioral therapy has been described (Klonoff et al., 1983), with the recommendation that psychodynamic considerations be addressed in a combined format.

Reich and Gottfried (1983) described a large group of patients with factitious complaints, virtually all of whom were said not to have Münchausen syndrome, sociopathy, or malingered behavior. The authors separated them from Münchausen patients on the basis of lack of known chronicity of the factitious illness behavior (although the patients were located by retrospective survey). These patients, seen from the point of view of internal medicine rather than psychiatry, were said to be immature, passive, and hypochondriacal, and none had major mental disorders. Thirty-three of 41 patients were confronted; none signed out of the hospital or became suicidal. About one-third acknowledged causing their disorders. Many more were said to have improved after confrontation. The authors note several differences between the clinical course of this group and that commonly predicted in the psychiatric literature.

Because of the danger that the patient represents to himself (or to children in some cases), the possibility of risk from unneeded diagnostic procedures, and financial losses to the health care system, most authors feel that searching the patient, his belongings, and his room for evidence or instruments of self-harm is both ethically and legally justified.

300.16 Factitious Disorder with Psychological Symptoms

Psychiatric or psychological presentation of factitious disorder is rare, although it does occur. It should be treated with the same general methods as just described for physical presentation, and may afford greater opportunity for psychiatric intervention.

This diagnostic group is sometimes erroneously substituted for the older concept of "Ganser's syndrome." Ganser's syndrome, however, is clearly not under voluntary control and should be treated with a combination of environmental change (when possible—its presentation is often in prisoners), support, and temporary use of antipsychotic medication. Antipsychotic medication or other biological treatment for factitious disorders, except insofar as some patients have significant depression, has not been effective.

300.19 Factitious Disorder Not Otherwise Specified

The treatment of patients who fall within this residual category should be based upon control of patient-induced illness or injury and the underlying psychopathology, using the guidelines just described. It should particularly be noted that patients who are malingering or who have somatoform disorders (q.v.) should not be placed in the 300.19 category and should not be treated as if they have a factitious disorder.

Chapter 24

Impulse Control Disorders Not Elsewhere Classified

312.34 Intermittent Explosive Disorder
This disorder may be seen as a lack of modulation of anger or, perhaps in a separate group of patients, as a seizure-like condition of idiosyncratic behavior which cannot be placed as easily on a spectrum of "normal" to "abnormal" impulse control.

For the patient seen as having difficulty with some aspect of recognition or modulation of affect or behavior, treatment may include biofeedback, desensitization, group therapy, and competent counseling which encourages careful exploration of one's behavior (such as by keeping a diary of explosive impulses, the events that precede them, and the behaviors that follow). For therapists taking this view—ordinarily nonmedical clinicians—the use of medication is controversial. Indeed, a few such patients have "paradoxical" reactions to the benzodiazepines or alcohol, with a concomitant rage response.

Those who view this disorder, or at least certain syndrome complexes within it, as related to seizure phenomena (Elliott, 1978) or episodic dyscontrol (Monroe, 1981) recommend a careful neurological workup and a combination of biological and psychotherapeutic treatment. Specialized anticonvulsive treatment should be considered, even in the absence of positive neurological findings.

Carbamazepine is often the initial drug of choice, prescribed according to therapeutic blood levels (Stone et al., 1986). Baseline blood count and blood chemistries are recommended. The clinicians should monitor the blood count, especially during early treatment. A transient, mild leukopenia should be expected, but should resolve itself quickly. Phenytoin was found to be potentially useful in a review by Finkel (1984). Combinations of the more common anticonvulsants, with or without other drugs (e.g., thioridazine), have also been tried, with limited success. In syndromes accompanied by organic hallucinosis, a high-potency antipsychotic is usually effective in low doses.

Propranolol has long been suggested by Elliott (1978) and others. Most recently, Jenkins and Maruta (1987) discussed eight cases of Intermittent Explosive Disorder, five of whom experienced substantial improvement with propranolol. Metoprolol, a selective beta-1-adrenoreceptor blocker, may be more specific (Mattes, 1985). Both drugs are prescribed in their usual medical range and require the usual cautions for beta-blockers. Propranolol has been combined with antidepressants (Elliott, 1978); however, controlled studies are lacking. It may be more useful in patients with a demonstrated central nervous system lesion.

It goes without saying that episodic behaviors should receive careful neurologic evaluation before one assumes that they represent Intermittent Explosive Disorder. There are also a number of systemic causes to consider, such as reactive hypoglycemia (Virkkunen, 1984). The treatments for those conditions are quite different, and should not be delayed by misdiagnosis.

Lithium carbonate is often prescribed for mood or behavioral instability (cf., the "emotionally unstable character disorder" of Rifkin et al., 1972). Tupin and colleagues (1972) found it effective for decreasing violence in prisoners. Consistent usefulness, however, in treating Intermittent Explosive Disorder has not been shown (Reid & Gutnik, 1982). Stereotaxic surgery has shown promise in experimental animals; however, its study in humans for this psychiatric (as differentiated from neurologic) disorder has been severely limited.

Psychotherapy. For many patients, the discovery that one's episodic violence is "organic" and can be decreased or eliminated with medication may, ironically, limit the success of treatment. Psychiatric or neurologic disorders with behavioral symptoms are almost never completely treated using biological means.

Psychotherapy defines and deals with secondary gain. It helps the patient who must adapt to life as a nonviolent person, which requires different coping skills and mechanisms than were previously employed. The patient's family is likely to have been in some sort of precarious equilibrium before treatment, which will require stabilization as one member—the patient—changes.

Psychology can also address depression related to the loss of symptoms and a particular kind of violent "identity." Finally, one must address the hope that one is "cured" and unconscious wishes not to be cured, which often lead to medication noncompliance.

Legal Considerations. Before treating patients with Intermittent Explosive Disorder, or other syndromes in which violent behavior is a known danger, the patient and his family should be apprised of the benefits and risks of outpatient vs. inpatient care, compliance vs. noncompliance, and the like. Everyone should understand that confidentiality will take a back seat to the safety of the patient, his family, clinic staff, or others.

There should be clear communication with family physicians, hospital staff, employers, the State Department of Motor Vehicles, and so forth. Some of these need not be detailed; however, it is foolhardy to accept and treat a patient whom one knows to be potentially dangerous without some attention to the reasonable warning of foreseeable victims. Many clinicians encourage the patient and his family to notify the appropriate individuals or agencies; however, certain reporting by the psychiatrist himself/herself may be required by law.

312.32 Kleptomania

The traditional treatment of Kleptomania is psychotherapy within which underlying causes for the irresistible impulse may be discovered. In some patients, reported as cases rather than controlled studies, discovery of the psychodynamics alone is sufficient to allow behavioral change. When the onset of the disorder is not acute or associated with some identifiable event, however, reports of therapeutic success become less common and treatment outcomes rely more upon changing one's symptoms to more acceptable defense mechanisms than upon outright cure.

Guilt and the need to be caught and punished are common, fairly accessible dynamics. Others are far more subtle, including efforts to find objects that help the patient maintain control over his destructive aggression (Cierpka, 1986) or psychologically nourishing self-objects (Tolpin, 1983). Behavioral treatment using covert sensitization (described in Chapter 21 in the section on Pedophilia) was reported by Glover (1985).

The presence of underlying depression in many shoplifting women not specifically diagnosed as having Kleptomania has led to the successful use of antidepressants (notably MAO inhibitors) in some patients (Robey, 1981).

312.31 Pathological Gambling

Treatment approaches to Pathological Gambling often equate this disorder with addiction, particularly addiction to alcohol. The patient almost invariably presents near the end of a long, downhill course of an illness which has been destructive to himself and his family. Whenever possible, treatment should employ techniques consistent with the seriousness of the patient's condition, that is, multifaceted programs which remove the patient from his environment and/or keep him from further injuring (usually financially) others.

Kellner (1982b) describes the highly structured residential programs available in many centers. These initially treat the crisis in which the patient finds himself, and then try to provide an accepting milieu in which firm and consistent efforts can be made to deal with personal, family, financial, and social issues. Among the specific topics that must be addressed are unrealistic expectations (both positive and negative) about the treatment program. The patient may also place undue emphasis on unrealistic or nonconstructive issues such as the hopelessness of getting out of debt or the belief that additional money will solve all his/her problems.

Taber and colleagues (1987) reported total abstinence in almost half the patients treated at a comprehensive program, six months after completion. The same group describes their "Brecksville unit" in which abstinence, reduction of the urge to gamble, and restoration of social functioning were the principal objectives (Russo et al., 1984). This and similar programs are residential or inpatient, and generally last about four weeks. Aftercare, particularly regular meetings with Gamblers Anonymous, is critical to continuing recovery. Control rather than cure is the goal (Rankin, 1982).

Gamblers Anonymous now has chapters in most cities, operating along lines similar to Alcoholics Anonymous. Family involvement should be pursued at some level of the treatment, in terms of long-term goals and to alleviate some of the family's suffering.

Psychodynamic approaches to gambling generally address the obsessive, neurotic characteristics related to the winning of symbolic objects and love, challenge and mastery. Behavioral approaches, particularly adversive conditioning, are based upon the tremendous reinforcing characteristic of gambling for the patient. Although the gambling itself, by the time treatment is sought, is not particularly pleasurable, it has provided reinforcement on a variable ratio, variable intensity schedule which requires specialized behavioral techniques to extinguish. Neither psychodynamic nor behavioral treatment programs have proved their efficacy for patients who fill the criteria for a diagnosis of Pathological Gambling; however, the behavioral technique of imaginal desensitization showed some promise in a study by McConaghy and colleagues (1983).

Several authors have pointed out the increased prevalence of affective disorders, suicidal behavior, substance abuse, and sexual dysfunction in pathological gamblers. These should be considered in any comprehensive treatment strategy (Daghestani, 1987; McCormick et al., 1984; Ramirez et al., 1983).

No matter what the approach, treatment should include attention not only to individual concerns but to the patient's family environment, social and vocational situation, and debts. It must be structured so that follow-up in these categories can be maintained. The clinician should be aware of both superficial and more lasting contributors to the symptoms, such as depression and particular life stresses.

312.33 Pyromania

The characteristics of neurotic defensive structure in Pyromania appear similar to those of Kleptomania; however, the causative psychodynamics and the age of the patient may be quite different. The obvious danger to others often dictates psychiatric or social control during treatment. In inpatient settings, safety of others must be considered paramount. The patient with this disorder is less likely than one who gambles or steals to be released on probation pending outpatient treatment.

Kellner (1982b) discusses this and other disorders of impulse control in the context of acceptance by the therapist; formation of the therapeutic relationship; exploration of the affectual, cognitive, and behavioral characteristics of pyromanic fantasies and acts; and therapeutic intervention to change beliefs, decrease situational factors (such as tension, by desensitization), and cope with unavoidable affects (such as rage). These principles are common to many other impulse disorders, not only those discussed in this chapter. Underlying or coexisting disorders should be sought and treated. Pyromania secondary to psychotic illness should be treated with neuroleptics.

Juvenile Firesetting. Most of the treatment literature addresses children and young adolescents, who make up the majority of firesetters.

There are a number of case reports of successful behavioral treatment, including satiation (in which the child is given supervised opportunity to light as many matches as he wishes) (Wolff, 1984), "negative practice with corrective consequences" (Kolko, 1983), and combination programs. The latter often include substitute behaviors, increased awareness of consequences (e.g., by visiting hospital burn units), and relaxation training (Koles & Jenson, 1985).

Many treatment techniques attempt to interrupt firesetting behavior by correlating events, feelings, and behavior, sometimes graphically (Bumpass, Brix, & Preston, 1985). These are often part of community-based programs, which treat more firesetters than most mental health clinics and are frequently quite successful. They usually stress the parents' teaching children how to appropriately ignite and extinguish fires, and allowing children to assist (under adult supervision) in igniting barbecues or fireplaces (Baizerman & Emshoff, 1984).

Issues of mastery in which the child creates a situation he believes he can control, and then panics when he cannot, can often be successfully addressed by having the parent or therapist start a fire, put it out (thus controlling the situation), and help the child predict that which is controllable and that which is not (Dalton, Haslett, & Baul, 1986).

312.39 Trichotillomania

Trichotillomania (compulsive hair-pulling) is seen in both children and adults. It has at various times been treated, with appropriate biological or psychological therapies, as a variant of depressive illness (Krishnan, Davidson, & Miller, 1984), a compulsive disorder (Snyder, 1980) and even a symptom of psychosis (Sticher, Abramovits, & Newcomer, 1980). Antidepressants are effective in some cases, based upon either the affective or compulsive viewpoint.

The majority of clinical successes, in children and adults, appear to be associated with simple behavioral techniques such as "habit reversal" (Rosenbaum, 1982), relaxation training, competing response training (De Luca & Holborn, 1984), and mild aversive therapy (Stevens, 1984). Simple hypnotic suggestion has been effective as well.

312.39 Impulse Control Disorder Not Otherwise Specified

This residual category applies to a wide variety of patients. After careful differential diagnosis, with the ruling out of other psychiatric illness and organic causes (particularly for older patients), treatment should be based upon the presenting symptoms and underlying causes as they appear to the psychiatrist. Because of the variety of treatments recommended for different impulse control disorders in this section, ranging from the multifaceted milieu treatment of Pathological Gambling to biological management of some Intermittent Explosive Disorders, the clinician should consider consultation with and/or referral to a colleague who works often with similar patients.

Chapter 25

Adjustment Disorders

General Treatment Principles
By definition, all these disorders are "maladaptive reactions" to identifiable psychosocial stressors, which occur within a few weeks of the stressor and have persisted for less than six months (American Psychiatric Association, 1987). The tasks of treatment are to deal with acute symptoms and to promote either a return to a healthy premorbid state or effective coping with a chronic stressor.

The symptoms are expected to remit or disappear once the stressor is gone, or to evolve into a more permanent (effective or ineffective) coping mechanism if the stressor persists. Any remaining symptoms or disorders should be dealt with according to guidelines found elsewhere in this book.

In a number of the disorders, support is important while the patient draws upon his or her own resources for improvement and growth. Support and active psychotherapeutic involvement may also prevent regressive or disabling resolution of the adjustment disorder.

Psychotherapeutic approaches most commonly indicated are crisis intervention, brief psychotherapy, behavioral therapy, counseling, and education. Brief environmental change may be helpful; however, simplistic advice such as "take a few days of vacation" is insufficient for patients who meet the criteria for these diagnoses. Some specific guidelines for brief dynamic psychotherapy, particularly for patients who need more than transient support, are presented by Horowitz (1986).

Group therapy, particularly that which focuses on enhancing self-image while showing the patient how to improve within a supportive environment, may be helpful. Patients with adjustment disorders often need individual attention, although it need not be intensive in nature. For those patients whose stressors continue (e.g., persons with a chronic illness), a consistent group therapy environment in which transient problems can be effectively resolved may be very useful.

Although much of treatment involves the patient alone, family members are often concerned and can benefit from reassurance, with the patient's permission, concerning the treatability and transience of the disorder. This is best done in a conjoint or family session soon after the initial evaluation.

Pharmacotherapy of adjustment disorders should not be emphasized. A number of physicians and pharmaceutical companies suggest anxiolytic agents and occasionally antidepressants. Their prescription, however, may rob the patient of the opportunity to use—or learn to use—his or her own emotional resources to deal with the crisis or stressor, and to feel good about it. In addition, the use of medications provides the patient with an opportunity to see himself as sicker than he actually is, decreases the amount of meaningful communication between doctor and patient, may promote masking of symptoms or feelings, and exposes the patient to the risks of side effects or medication abuse.

It is common practice for nonmedical psychotherapists to ask for a medical consultation for the purpose of obtaining medications for uncomfortable patients. In such instances, if the diagnosis is Adjustment Disorder, the psychiatrist should consider whether there is a temporary need for medication, whether there is no real need, or whether the diagnosis is inaccurate. If the patient appears to require chronic medication, the clinician should entertain the possibility of either an erroneous original diagnosis or an evolving of the adjustment disorder toward a chronic, pathological resolution.

Responses to Medical Conditions. Medical illness or injury is often a precipitating stressor. Adjustment to loss or fear of loss is the usual dynamic, and can be seen in a wide variety of medical settings. There are often time constraints for treatment, such as the patient's expected hospital stay or an approaching date for surgery. Psychotherapy skills, relaxation techniques (including hypnosis), and often the ability to explain more about the illness or medical procedure involved (as might be done by a psychiatrist or nurse psychotherapist) are all helpful. Even the use of selected reading material as an adjunct to treatment can help, although one should not substitute a few books or pamphlets for the therapeutic relationship.

Consultation for medically related adjustment disorders should not usually lead to medication. From time to time, however, rapid alleviation of acute symptoms of anxiety, depression, or even psychosis cannot be accomplished without psychoactive drugs. Consideration should be given to interactions with medications already being prescribed, and to effects of the psychotropic on the primary illness. It should be remembered that most of the medications used for treatment of depression or psychotic symptoms do not act quickly. In some cases, stimulants, such as amphetamines or methylphenidate, given in small doses are helpful, particularly for their rapid action in elderly patients.

A large part of the consultative treatment of medical patients is communication to the referring physician (and the ward staff if the patient is in a hospital). A concise outline of the psychiatrist's findings, prescribed treatment, and recommendations for other caregivers should be placed in the chart. They should not be vague or full of jargon, but should be written with the understanding that the psychiatrist may not be personally involved in the next steps of the patient's care.

Unusual Grief Reactions. Although Uncomplicated Bereavement (V62.82) is discussed elsewhere, it is appropriate to consider "complicated" bereavement or "aberrant grief reaction" in the section on adjustment disorders. The principles discussed often apply to other forms of loss, including divorce or loss of part of one's body, as well.

If grief remains unresolved for a particularly long time, with persistent yearning, overidentification with the deceased, and/or inability to express sadness or rage, then Uncomplicated Bereavement may not be an appropriate diagnosis and some sort of grief-resolution therapy should be offered. This may include helping the patient to make a decision to grieve, techniques of guided imagery or guided mourning (Mawson et al., 1981), and helping construct a life and an identity in the absence of the lost object.

Brief psychotherapy is the treatment of choice and has been described for bereavement by Horowitz and colleagues (1984). Self-help groups are often useful for certain kinds of loss, such as the death of a child, divorce, or amputation (Videka-Sherman & Lieberman, 1985).

Essa (1986) describes psychotherapeutic intervention for grief in elderly patients.

309.24 Adjustment Disorder with Anxious Mood

In addition to the principles outlined in the preceding General Treatment Principles, reassuring the patient that the symptoms are transient and that the clinician and patient together can alleviate them will be useful. Nonintrusive support, crisis intervention techniques, relaxation, meditation, hypnosis, or biofeedback may be used by those therapists experienced in one of these other techniques. Temporary antianxiety medication, preferably a benzodiazepine, may be considered. Emphasis on the patient's ability to weather the stress, as well as praise for his or her ability to strengthen coping mechanisms, is helpful.

309.00 Adjustment Disorder with Depressed Mood

Patients with depressive symptoms are often more uncomfortable than those with other adjustment disorders, may appear more disabled, may experience more behavioral change (e.g., sleep disturbance, lack of energy), may appear more regressed, and may present with suicidal ideation. Unless the patient has other symptoms of major affective or bipolar disorder (in which case the Adjustment Disorder diagnosis is probably inappropriate)—for example, vegetative signs or a positive dexamethasone suppression test—antidepressant medication should not be used. Antianxiety medications, including alprazolam, should be avoided as well, except perhaps short-acting preparations for sleep.

Support and availability of the clinician, with reassurance that the current experience is probably transient, are important for these patients. Simple, practical recommendations—not necessarily pharmacologic ones—for complaints of sleeplessness, lack of energy, and the like often have good results.

The patient should be asked about suicidal thoughts, and any suicidal ideation or behavior openly discussed. In Adjustment Disorder patients, as opposed to those with more serious depression, thoughts of suicide are more likely to be anxiety-producing and to be efforts at resolution in fantasy of real problems. Nevertheless, the clinician must assure the patient that this topic can be discussed as any other, and that in the unlikely event that further control or treatment should be necessary, it is readily available.

309.30 Adjustment Disorder with Disturbance of Conduct

It is important for the clinician, the patient, and the patient's family to understand the difference between this disorder and other, more chronic, antisocial conditions (e.g., Antisocial Personality Disorder). It may also be useful to point out that the treatment of antisocial behaviors at the time of their presentation as an Adjustment Disorder lowers the probability that the antisocial symptoms will continue as a chronic pattern of coping or adaptation after the initial stress is removed (or as the chronic stress continues).

Countertransference issues and the temptation of some therapists to take a harsh approach to persons with this disorder should be carefully monitored. In spite of the inconvenience or injury which has been caused to others, acceptance and attempts to have the patient understand that his or her symptoms are characteristics of his difficulty adjusting—and not indications of some deep inner criminality, character disorder, or evil—are very important. This allows the patient to see treatment as something logical and accomplishable, whose explorations and anxieties can be tolerated.

Continuing responsibility for one's own actions is also in order. The therapist's acceptance of the *patient* and reassurance for his or her fragile condition do not imply acceptance of the antisocial *acts* that place people and property in jeopardy. Although the psychiatrist may support the patient in court, for example, under most circumstances these conditions should not be allowed to exonerate him altogether.

309.40 Adjustment Disorder with Mixed Disturbance of Emotions and Conduct

This disorder should be treated using the principles already outlined, both at the beginning of this chapter and within the paragraphs on individual disorders. It should be noted that treatment for one portion of the disorder (e.g., prescription of benzodiazepines for anxiety) may have either a positive or an adverse effect on some other group of symptoms (e.g., recklessness or self-destructive behavior). The risks and benefits of each must be weighed. The self-destructive nature of many reckless or antisocial-appearing acts should not be overlooked.

309.28 Adjustment Disorder with Mixed Emotional Features

The principles outlined earlier in this chapter address this disorder.

326 The Treatment of Psychiatric Disorders

309.82 Adjustment Disorder with Physical Complaints
In addition to the General Treatment Principles outlined earlier, the clinician should think of the physical complaints in much the same way as emotional features of Adjustment Disorder. That is, their presence should be acknowledged, along with the dysphoria they generate, without elevating them to the level of Axis III disorders. Once the psychiatrist is confident that no organic disease is present, prescriptions and referral for additional medical evaluation or treatment should be strictly limited.

Some of the psychotherapy techniques found in the section on somatoform disorders, particularly ways in which therapy can focus on emotional issues and feelings rather than the physical complaints, help both patient and clinician attend to the real issues: clarifying stressors, improving coping skills, and emotional adaptation.

309.83 Adjustment Disorder with Withdrawal
In addition to the General Treatment Principles outlined earlier, the clinician should be aware that withdrawal lends itself to isolation from sources of growth and support, and thus may increase the probability that the Adjustment Disorder will evolve into chronic avoidance or depression. The patient should be encouraged, perhaps by "prescription," to have a certain amount of contact with others. The family can continue at home the psychotherapist's therapeutic pressure and reassurance.

309.23 Adjustment Disorder with Work (or Academic) Inhibition
In addition to the earlier General Treatment Principles, it should be noted that disorders involving work or academic inhibition may have effects which last beyond the duration of the psychiatric symptoms themselves. That is, one's behavior on the job or in class may endanger or postpone career progress.

In such cases, brief, supportive, goal-directed counseling (such as that found in many student health centers and some employee assistance programs) should include encouragement to discuss current difficulties with the teacher or employer in person. This may clarify misperceptions about, for example, the way one has been treated on the job and help separate the real-world situation from distressing fantasies experienced with anxiety or depression.

Although treatment may address specific work or school behaviors or issues, the therapist should not allow the patient to avoid eventual responsibility for overall performance. If problems continue or appear to be disabling, the diagnosis should be changed.

309.90 Adjustment Disorder Not Otherwise Specified
Disorders that fall into this residual category should be treated according to the above suggestions, their presenting symptoms, the temporary or chronic stressors involved, and the environmental and psychodynamic characteristics that are likely to have an influence upon the eventual resolution of the condition. When the disorder does not fit one of the several "defined" adjustment disorders, the possibility of erroneous diagnosis should be explored.

Chapter 26

Psychological Factors Affecting Physical Condition

316.00 Psychological Factors Affecting Physical Condition
The psychological factors, accompanying symptoms, and treatment approaches vary widely, depending upon the patient's emotional characteristics and the specific physical disorder specified on Axis III. Some principles for intervention of the psychiatrist or other mental health professional, or psychiatrically oriented approaches by the attending physician, can be described, however. In each, the therapist should be a consistent, powerful ally of the patient. The family environment must not be neglected; formal family therapy may be important to the lasting alleviation of the disorder.

For purposes of this discussion, Psychological Factors Affecting Physical Condition will be divided into three sometimes overlapping groups:

1. Those in which the psychologically meaningful stimulus or process is acute and is followed by physical complications which are acute and short-lived;
2. Those in which the psychologically meaningful stimulus or process is acute, but the resultant physical complications are more lasting or chronic;

3. Those in which the psychological precipitating process is either ongoing or intermittent over a long period, and thus for which the physical symptoms or complications are chronic and/or recurrent.

It will be noted that the first of these is phenomenologically similar to the adjustment disorders discussed in the last section.

1. Acute Psychologically Meaningful Event with Acute Physical Reaction. One example of such a situation might be an emotional reaction to pending surgery, which increases the probability of medical or surgical complications. Another might be an emotional reaction to isolation and threat of death while one is being treated in an intensive care unit.

Psychiatric approaches vary widely, depending on presentation and individual needs; however, one can generally recommend a consultation-liaison approach. This may include suggestions to the treating staff about careful explanation of procedures, discussion of events that occurred prior to onset (Theorell, 1980), environmental changes within the health-care facility, increasing sensory stimulation and information available to an isolated or deprived patient, or small doses of psychotropic medication, each as appropriate to the case at hand.

2. Acute Psychologically Meaningful Physical or Emotional Stimuli Precipitating or Worsening a Chronic Physical Condition. Such a clinical situation may evolve from the more acute setting discussed above. Examples include some cases of psychogenic amenorrhea which begin with apparently acute stimuli and which may remit after brief psychiatric intervention (Khuri & Gehi, 1981). Some conditions may appear similar to Post-traumatic Stress Disorder (q.v.).

Treatment is often more complex than the relatively straightforward consultation-liaison or brief counseling approaches to acute, brief reactions (above). The ongoing nature of the physical symptoms may imply greater depth of psychopathology, a more pervasive precipitating trauma, and/or more deeply embedded symptoms by the time the patient is seen by the psychiatrist.

Ross, Schultz, and Edelstein (1982) described cases in which incomplete early treatment of psychologically significant stressors and the symptoms precipitated led to both medical and psychological problems in the future. The abilities of a consultation-liaison team to have an impact on several levels of medical care and to follow up patients whom they have seen are important in this regard. The specific treatment approach may still be relatively brief and nonintensive, with symptom removal by a variety of means (e.g., additional psychotherapy, biofeedback) and ongoing support frequently leading to good resolution, especially in cases of relatively acute onset and clear-cut stressors.

3. Psychologically Significant Events or Residua Which Continue to Influence, Chronically or Intermittently, the Physical Condition of the Patient. This group of patients includes those who fall most clearly into the classic "psychosomatic" bailiwick. Our understanding of the psychodynamics of some of the disorders is quite good; others have only recently been added to the seven whose developmental characteristics were originally suggested by Franz Alexander (1950).

Karasu (1979) points out that psychosomatic patients present a number of barriers to traditional psychodynamic treatment. These include the complexity of the influences between the psyche and the rest of the self, routinely profound resistance and denial, and countertransference reactions within the psychotherapist. He describes two "phases" of psychotherapy that should precede a therapeutic alliance: the "health alliance," in which the therapist has a doctor–patient relationship with the patient and is intimately involved with medical aspects of his illness; and the "life alliance," in which, as the medical condition improves, the therapist slowly becomes a friend or teacher.

Karasu notes that these preparatory phases may last months or years before the patient becomes accessible to a more psychoanalytic approach. Bräutigan (1979) also notes the necessity for lengthy treatment, perhaps including preverbal (e.g., movement, art) therapies, prior to, for example, an outpatient group. Bräutigan particularly recommends group therapy and notes that shortcuts are to be avoided while one tries to narrow the discrepancy between the patient's self-image and his or her ideal. Karasu and Bräutigan both note the need for flexibility of therapeutic approach, and the likely failure of the rigid psychotherapist who assumes that the psychosomatic patient will respond as a neurotic one.

Specific gains may be seen when psychotherapy is added to medical treatment. These vary with a number of factors, including the medical illness itself. For example, patients with asthma often respond well to psychotherapy aimed at altering their attitudes toward the illness, whether individually or in groups. Essential hypertension, on the other hand, has shown little response to psychiatric intervention whether or not it addresses theoretical underlying or precipitating psychodynamics.

Much treatment, such as supportive therapy for a brittle diabetic, is similar to that for patients with chronic Adjustment Disorder from an illness-stressor. Modifying patterns of communication and relationships, altering behavioral patterns, broadening the patient's perception of external and internal situations, and use of biofeedback or other conditioning techniques may be helpful for specific goals (Cohen, 1979). These should be offered in a biopsychosocial context (Kimball, 1981). In all consultation-liaison relationships there should be good communication between the psychiatrist and the treating physician (Strain, 1981).

Wolpe (1980) is among those who established that learned responses are a significant factor in most psychosomatic disorders, and who discussed ways to utilize this fact in behavior therapy. An initial behavior analysis to establish a correlation between psychological factors and somatic illness (or exacerbation thereof) should be exhaustive. Following this, any of a number of methods (e.g., systematic desensitization, biofeedback) may be effective in many patients. Asthmatics appear to respond particularly well to desensitization aimed at the asthma attack, the environment surrounding attacks, and situations that produce key stresses.

Relaxation and other techniques have been useful for symptomatic relief of headache and hypertension; however, the effects of any behavioral approaches on the long-term treatment of hypertension are still in question. Catharsis, assertiveness training, and even simple insight have been found helpful in some psychogenic dermatologic reactions.

Chapter 27

Personality Disorders

General Treatment Principles
For the most part, a personality disorder in and of itself does not produce discomfort; the diagnostic concept of personality disorders is designed to describe the character matrix upon which Axis I disorders may appear. Treatment usually alleviates peripheral symptoms, decreases social or emotional disability, or deals with some aspect of society's need for management of, for example, the antisocial person. For some disorders, treatment is rarely an issue; for others, reliable strategies have not been developed.

The depth of pathology is such that any concept of "cure" requires marked restructuring of very basic developmental characteristics. This approach has been studied for several years for some of the personality disorders but such attempts involve highly specialized, enormously energy-consuming therapies. Biological approaches (e.g., pharmacotherapy) may be useful for some symptoms of some disorders, and for some Axis I disorders overlaid upon personality disorders; however, none is globally helpful.

Countertransference and related feelings in the psychiatrist or psychotherapist are major issues in the treatment of the personality disorders. The frustration of dealing with treatment-resistant and/or primitive patients who (unless dismissed by the therapist) may be seen over many years is obvious. Less obvious is the problem of the therapist's true countertransference, seeing in the patient frightening or distasteful aspects of his or her own angry, sexual, or dependent impulses.

Three kinds of treatment are considered here. One may treat symptoms which arise because of vulnerability related to the personality disorder, but which are indistinguishable from the Axis I disorders addressed elsewhere in the text. The treatment of depressions or adjustment disorders, for example, should proceed as already discussed, with consideration given to the personality disorder's effect. Second, symptoms related to the personality disorder but not expressed in Axis I criteria, such as the impulsiveness and lability of many borderline patients, may be a focus of treatment. Finally, one may attempt to restructure the personality itself (or at least the manifest defensive style).

27A: CLUSTER A

301.00 Paranoid Personality Disorder

Individuals with paranoid personality rarely come to treatment unless they develop an Axis I disorder. Those who do present to the psychiatrist may do so to prove to others that "there is nothing wrong with me," or may consult the clinician as a peer or colleague about some problem the patient is perceiving as external (e.g., a woman who calls for assistance in creating a psychological profile of her ex-husband so that the police can arrest him for—imagined—harassment). Although many therapists would choose not to continue what appears to be an unrewarding interaction with such a person, there may be some value in allowing a benign relationship to form within which future, perhaps more serious, problems may be handled. The relationship should be a professional one; the temptation to befriend or "humor" the patient should be resisted.

Pharmacotherapy is not indicated unless psychotic decompensation appears to be approaching. When the patient feels anxiety about loss of control, he or she may accept, and benefit from, low doses of neuroleptics from a physician for whom there is some trust. The patient should never be treated surreptitiously.

301.20 Schizoid Personality Disorder

These patients rarely come to treatment in the absence of some form of decompensation, which may be triggered by unavoidable shifts in the external environment (e.g., serious illness). Crisis treatment should be symptomatic.

Anecdotal experience in psychotherapy, particularly recent work in the understanding and restructuring of primitive developmental phenomena, suggests intensive psychotherapy; however, it is available to few patients. Appel (1974) suggests that therapeutic goals include providing a sense of optimism that the patient's basic needs can be met without encountering overwhelming "collapse or supplication." The most useful therapeutic interaction is consistent and supportive, with clear rules, an ability for the patient to set therapeutic distance as needed, and some tolerance for acting out.

Medications are generally not useful except as temporary aids in cases of extraordinary anxiety. Antidepressants should not be prescribed in the absence of clinical signs of an Axis I affective disorder. Neuroleptics tend not to be useful unless signs of psychotic decompensation appear.

301.22 Schizotypal Personality Disorder

There is considerable psychotherapeutic experience with schizotypal patients. Reports frequently discuss schizotypal and "borderline" patients together, one author (Stone, 1985a) noting that the two are similar, and that schizotypal personality was derived from the "borderline schizophrenia" concept.

Analytically oriented psychotherapy is considered useful, provided the patient meets the usual criteria for this form of therapy, including likable demeanor, autoplastic defenses, high motivation, psychological-mindedness, genuine concern, good moral sense, self-discipline, and low impulsivity (Stone, 1985b). The therapy is lengthy, and—as with many personality-disordered patients—fraught with problems of transference and countertransference.

Supportive and educational aspects of therapy must often be allowed to intervene in the psychodynamic work. Because of the difficulty with social skills and comfort, group therapy and behavior modification are often useful. The principles discussed in the section on Borderline Personality (p. 339) often apply.

Schizotypal patients often present with symptoms for which medication is indicated, and frequently are treated in inpatient settings. As with borderline patients, low doses of high-potency neuroleptics such as thiothixene or haloperidol are often effective, even in the absence of frank psychosis (Goldberg et al., 1986; Serban & Siegel, 1984). Medication compliance tends to be relatively poor; even in hospital settings patients appear highly sensitive to side effects (Hymowitz et al., 1986).

Response to tricyclic antidepressants is usually disappointing (Soloff et al., 1986b). There are anecdotal reports of response to MAO inhibitors, although treatment compliance may be an even larger issue with these drugs. Although alprazolam may seem the logical choice because of its anxiolytic properties and good patient acceptance, there is little or no evidence of lasting benefit.

Treatment of superficial symptoms, including acute psychosis or depression, is often successful. Outcome for the personality disorder itself is enhanced when the patient is able to remain in lengthy, restorative therapy; however, the overall prognosis must be guarded. Patients tend to do considerably better than schizophrenics in long-term follow-up studies, but worse than patients with major affective disorders (McGlashan, 1986; Plakun, Burkhardt, & Muller, 1985).

27B: CLUSTER B

301.70 Antisocial Personality Disorder

The importance of differentiating Antisocial Personality from other psychiatric diagnoses in nonillness conditions (e.g., Adult Antisocial Behavior, V71.01) cannot be overstated. Nevertheless, clinicians often treat antisocial symptoms and behaviors as if they represent the personality disorder itself. This approach interferes with adequate treatment planning and often leads to poor response (Reid, 1981a; Reid, 1986).

It is a truism that most characterologically antisocial persons do not actively seek therapy; however, they may come to treatment in a variety of ways, the most familiar being within a forensic setting. Even without internal motivation, it may be possible for the therapist to find reasons to keep the patient working in treatment (e.g., in order to accomplish release from incarceration). Under a few circumstances the patient may begin to experience some form of dysphoria, usually either depression or temporary anxiety about some life situation. The former may arise late in the natural course of the personality disorder, as a result of containment in a hospital or prison in which self-stimulation is impossible, or late in psychotherapy (Reid, 1981b).

Insight-oriented treatment of sufficient intensity and duration to penetrate the psychopathic defensive structure requires extraordinary dedication of patient and therapist. The former is likely to be unwilling to take on this task; the latter may not wish to spend his or her time treating such a patient instead of one with some other disturbance.

For those patients who do become engaged in treatment, the most reliable sign of progress is the development of true, dysphoric affect. The first affect seen is often depression, which is both surprising and uncomfortable for the patient (who is not used to experiencing such feelings). At this point, the therapist should become supportive and empathic, helping the patient to understand that the discomfort is a sign of progress, that it is bearable, and that the patient and therapist will work together to understand it, provided the patient chooses not to escape therapy. This depression is probably separate from the genetic relationship between antisocial and affective syndromes described by Reich (1985). Countertransference issues are very important, with powerful feelings of both seduction and revulsion in the therapist. Consultation or supervision is highly recommended (Lion, 1981).

Hospital Treatment. Definitive inpatient treatment must be carried on a specialized unit. There should be no patients with nonantisocial diagnoses, and staff must be well experienced in the care of characterologically disordered patients.

Successful inpatient programs involve long-term, strictly structured hierarchical settings in which every aspect of the patient's life affects, and is affected by, his progress. Some programs control the patient's administrative status as well as other parts of his life from the day he enters the hospital. He begins with very few privileges except that of being treated as a human being.

Carney (1978) notes four particular deficits in the truly psychopathic patient which must be addressed during such intensive residential treatment: the inability to trust, to fantasize, to feel affect, and to learn from experience. As the patient slowly moves through a hierarchy of levels and privileges, he acquires more and more self-esteem, awareness of his emotional life, and social and interpersonal competence, leading to lessened need for the antisocial character style.

In addition to the rigorous structure, there should always be time for reflection. Particularly during early stages, the patient needs a place to become "emotional" without exposing himself completely to others. Later in the program, sharing one's feelings is a necessary part of treatment (Reid, 1985). Consistent support, short of coddling, is extremely important; the very basic fragility of these patients' self-images must be recognized in spite of their tough exteriors.

Because such programs are uniformly on closed units, and often part of correctional systems rather than hospitals, staff members often have the dual role of therapist and jailer. Even the correctional staff should be chosen for sensitivity and absence of sadistic characteristics.

Communication among staff for mutual support and consistent treatment approaches is critical. Many institutions use the same staff for both inpatient and outpatient treatment; the period of transition between the hospital and community should be monitored especially carefully. Control over discharge, such as by means of close relationships between treating staff and the paroling authority, is important.

Unfortunately, there are few programs that meet the above standards. Those that do exist are moderately expensive (although far less so than ineffective incarceration), take years to complete, and tend to have good results, particularly if the patient receives community follow-up by the same treatment team. The reader may wish to consult the work of George Stürup for more detailed program descriptions (Stürup & Reid, 1981).

Most programs for women are considerably less advanced and tend to address more correctional than therapeutic issues (Benedek, 1981).

Patients with antisocial and aggressive personality styles are quite difficult to treat on ordinary psychiatric units. Staff are reluctant to admit and work with them (Willner & Radiner, 1983); their symptoms generally do not remit (even superficial ones); and they are often destructive to the milieu and other patients.

Medications. Medications have in general not proved helpful. They are sometimes prescribed for specific symptoms, but those symptoms in patients with antisocial personality are usually situational (e.g., anxiety, depression) and thus better treated with brief counseling.

Several medications have been studied to address aggressive behavior in Antisocial Personality Disorder and other diagnoses. Lithium carbonate has decreased fighting in some prison populations (Tupin et al., 1972). Methylphenidate has been suggested for patients whose Antisocial Personality Disorder is felt to be linked to childhood Attention-deficit Hyperactivity Disorder (Stringer & Josef, 1983). These should not be considered routine treatments.

One exception to this general premise is the treatment of severe depression, which occasionally develops in older patients and in patients whose treatment has led to a restructuring of the Antisocial Personality. These patients may benefit from antidepressant medication, and are sometimes suicidal. There are no reported controlled studies of the use of antidepressants for such patients, however.

Family. The patient's family deserves educational counseling. The patient usually appears superficially normal, but causes (or encounters) repeated problems which are often confusing for family members. This confusion, the guilt, the temptation to make restitution for his criminal acts, and the frustration of working with someone who is apparently quite ill but refuses treatment (or for whom treatment is not offered) should be discussed openly with family members. Family members may find it helpful to read Cleckley's *The Mask of Sanity* (1976).

Other Treatment Approaches. Treatment programs in correctional settings are usually not aimed at changing personality disorders, although they may be valuable for treating schizophrenic, affective, and substance abuse disorders (Shively & Petrich, 1985). Substance abuse treatment programs often address antisocial behavior, but should not be confused with comprehensive programs for Antisocial Personality (Rosenthal, 1984; Woody et al., 1985).

Some specialized community programs, particularly those patterned after the Probationed Offender's Rehabilitation and his Treatment (P.O.R.T.) program designed by Francis Tyce, provide a modern, successful alternative for many nonmentally ill offenders. Although not specifically designed for Antisocial Personality, they share some characteristics with the longer, more intensive residential approaches just described (e.g., hierarchical structures). The offender is expected to become employed or enroll in full-time school, be responsible for his own behavior and that of his peers in the program, arrange restitution to victims, and engage completely in a program that lasts about six months.

These programs should not be confused with "halfway houses." Although the doors are not locked, many antisocial individuals find the pressures of responsibility, affect, and noncriminal lifestyles to be highly stressful; up to 50% drop out.

Wilderness. Another treatment modality, helpful for antisocial people but not specifically designed for Antisocial Personality, is the specialized wilderness program with challenging physical and social settings designed specifically for adolescent and adult offenders. Such programs usually consist of three phases, which take about three weeks to complete: orientation and learning about the survival and interpersonal skills that will be required; a wilderness trip with several offenders and a few counselors working together to achieve a complex physical goal in a natural setting; and a "solo" phase during which the individual experiences himself and the wilderness alone.

Some such programs include only the wilderness component, with little or no follow-up. Others provide as much as a year of residential activity designed to increase personal and social competence and prepare the patient for reentering his community. A few similar programs use urban settings instead of wilderness. Recidivism rates are considerably better than those for incarceration, or for "easy" or nonspecialized wilderness trips (e.g., ordinary camping trips).

301.83 Borderline Personality Disorder

In spite of its relatively recent classification, the diagnosis of "Borderline Personality" has become one of the most common for psychiatric patients. It has the largest literature of any personality disorder, with a huge variety of treatment approaches and concepts for superficial symptoms, the disorder itself, and Axis I symptoms overlaid upon Borderline Personality. The following summary is necessarily limited in scope.

Crisis, Superficial Symptoms. Patients with Borderline Personality Disorder may present with virtually any psychiatric symptom seen in the Axis I disorders. The hallmarks of crisis and symptomatic treatment must be one's understanding of their defensive purpose, the patient's vulnerability to relapse or other symptoms, and the extraordinary transference and other aspects of the therapeutic relationship. The word "containment" is often used to describe one of the needs of the borderline patient, relating sometimes to the psychodynamic need for ego containment, and by other writers to a reassuring control of symptoms and environment which can be a focus of treatment.

Clear and consistent therapeutic rules are sometimes effective for patients whose treatment is continuously disrupted by crises (often with a resistive purpose). The rules must be ones that the therapist can keep, however, and not ones that merely invite escalation by the patient (as might occur if the therapist says "I refuse to rehospitalize you").

The therapist's *expectation* that the patient will succeed—socially or vocationally, for example—is important. In this regard, although the therapist may be tempted to be available at all times for the patient's crises, he or she should support the patient's strengths as well (e.g., a good work record, staying out of the hospital for several months, or even merely keeping therapy appointments). Although the first consideration for many patients and their therapists in a crisis is sometimes a return to the hospital, alternatives should be presented (e.g., changes in the treatment contract, increasing the intensity of outpatient support, or considering halfway houses or day hospitals).

The hospital emergency room frequently enters into the treatment of any borderline patient. Beresin and Gordon (1981) note that the emergency room can be a source of empathic reassurance, crisis intervention, and education in spite of its drawback for psychiatric assessment and treatment. There is no lasting working alliance in the emergency room (although there may be an institutional "transference"); support is paramount and interpretation should be absent. Any medication should be directed at specific symptoms or at crisis management.

Disposition of the patient is difficult, with power struggles often being part of the negotiations. Immediate return to the ongoing outpatient therapist or mental health center, if any, is important. The emergency clinician must be careful not to reinforce dilution of therapy or "splitting" in patients who are already being treated elsewhere but who turn to the emergency room in crisis.

Short-term Hospitalization. Some indications for short-term hospitalization include protection of the patient (e.g., from potential suicide), need for comprehensive assessment, preparation for outpatient psychotherapy, resolution of a therapeutic *impasse*, and restoration of impaired reality testing (Koenigsberg, 1984). Short-term hospitalization has little effect on underlying development deficits (Simon, 1986). Nevertheless, an understanding of the borderline syndrome provides the basis for practical approaches that may be helpful to these and other patients.

Nursing staff face a particular challenge from these patients. The psychiatrist should be aware of the hour-to-hour and day-to-day treatment dilemmas that arise among members of the inpatient treatment team (Kaplan, 1986). Acute-care psychiatric hospitals and general hospitals with psychiatric units should assess the impact of borderline patients on the treatment milieu, and decide whether or not to tailor their functions to fit the unusual needs of these patients, such as by creating an especially intensive, containing milieu (Greben, 1983; Johansen, 1983).

The short-term milieu should be a model for self-regulation of regression and impulsive behavior. Intensive protection and infantilization with, for example, one-to-one observation is often destructive to the patient's progress and sets up struggles which may lead to countertherapeutic actions by both staff and patient. The treatment plan should include very early establishment of modest, focused goals for short-term gains; careful orientation and assessment of the patient's needs and abilities to participate in treatment; monitoring of patterns of interaction with staff and other patients; and early identification of issues that may disrupt treatment so that they can be discussed with patient, staff, family, and the like (Viner, 1986). The hospital must not potentiate the tremendous regressive potential of these patients; the situation should be "dependable," not "dependent" (Peteet & Gutheil, 1979).

A few programs offer short-term residential alternatives to actual hospitalization for chronic psychiatric patients, including borderline patients. One, the La Posada program, combines crisis intervention with halfway house methods to enhance independent functioning and counteract regressive behavior. The setting is highly structured and includes group and individual therapy, as well as expectations of appropriate behavior and responsibility. Patients begin outpatient and/or day treatment prior to discharge (Weisman, 1985).

Open-ended therapeutic programs should be avoided for acutely hospitalized borderline patients. Structuring of activities, objectives, and even time sequences (past, present, and future) is important and helps to address the excessive permissiveness commonly found in staff or therapist (Nurnberg & Feldman, 1983).

Long-term Hospitalization and Residential Treatment. For many patients, any attempt at structural change of Borderline Personality involves care in a specialized residential environment. Such units should not confuse the major psychodynamic issues of the borderline patient with those more typical of frankly psychotic, severely depressed, or neurotic patients. Many of the concepts discussed below apply as well to severely narcissistic patients, however. Many of the psychotherapeutic approaches found in the long-term hospital environment are discussed later in the psychotherapy sections.

One of the most important purposes of active long-term treatment is preparation for and beginning of major structural change. Patients with long-standing withdrawal (sometimes to a virtually psychotic extent), agitation and/or impulsive violence, or intractable depression and self-destructive behavior are candidates. Long-term hospitalization allows establishment of a much more consistent and realistic therapeutic community than is possible in acute-care hospitals. The well-established inpatient community can provide important containment and a caring, flexible "family" (with the accompanying transference implications). It illustrates but also attenuates interpersonal and social problems, and serves as an important adjunct to individual psychotherapy (Stern, Fromm, & Sacksteder, 1986).

Group and individual psychotherapy with qualified clinicians is imperative for treatment success (see below). Stabilization of the patient and preparation for outpatient care—particularly transition to an appropriate aftercare system—is often the ultimate objective (Rosenbluth,

1987). The long-term treatment program should be seen as an environment in which the patient experiences development, and in which staff (particularly the primary therapist) consistently accompany and empathize with the patient (Chessick, 1982).

Short-term Psychotherapy. For most patients, support, often sporadic and crisis-oriented, will be a frequent treatment modality, even during exploratory psychotherapy. The usual supportive techniques include education, clarification, direct comments, genuineness, sympathy, and establishment of limits.

The treatment orientation should include flexibility, a *realistic* therapeutic contract, and consideration for the patient's fragility. Therapists who are rigid in their expectations are likely to be disappointed, and feel helpless and enraged when the patient does not improve (Silver, 1985). Errors are easily made by premature confrontation or transference interpretation, inappropriate management of countertherapeutic or destructive behaviors, and misunderstanding of the patient's "attachment to pain" (Sederer & Thorbeck, 1986).

Rapid mood shifts make suicidal behavior common and dangerous. Although many such behaviors are interpreted as "acting-out" and often irritate and frustrate the therapist more than they physically injure the patient, the therapist must accept the fact that the patient's suicidal threats and behaviors are a very effective tool for manipulation and resistance; they cannot be ignored. Suicide potential should be particularly evaluated in the presence of poor reality-testing or incipient psychosis.

Intensive Therapies and Psychoanalysis. Given a qualified and experienced therapist, structural change is a reasonable goal for some patients. Recent shifts in theoretical emphasis from drive theory to object relations theories and self psychology encourage many psychiatrists to consider psychotherapy for those with Borderline and Narcissistic character traits (Silver, 1983). Clinical indications that intensive exploration may be successful include consistent motivation, limited impulsivity, "psychological mindedness," tolerance for interpersonal relationships, the ability to soothe oneself emotionally, reasonable likeableness, a preponderance of autoplastic defenses, some general concern for change and empathy, and sufficient self-discipline to adhere to the therapeutic contract and schedule.

Patients who are particularly vengeful or who have been severely exploited or abused are relatively poorer candidates (Silver, 1983; Stone, 1985b). Uncontrolled substance abuse and paraphilias traditionally predict poor response. Intractable acting-out renders the patient unavailable for outpatient therapy. Some of these relative contraindications can be circumvented if the patient can be treated in a long-term residential setting.

Stone (1987) stresses that one of the most important transactions in reconstructive therapy involves the therapist's ability to recognize his own reactions, to understand the source of his countertransference within the patient's psyche, and to translate this understanding for the patient. This important use of countertransference brings out feelings (especially angry ones) which the patient has, but disowns.

The treatment itself includes strong relationships between patient and therapist, within which the patient can move as needed from extreme closeness to considerable distance, but which encourages separation-individuation and tolerance for therapeutic interventions (Horwitz, 1985). Early in the work, content deserves more active attention than process, and negative feelings toward the therapist-object should be made as conscious as possible (Waldinger, 1987). Throughout treatment, the therapist will need to insert support and "real" intervention, often followed by observation or interpretation of the situation which gave rise to the need for such actions.

There are many controversies within the literature and among clinicians with regard to proper therapeutic stance, the order of addressing various psychodynamic issues, tolerance for various behaviors of the patient, and the like. The reader is referred to references cited for further discussion.

Diagnostic continua or spectra, particularly between Borderline and Narcissistic Personality Disorders and between character pathology and neurosis, have suggested that many borderline patients who are successful in psychotherapy or psychoanalysis begin to look increasingly narcissistic. This is considered by Adler (1980) to be a goal of treatment for such patients, and the antithesis of retreat into schizoid isolation.

The treatment of Narcissistic Personality Disorder (q.v.) is often discussed with, and compared to, the treatment of Borderline Personality Disorder. Adler (1986) agrees with most other clinicians that the first few months of psychotherapy consist largely of support and empathy, early clarification of countertransference, and awareness of the power of the patient's issues of anger and aloneness. Success in this phase leads to attempts at optimal frustration within the psychotherapy, and the experiencing of self-object transferences with the therapist.

In spite of the extensive literature and interesting discussion among clinicians about the psychotherapeutic treatment of Borderline Personality Disorder, there remains little in the way of nonanecdotal description of treatment techniques to guide the psychotherapist (Frosch, 1983). In Silver's words (1983), such treatment may still be considered "therapeutic heroics."

Group Therapy. A wide variety of group therapy experiences may be helpful for borderline patients. Some are practical and related to day-to-day issues, such as parenting skills and experiences groups (Holman, 1985). Others are quite intensive, offering consistent, analytically oriented environments for reality testing, growth, and change (Kretsch, Goren, & Wasserman, 1987; Macaskill, 1982). The importance of group involvement in long-term inpatient settings, both as a part of a therapeutic community and as a vehicle for internal exploration, has already been addressed.

Medications. Unlike the case with some other personality disorders, judicious choice of medication can affect the course of Borderline Personality Disorder. On the other hand, like hysteroid and schizotypal patients, the borderline individual is often inordinately sensitive to side effects, poorly compliant, and exhibits capricious-appearing vacillations of symptoms—even metamorphoses—that are distressing to the ordered style of many biological psychiatrists.

Antipsychotic medications are the ones most often considered, and may be prescribed either for the occasional acute psychosis seen in these patients or for their chronic (especially schizotypal) symptoms. For acute psychosis, routine doses of high-potency neuroleptics such as thiothixene or haloperidol are used (see Chapter 14).

Schizotypal symptoms (i.e., near-psychotic eccentricities and anxieties) are the next most frequently considered indication. Low doses are sufficient. Thiothixene in the general range of 6–12 mg per day is sometimes found to be superior to haloperidol; however, both appear to address cognitive disturbance, derealization, ideas of reference, anxiety, and even depression in borderline patients (see below) (Goldberg et al., 1986; Serban & Siegel, 1984). Addition of adjunctive drugs has not been well studied. An understanding of the psychodynamic meaning of medication, particularly in patients engaged in psychotherapy, should include considering pills as transitional objects (Adelman, 1985).

The use of antidepressants in Borderline Personality is often disappointing. At least one series of double-blind comparisons indicated uniformly better results from neuroleptics than from tricyclic antidepressants in reducing overall symptom severity (Soloff et al., 1986a,b). Cole and colleagues (1984), however, found that tricyclics were effective for borderline patients with specific symptoms of major depression. These studies reflect the general clinical feeling that severe depressive symptoms in borderline patients should be treated with antidepressants, in spite of a relative dearth of research support. There is at least one report of severe adverse reactions to tricyclic antidepressants in borderline patients, including increased suicide threats, assaultive behavior, and paranoid ideation (Soloff, 1986c).

Many other medications may be prescribed for specific symptoms or syndromes, although the response in borderline patients may not be as good as that expected in patients with uncomplicated Axis I disorders. Thus, patients with hypomanic symptoms may respond to lithium, some depressed or primitively self-destructive patients to MAO inhibitors, and so forth. Gardner and Cowdry (1986) reported some decrease in behavioral dyscontrol when carbamazepine was prescribed for borderline women with intractable impulsiveness.

Medication should never been given without adequate psychosocial intervention. Repeated use of medication for patients' frequent complaints of anxiety may sometimes be necessary, but should be viewed with caution.

Outcome and Follow-up. Many of the indicators for psychotherapeutic or psychoanalytic success discussed above are associated with relatively better outcome for the patient, and sometimes a good prognosis. Woollcott (1985) proposes a similar list of prognostic indicators for psychotherapy. Waldinger and Gunderson (1984) examined the outcome of 78 borderline patients of some 11 experienced psychotherapists. They came to the general conclusion that the longer patients stayed in treatment, the more they improved. In addition, the more prior treatment the patient had, the better the therapeutic outcome.

This finding is particularly important, since many patients stop therapy prematurely and both patient and therapist may be pessimistic about the future. Subsequent psychotherapy often builds upon the last experience, when the patient is ready for another "step" in his or her growth. Many of the patients in the Waldinger and Gunderson study did not complete treatment, but had made considerable gains in ego function, behavior, object relatedness, and sense of self.

Stone (1987) traced a large number of borderline patients 10 to 23 years after referral for psychoanalytic psychotherapy. He reported that 40% showed "clinical recovery," often after five to 10 years of treatment. Two-thirds had at least a "good" outcome. It may be noted that these patients were treated by very experienced psychotherapists.

301.50 Histrionic Personality Disorder

According to *DSM-III-R*, Histrionic Personality Disorder is identical to "hysterical personality." Kernberg (1986b), however, differentiates the two in a recent psychiatry textbook. To make matters more confusing, psychiatry and the public have various definitions of "hysterical," which are nicely differentiated by Chodoff (1982). For purposes of this chapter, we will refer to patients who meet *DSM-III-R* criteria for Histrionic Personality Disorder and to symptoms they are likely to present.

Although medications may be indicated for acute psychotic or depressive symptoms, most superficial and characterologic symptoms are best addressed with psychotherapy. Hysterical neurosis should be differentiated from hysterical or Histrionic Personality, the personality disorder being considerably more complicated to treat. Sometimes this differentiation cannot be made until the patient has revealed the character pathology in several weeks or months of psychoanalytically oriented psychotherapy.

Specific topics to be addressed, or which present particular problems in therapy, cannot be comprehensively addressed in this text, but include early, stormy, and intense transference with erotic-seeming (but not truly erotic) defenses guarding against awareness of great dependency. Patients are often quite seductive, in the sense that they appear to be working on important therapeutic issues and forming positive transferences, while becoming angry at the therapist's lack of total, giving presence. The therapist's skill at knowing when to give and when to judiciously frustrate the patient is critically important.

Kernberg (1986b) feels that Histrionic Personality is likely to worsen without psychotherapy, while hysterical personality may gradually improve as the patient adjusts with age. He suggests prompt treatment, even if severe pathology, intractable acting-out, or antisocial features limit the therapist's interventions to support and superficial exploration.

The therapist should be aware that the reactive aspects of the disorder often lead to anxious, depressive, or other overreactions to minor emotional or external events. Brief counseling techniques should thus be available, even for the patient engaged in ongoing psychotherapy. Dramatic, impulsive, often poorly-thought-out suicidal behavior is frequently seen. Although it may accurately be interpreted as manipulative or "gesture," such behavior must always be taken seriously, particularly if one is not familiar with the patient. For those with whom the therapist is quite familiar, the principles of availability, consistency, and firmness outlined in the section on Borderline Personality Disorder may be helpful.

301.81 Narcissistic Personality Disorder

The "spectrum" of narcissistic disorders to which Adler (1986) refers has been touched upon in earlier sections of this chapter. Here, we will refer to the many levels at which the patient may have problems with narcissistic needs and expectations, and the accompanying levels of adaptation found (from severe impairment to great social success). The goals of restructuring therapies are increased empathy for others and toward the self; decreased regression in the face of rebuff, failure, or separation; a capacity for flexible detachment and distancing oneself; the ability to feel gratified when working alone; the ability to give without personal gain; and the capacity to truly mourn an important loss (Nurnberg, 1984).

One of the issues in the psychotherapeutic treatment of the successful narcissistic patient is whether or not he or she has a personality disorder. Ledermann (1982) points out the danger of underdiagnosing these patients, and then discusses their psychoanalysis in much the same way as that of other serious personality disorders. The patient eventually becomes able to integrate his disowned or split-off impulses, experience them as not absolute, and tolerate a world in which love and hate, black and white, can coexist.

Battegay (1985) recognizes a need for a modified psychoanalytic approach, however, in which empathy is important during periods of depression. Ganzarain (1982) discusses opportunities that may be available in group, as opposed to individual, psychotherapy which help the patient consider overcoming his grandiose wish to be his own provider, depending upon no one.

The understanding, and eventual interpretation and working-through, of the grandiose self is the primary task of psychoanalytically oriented treatment. This is often seen in the transference, in which the "real" aspects of the therapeutic relationship are missing and the patient seems emotionally unavailable (Kernberg, 1986a).

The concept of mourning is important to change in narcissistic patients. Protection against significant loss, of real objects, is the major purpose of narcissistic character structure. Warnes (1984) describes a poignant termination phase in which the activation of profound mourning led to structural change.

Nonintensive Treatment. Treatment of reactive or superficial symptoms should progress largely upon the lines discussed for the Axis I disorders and symptoms, with an understanding of the underlying personality disorder. Symptom fluctuations and suicide dangers are of less concern than with Borderline Personality Disorder. The hiding of the patient's pathology through normal-appearing narcissistic defenses and behavior is common; however, the purpose of short-term or crisis treatment is the shoring up of existing defenses, not the restructuring of narcissistic character.

27C: CLUSTER C

301.82 Avoidant Personality Disorder

There have been no research reports of treatment of this disorder since its inclusion in the original *DSM-III*. A few authors suggest differences between the avoidant patient and the schizoid patient (the latter possessing a deficit in relating ability, rather than a defense against relating) or the borderline patient; however, most clinical recommendations are similar to those for Schizoid Personality Disorder.

Most patients never come to treatment because of the security of their "neurotic equilibrium," which would be upset by any change in symptoms. For those who do, initial supportive care and enhancement of self-image may allow some tentative exploration of interactions with others and with the environment within the safety of the therapeutic relationship.

Group therapy offers opportunities to explore growth within a protected setting. A number of behavioral treatments (e.g., desensitization) offer the patient control over progress and change. In addition, specific treatments for symptoms or signs of Axis I disorders such as anxiety or phobia should prove useful, while allowing the patient to retain ego-syntonic avoidance defenses. Psychoanalytically oriented techniques such as those earlier described for the personality disorders probably represent the treatment of choice for a few patients.

301.60 Dependent Personality Disorder

As with many of the other personality disorders, patients with this diagnosis are unlikely to seek treatment. They may, however, wish to explore reasons for lack of social or vocational success, and may suffer considerable loss when an important figure leaves them in one way or another. Referrals of dependent patients within a consultation-liaison framework are common; however, many of these patients' characteristics are related to a medical illness within a hospital setting and do not fill DSM-III-R criteria for Dependent Personality Disorder.

The primary therapeutic modality is psychotherapy. Early in therapy, the clinician should accept much of the same dependence that the patient feels toward others in his or her life. Symptoms and psychodynamics can then be discussed firsthand, rather than as reports of feelings about others. The therapist's support of the patient's individuation from others (and now from the therapist as well) should include practical issues such as jobs and housing.

Failure of the highly gratifying dependent style may give rise to anxiety, depression, or other symptoms. These may be superficially treated using suggestions given elsewhere in this book; however, caution should be exercised when considering medication. Anxiolytics are likely to be abused, and antidepressants are inappropriate for reactive symptoms such as these. Behavioral interventions or practical, directive counseling approaches are more likely to help, and less likely to add to the patient's problems in the long run.

One should, however, take these reactive symptoms seriously, since severely dependent patients harbor a potential for overwhelming despondency or rage against the self or others (Kiev, 1976). Profound loss or intense affect in these patients should lead the therapist to consider protective measures such as hospitalization, with which the patient can be contained to some extent and definitive therapy for Axis I symptoms carried out in a controlled setting.

Termination of individual or group psychotherapy is a delicate task, and should be a joint decision. The therapist should be flexible, allowing the patient to return as needed, within reason. Frustration of lingering dependent needs, which one might consider in other kinds of patients to be a therapeutic motivating factor, may have countertherapeutic effects (Malinow, 1981).

301.40 Obsessive Compulsive Personality Disorder

Patients with Obsessive Compulsive Personality Disorder who seek treatment usually do so because the usefulness of this usually effective character style has been compromised. Common symptoms are those of Axis I diagnoses of Obsessive Compulsive Disorder, Affective Disorder, or occasionally Paranoia. The patient is often quite anxious, and motivated for psychotherapy. The short-term treatments for Obsessive Compulsive Disorder described elsewhere in this text are often effective. Behavioral and psychotherapeutic treatments for depression or anxiety, or anxiolytic medication, are usually effective. Reconstitution of the previously effective personality disorder usually preempts any need for tricyclic antidepressants or longer-term care.

For motivated patients, the definitive treatment is insight-oriented or psychoanalytic psychotherapy. Needs for control and related fears of destructive impulses are important issues at all levels of treatment, from simple scheduling requests, to intellectualization and rationalization, to other resistances against fantasy and free association. Many of the characteristics that lead to a successful life for such a patient and that appear to the inexperienced therapist to create an excellent therapy candidate are actually symptoms that can become serious impediments to treatment (Tarachow, 1963).

The therapist must avoid competing with the patient and should be able to tolerate his verbal attacks, retaining a therapeutic posture rather than allowing sessions to deteriorate into intellectual discussions or nonproductive interchange. Patients who show signs of deteriorating should probably be treated less intensively and more actively. In some cases, cognitive therapy may be tried (Quality Assurance Project, 1985). Although many patients will have read a psychiatry text and may request specific medications or therapies, the clinician's treatment decisions should be continued, and the patient's behavior observed or interpreted as resistance.

301.84 Passive Aggressive Personality Disorder

Treatment of these patients is similar to, but may be less rewarding than, the treatment of the patient with Dependent Personality Disorder. Psychotherapy is likely to be frustrating; however, the fact that the passive-aggressive symptoms often severely interfere with work or social goals may motivate the patient to participate long enough to form a therapeutic alliance. Clear rules of therapy must be outlined; those that involve schedules, billing, and the like should be provided in writing. This prevents spending inordinate amounts of time arguing over something that the patient calls forgetfulness, but the therapist calls (sometimes pejoratively) resistance. Passive-aggressive patients respond to the therapist much as they respond to others in their lives, whom they often perceive to be unfairly demanding.

Presenting symptoms of either failure of the passive-aggressive coping style or problems with the patient's environment guide initial interventions toward Axis I-like symptoms, usually of anxiety or depression. Although it is tempting to use their distress as fuel for commitment to psychotherapy, patients who cannot escape their defensive binds or environmental situations through their usual passive-aggressive resources may escalate their defensive behavior, even to the point of suicide attempts. When possible, one should not confuse passive-aggressive sources of self-destructive behavior with major affective disorder, and should avoid antidepressants. Protective hospitalization is occasionally required; the patient has now thrown down a gauntlet of confrontation or panic, which the therapist should not firmly challenge.

In this and other treatment situations, countertransference and related issues must be carefully considered. One commonly hears the term "passive-aggressive" used to connote manipulative or frustrating patients in a way that is punishing or derisive. Although the clinician may feel angry, he or she should be flexible and remember that the patient's behavior, even if apparently voluntary, is defending against severe anxiety or deterioration. On the other hand, if the therapist's "giving in" is seen as ambivalence or abandoning of therapeutic interest, the patient may feel bereft and the therapeutic alliance may be injured.

Directive and behavioral techniques, such as assertiveness training, offer concrete ways to address the patient (Perry & Flannery, 1982). These should be considered symptomatic treatment, however, except when added to a comprehensive plan for long-term psychotherapy.

301.90 Personality Disorder Not Otherwise Specified

Patients who qualify for this residual category should be treated based upon the clinician's estimate of presenting symptoms, personality dynamics, and developmental level, and interactions among them.

Chapter 28

V Codes for Conditions Not Attributable to a Mental Disorder That Are a Focus of Attention or Treatment

V62.30 Academic Problem
Treatment of this disorder in the absence of any other diagnosable mental disorder should be based upon simple counseling with exploration of possible family or environmental stresses. As with many of the other V Code conditions, one should be aware of the dangers of overdiagnosis and mislabeling of conditions not attributable to a mental disorder.

V71.01 Adult Antisocial Behavior
Few treatment approaches are effective for repeated antisocial behavior which is not due to one of the mental disorders already discussed (including a reactive Adjustment Disorder). Individual and group psychotherapy alone have poor records of success, as do all of the biological therapies, ordinary psychiatric hospitalization, or simple incarceration.

Inpatient hospitalization at institutions such as those discussed under Antisocial Personality Disorder may be successful for some patients; however, the majority of patients with adult antisocial behavior do not commit crimes sufficient to allow their being sentenced to several years of maximum security treatment. For many of these people, the community and wilderness treatment programs discussed under Antisocial Personality Disorder have met with some success and are quite cost-effective (Cytrynbaum & Ken, 1975; Kimball, 1979; Reid & Matthews, 1980; Reid & Solomon, 1981).

V40.00 Borderline Intellectual Functioning

This category, which is made up of the majority of individuals society calls "mentally retarded," does not represent true mental retardation (Strider & Menolascino, 1981). For the most part, these people have few serious difficulties in society; however, they may be prone to problems in those areas in which one's cognitive abilities or fund of knowledge are important for coping with personal or environmental problems. Supportive treatment, along with relevant education for the patient when such problems or crises develop, is almost always helpful. One may wish to counsel the family as well and to be sure that the patient knows of available help from social agencies (e.g., employment counseling for a worker who has lost his job).

Much of the frustration of the person with Borderline Intellectual Functioning is related to how he or she is treated by an uninformed or prejudiced public. Discussions with community, school, or work officials may be helpful. When problems are more troublesome (as in a person with an accompanying Conduct Disorder), flexible, practical therapeutic measures should be employed rather than traditional approaches such as individual or group psychotherapy (although some group therapy is highly effective). Institutionalization or other infantilizing procedures are never necessary for the treatment of Borderline Intellectual Functioning per se.

V71.02 Childhood or Adolescent Antisocial Behavior

The treatment of many of these behaviors is discussed earlier in the text, in both the section on Disorders Usually First Evident in Infancy, Childhood, or Adolescence and the section on Antisocial Personality Disorder (although persons of this age should never be given the diagnosis of Antisocial Personality Disorder). It is important that children or adolescents not be given this diagnosis if their antisocial behavior forms a pattern that can be diagnosed elsewhere in the *DSM-III-R*.

Unfortunately, it has become common for children or adolescents with simple antisocial behavior to be placed in psychiatric hospitals. In some cases, this is because of well-meaning parents, judges, or probation officers who feel that psychiatric hospitalization is preferable to juvenile detention or jail. In others, it seems related to the marketing of adolescent hospital beds by enthusiastic providers. In either case, adding an indelible record of psychiatric hospitalization and fostering a "sick" self-image is rarely helpful in the long run. In addition, the brief hospitalization usually available in acute-care hospitals does not adequately address many kinds of delinquency. Specialized programs for conduct disorders may be effective.

V65.20 Malingering

Since by definition there is no primary illness to treat once malingering has been established, there remain only a couple of issues of management of the patient who is felt to be voluntarily misrepresenting his or her symptoms for some conscious reason not associated with factitious illness (e.g., to obtain money, avoid work, or avoid responsibility for criminal behavior). The most obvious of these is to offer understanding and counsel to the person who feels that he or she must use this dishonest course of action. Education with respect to social agencies available to help with financial problems, the possible consequences of one's dishonesty, or even the fact that faking an illness really *is* dishonest, and a serious misuse of resources may be beneficial.

The temptation to tell someone about the malingering should be resisted. In addition to the possibility that the patient is not malingering, this author would disagree with Getto (1982) that one of the treatment goals is to make the malingering "diagnosis" available to legal, health, and social agencies with which the patient may have contact. The physician who does this runs considerable risk of breach of ethics and could under some circumstances be liable for slander or libel. It seems more prudent, if less gratifying, to note in the record that one is unable to find any medical or psychological basis for the individual's complaints.

V61.10 Marital Problem

In the absence of other mental disorder, including Adjustment Disorder, the goals of the therapist are generally to provide information and counseling, be an objective observer, recognize problems in communication and facilitate their resolution, and avoid overdiagnosis. To some extent, the therapist may wish to become a negotiator; however, most authors recommend against placing oneself in the position of "referee."

The question of whether a therapist should assist with the completion of a separation or divorce, when he or she feels that it is appropriate or inevitable, may arise. The clinician should be certain that such decisions are made by one or both members of the couple, and not by the therapist, before proceeding. Although patients may describe symptoms that make the diagnosis of Axis I disorders tempting, in themselves or in their partners, marital problems in their normal course should be treated without extensive diagnosis or overtreatment.

Some therapists treat both husband and wife individually, or provide both conjoint and individual counseling. This approach is usually ill-advised and fraught with opportunities for misunderstanding and conflict of interest. An additional therapist should be chosen for each person if individual work is needed.

V15.81 Noncompliance with Medical Treatment

Noncompliance in the absence of any of the mental disorders already described may be treated with education (about one's illness or the treatment involved) or counseling. Since the patient generally has a right not to comply (except in some narrowly circumscribed legal situations), counseling with family members or with frustrated medical staff who are having difficulty accepting the patient's decision may be indirectly helpful. For example, a clinician may ease tensions between nursing staff and the patient which might adversely affect other aspects of the patient's care.

V62.20 Occupational Problems

The same basic treatment principles apply as were mentioned above under Academic Problem (V62.30). One may also wish to consider some of the issues discussed in the chapter on Adjustment Disorders.

V61.20 Parent-Child Problem

The general principles of counseling in parent-child problems are occasionally similar to those of marital problems; however, practical issues, psychodynamics, and the fact that one member of the parent-child dyad is a child make specific issues quite different. The variety of potential conflicts and problems that may arise and the intricacy of family therapies involved make complete discussion impossible in this section. Helpful information may be found in the section on Disorders Usually First Evident in Infancy, Childhood, or Adolescence, and in other texts. Specific training and experience in child psychiatry are recommended.

V62.81 Other Interpersonal Problems

These conditions should be addressed according to the presenting complaints and situations as perceived by the clinician. General principles of education, counseling, and avoidance of overdiagnosis apply.

V61.80 Other Specified Family Circumstances
These conditions should be addressed according to the presenting complaints and situations as perceived by the clinician. General principles of education, counseling, and avoidance of overdiagnosis apply.

V62.89 Phase of Life Problem or Other Life Circumstance Problem
The tremendous variety of problems that might fall into this category is too broad to address completely. The educational and counseling principles already discussed should suffice for most cases. The therapist should be alert for countertransference and related issues; for example, those of a young therapist treating an older patient with concerns about retirement, or a therapist with particular values who attempts to give objective counseling to a patient with opposing views.

V62.82 Uncomplicated Bereavement
The psychiatrist (or more frequently the family physician) may be consulted about some of the more striking symptoms of normal grief. One pitfall of treatment is overdiagnosis. The patient should not be told, or treated as if, he has an aberrant grief reaction or serious depression unless he does not qualify for this V Code condition. Support and guidance may be given, however, with reassurance that the feelings are normal and should not be avoided. The therapist should show approval of the many feelings experienced by the grieving person, including anger for the lost object.

Counseling for the individual and for well-meaning family or friends should include a caveat against overprotection. That is, such activities as attending funeral and memorial services, returning to the home where the deceased lived, and putting away his or her possessions (and, with them, memories) should be encouraged for grieving individuals of all ages. The clinician should make it clear that he or she is available, but need not be intrusive.

Treatment for aberrant or unresolved grief, with persistent yearning, overidentification with the deceased, and/or inability to express sadness or rage, is addressed in the chapter on Adjustment Disorders.

References for Section IV

Abel, G. G., Becker, J. V., Cunningham-Rather, J., et al.: *The Treatment of Child Molesters.* Behavioral Medicine Laboratory, P. O. Box AF, Emory University, Atlanta, Georgia, 30322. Published 1984.

Achte, K., Lonnqvist, J., Kuusi, K., et al.: Outcome studies on schizophrenic psychoses in Helsinki. *Psychopathology,* 19(1-2):60-67, 1986.

Adelman, S. A.: Pills as transitional objects: A dynamic understanding of the use of medication in psychotherapy. *Psychiatry,* 48(3):246-253, 1985.

Adler, G.: A treatment framework for adult patients with borderline and narcissistic personality disorders. *Bulletin of the Menninger Clinic,* 44(2):171-180, 1980.

Adler, G.: Psychotherapy of the narcissistic personality disorder patient: Two contrasting approaches. *American Journal of Psychiatry,* 143(4):430-436, 1986.

Afchoff, J., Hoffman, K., & Pohl, H.: Re-entrainment of circadian rhythms after phase-shifts of the zeitgeber. *Chronobiologia,* 2(2):23-78, 1975.

Akiskal, H. S., Arana, G. W., Baldessarini, R. J., et al.: A clinical report of thymoleptic-responsive atypical paranoid psychoses. *American Journal of Psychiatry,* 140(9):1187-1190, 1983.

Alexander, F. G.: *Psychosomatic Medicine: Its Principles and Applications.* New York: Norton, 1950.

Alexander, P. E., & Alexander, D. D.: Alprazolam treatment for panic disorders. *Journal of Clinical Psychiatry,* 47(6):301-304, 1986.

Allen, J. G., Colson, D. B., Coyne, L., et al.: Problems to anticipate in treating difficult patients in a long-term psychiatric hospital. *Psychiatry,* 49(4):350-358, 1986.

Allen, C. B., Davis, B. M., & Davis, K. L.: Psychoendocrinology in clinical psychiatry. In R. E. Hales & A. J. Frances (Eds.), *Psychiatry Update, Annual Review, Volume 6.* Washington, D.C.: American Psychiatric Press, 1987, p. 198.

Allsopp, L. F., Huitson, A., Deering, R. B., et al.: Efficacy and tolerability of sustained-release clomipramine (Anafranil SR) in the treatment of phobias: A comparison with the conventional formulation of clomipramine (Anafranil). *Journal of Internal Medicine Research,* 13(4):203-208, 1985.

American Psychiatric Association: *Task Force Report #14: Electroconvulsive Therapy* (F. Frankel [Chairperson] et al.). Washington, D.C.: APA Board of Trustees, 1979.

American Psychiatric Association: *Diagnostic and Statistical Manual of Mental Disorders, Third Edition-Revised.* Washington, D.C.: American Psychiatric Press, 1987.

Ames, D., Burrows, G., Davies, B., et al.: A study of the dexamethasone suppression test in hospitalized depressed patients. *British Journal of Psychiatry*, 144:311–313, 1984.

Ananth, J.: Clomipramine: An antiobsessive drug. *Canadian Journal of Psychiatry*, 31(3):253–258, 1986.

Andrews, E., Bellard, J., & Walter-Ryan, W. G.: Monosymptomatic hypochondriacal psychosis manifesting as delusions of infestation: Case studies of treatment with haloperidol. *Journal of Clinical Psychiatry*, 47(4):188–190, 1986.

Ansseau, M., Doumont, A., Thiry, D., von Frenckell, R., et al.: Initial study of methylclonazepam in generalized anxiety disorder. Evidence for greater power in the crossover design. *Psychopharmacology* (Berlin), 87(2):130–135, 1985.

Appel, G.: An approach to the treatment of schizoid phenomena. *Psychoanalytic Review*, 61:99–113, 1974.

Arieti, S.: Psychotherapy of schizophrenia: New or revised procedures. *American Journal of Psychotherapy*, 34(4):464–476, 1980.

Astrup, C.: Querulent paranoia: A follow-up. *Neuropsychobiology*, 11(3):149–154, 1984.

Babiker, I. E.: Comparative efficacy of long-acting depot and oral neuroleptic medications in preventing schizophrenic recidivism. *Journal of Clinical Psychiatry*, 48(3):94–97, 1987.

Baizerman, M., & Emshoff, B.: Juvenile firesetting: Building a community-based prevention program. *Children Today*, 13(3):7–12, 1984.

Ban, T. A., Guy, W., & Wilson, W. H.: The psychopharmacological treatment of depression in the medically ill patient. *Canadian Journal of Psychiatry*, 29(6):461–466, 1984.

Bancroft, J., Davidson, D. W., Warner, T., et al.: Androgens and sexual behaviour in women using oral contraceptives. *Clinical Endocrinology* (Oxford), 12(4):327–340, 1980.

Bancroft, J., O'Carroll, R., McNeilly, A., et al.: The effects of bromocriptine on the sexual behaviour of hyperprolactinaemic men: A controlled case study. *Clinical Endocrinology* (Oxford), 21(2):131–137, 1984.

Bastani, J. B., & Kentsmith, D. K.: Psychotherapy with wives of sexual deviants. *American Journal of Psychotherapy*, 34(1):20–25, 1980.

Battegay, R.: The different narcissistic disturbances of personality and their psychotherapeutic approach. *Psychotherapy and Psychosomatics*, 44(1):46–53, 1985.

Baum, N.: Treatment of impotence. 1. Non-surgical methods. *Postgraduate Medicine*, 81(7):133–136, 1987.

Bayer, A. J., Bayer, E. M., Pathy, M. S. J., et al.: Double-blind controlled study of chlormethiazole and triazolam as hypnotics in the elderly. *Acta Psychiatrica Scandinavica*, 73(329):104–111, 1986.

Beck, A. T., Hollon, S. V., Young, J. E., et al.: Treatment of depression with cognitive therapy and amitriptyline. *Archives of General Psychiatry*, 42:142, 1985.

Benedek, E. T.: Treatment of the female offender: One facility's experience. In W. H. Reid (Ed.), *Treatment of Antisocial Syndromes*. New York: Van Nostrand Reinhold, 1981.

Benson, D. M., Stuss, D. T., Naeser, M. A., et al.: The long-term effects of prefrontal leukotomy. *Archives of Neurology*, 38:165–169, 1981.

Beresin, E., & Gordon, C.: Emergency ward management of the borderline patient. *General Hospital Psychiatry*, 3:237–244, 1981.

Bergman, B., Damber, J. E., Littbrand, B., et al.: Sexual function in prostatic cancer patients treated with radiotherapy, orchiectomy or estrogens. *British Journal of Urology*, 56(1):64–69, 1984.

Berlant, J. L.: Neuroleptics and reserpine in refractory psychoses. *Journal of Clinical Psychopharmacology*, 6(3):180–184, 1986.

Berlin, F. S., & Meinecke, C. F.: Treatment of sex offenders with antiandrogenic medication: Conceptualization, review of treatment modalities, and preliminary findings. *American Journal of Psychiatry*, 138(5):601–607, 1981.

Berman, E., & Wolpert, E. A.: Intractable manic-depressive psychosis with rapid cycling in an eighteen-year-old woman successfully treated with electroconvulsive therapy. *Journal of Nervous and Mental Disease*, 175(4):236–239, 1987.

Biehl, H., Maurer, K., Schubart, C., et al.: Prediction of outcome and utilization of medical services in a prospective study of first onset schizophrenics. Results of a prospective 5-year follow-up study. *European Archives of Psychiatry and Neurological Science*, 236(3):139–147, 1986.

Billiard, M.: The Kleine-Levin syndrome. In W. P. Koella (Ed.), *Sleep*. Basel: S. Karger, 1981, pp. 124–127.

Billiard, M., Guilleminault, C., & Dement, W. C.: A menstruation-linked periodic hypersomnia. *Neurology*, 25:436–443, 1975.

Bixler, E. O., Kales, J. D., Scharf, M. D., et al.: Incidence of sleep disorders in medical practice: A physician survey. In M. H. Chace, M. Mitler, & P. L. Walter (Eds.), *Sleep Research*. Los Angeles: UCLA BIS/BRI 5:160, 1976.

Blackwell, B.: Antidepressant drugs. In M. N. G. Dukes (Ed.), *Meyler's Side Effects of Drugs, Tenth Edition*. Amsterdam: Excerpta Medica, 1984.

Blackwell, B.: Side effects of antidepressant drugs. In R. E. Hales & A. J. Frances (Eds.), *Psychiatry Update, American Psychiatric Association Annual Review, Volume 6*. Washington, D.C.: American Psychiatric Press, 1987, pp. 724–745.

Bliss, E. L.: Multiple personalities. A report of fourteen cases with implications for schizophrenia and hysteria. *Archives of General Psychiatry*, 37(12):1388–1397, 1980.

Blue, F. R.: Use of directive therapy treatment of depersonalization neurosis. *Psychological Reports*, 45: 904–906, 1979.

Bootzin, R. R., & Nicassio, P. N.: Behavior treatments for insomnia. In M. Hersen, R. Eisler, & P. Miller (Eds.), *Progress in Behavior Modification*. New York: Academic Press, 1978.

Bradford, J. M., & Tawlak, A.: Sadistic homosexual pedophilia: Treatment with cyproterone acetate—a single case study. *Canadian Journal of Psychiatry*, 32(1):22–30, 1987.

Branbilla, F., Aguglia, D., Massironi, R., et al.: Neuropeptide therapies in chronic schizophrenia: Trh and vasopressin administration. *Neuropsychobiology* (Switzerland), 15(3–4):114–121, 1986.

Branchy, M. H., Branchy, L. B., & Richardson, M. A.: Effects of neuroleptic adjustment on clinical condition and tardive dyskinesia in schizophrenic patients. *American Journal of Psychiatry*, 138: 608–612, 1981.

Brantley, J. T., & Wise, T. N.: Antiandrogenic treatment of a gender-dysphoric transvestite. *Journal of Sex & Marital Therapy*, 11(2):109–112, 1985.

Braunstein, G. D.: Endocrine causes of impotence. Optimistic outlook for restoration of potency. *Postgraduate Medicine*, 74(4):207–217, 1983.

Bräutigan, W.: Aspects of therapy in psychosomatic medicine. *Psychotherapy and Psychosomatics*, 32:41–51, 1979.

Bridge, T. P., & Wyatt, R. J.: Paraphrenia: Paranoid states of late life. II. American Research. *Journal of the American Geriatric Society*, 28(5):201–205, 1980.

Brizer, D. A., Hartman, N., Sweeney, J., et al.: Effect of methadone plus neuroleptics on treatment-resistant chronic paranoid schizophrenia. *American Journal of Psychiatry*, 142(9):1106–1107, 1985.

Brown, L. S.: Confronting internalized oppression in sex therapy with lesbians. *Journal of Homosexuality*, 12(3–4):99–107, 1986.

Brownell, L. G., West, P., Sweatman, P., et al.: Protriptyline in obstructive sleep apnea. *New England Journal of Medicine*, 307: 1037–1042, 1982.

Bucci, L.: The negative symptoms of schizophrenia and the monoamine oxidase inhibitors. *Psychopharmacology* (Berlin), 91(1):104–108, 1987.

Buigues, J., & Vallejo, J.: Therapeutic response to phenelzine in patients with panic disorder and agoraphobia with panic attacks. *Journal of Clinical Psychiatry*, 48(2):55–59, 1987.

Bumpass, E. R., Brix, R. J., & Preston, B.: A community-based program for juvenile firesetters. *Hospital and Community Psychiatry,* 36(5):529-533, 1985.

Capponi, R., Hormazabal, L., & Schmid-Burgk, W.: Diclofensine and imipramine. A double-blind comparative trial in depressive out-patients. *Neuropsychobiology,* 14(4):173-180, 1985.

Carney, F.: Inpatient treatment programs. In W. H. Reid (Ed.), *The Psychopath: A Comprehensive Study of Antisocial Disorders and Behaviors.* New York: Brunner/Mazel, 1978.

Carpenter, W. T., Jr., & Heinrichs, D. W.: Intermittent psychotherapy of schizophrenia. In J. M. Kane (Ed.), *Drug Maintenance Strategies in Schizophrenia.* Washington, D.C.: American Psychiatric Press, 1984.

Carpenter, W. T., Jr., Heinrichs, D. W., & Hanlon, T. E.: Interpersonal and pharmacologic treatment in schizophrenia: A comparative study of new approaches. *Psychopharmacology Bulletin,* 22(3):854-859, 1986.

Casas, M., Alvarez, E., Duro, T., et al.: Antiandrogenic treatment of obsessive-compulsive neurosis. *Acta Psychiatrica Scandinavica,* 73(2):221-222, 1986.

Casley-Smith, J. R., Casley-Smith, J. R., Johnson, A. F., et al.: Benzo-pyrones and the treatment of chronic schizophrenic diseases. *Psychiatry Research,* 18(3):367-373, 1986.

Chandler, G. M., Burck, H. D., & Sampson, J. P., Jr.: A generic computer program for systematic desensitization: Description, construction, and case study. *Journal of Behavioral Therapy and Experimental Psychiatry,* 17(3):171-174, 1986.

Charney, D. S., & Heninger, G. R.: Noradrenergic function and the mechanism of action of antianxiety treatment. I and II: The effect of long-term alprazolam treatment; the effect of long-term imipramine treatment. *Archives of General Psychiatry,* 42(5):458-467, 473-481, 1985.

Charney, D. S., Woods, S. W., Goodman, W. K., et al.: Drug treatment of panic disorder: The comparative efficacy of imipramine, alprazolam and trazodone. *Journal of Clinical Psychiatry,* 47(12):580-586, 1986.

Chen, H. C., Hsie, M. T., & Shibuya, T. K.: Suanzaorentang vs. diazepam: A controlled double-blind study in anxiety. *International Journal of Clinical Pharmacology, Therapy & Toxicology* (West Germany), 24(12):646-650, 1986.

Chessick, R. D.: Intensive psychotherapy of a borderline patient. *Archives of General Psychiatry,* 39:413-419, 1982.

Chodoff, P.: The therapy of hysterical personality disorders. In J. H. Masserman (Ed.), *Current Psychiatric Therapies, Volume 21.* New York: Grune & Stratton, 1982, pp. 59-65.

Cierpka, M.: Zur psychodynamik der neurotisch bedingten kleptomanie. *Psychiatr Prax.,* 13(3):94-103, 1986.

Clark, B. G., Jue, S. G., Dawson, G. W., et al.: Loprazolam: A preliminary review of its pharmacodynamic and pharmacokinetic properties and therapeutic efficacy in insomnia. *Drugs* 31:500-516, 1986.

Cleckley, H: *The Mask of Sanity (5th ed.).* St. Louis: C. V. Mosby, 1976.

Climo, L. H.: Treatment-resistant catatonic stupor and combined lithium-neuroleptic therapy: A case report. *Journal of Clinical Psychopharmacology,* 5 (3):166-170, 1985.

Coccaro, E. F., & Siever, L. J.: Second generation antidepressants: A comparative review. *Journal of Clinical Pharmacology,* 25:241-260, 1985.

Cohen, L. J., Shapiro, E., Manson, J. E., et al.: The high cost of treating a psychiatric disorder as a medical/surgical illness. *Psychosomatics,* 26(5):453-455, 1985.

Cohen, S. I.: Updating the model for psychosomatic problems. *Psychotherapy and Psychosomatics,* 32:72-90, 1979.

Cole, J. O., Salomon, M., Gunderson, J., et al.: Drug therapy in borderline patients. *Comprehensive Psychiatry,* 25(3):249-262, 1984.

Cole, M.: Sex therapy—A critical appraisal. *British Journal of Psychiatry,* 147:337-351, 1985.

Coleman, R. M.: Periodic movements in sleep (nocturnal myoclonus) and restless leg syndrome. In C. Guilleminault (Ed.), *Sleeping and Waking Disorder: Indications and Techniques* (pp. 265-296). Menlo Park, CA: Addison-Wesley, 1982.

Coleman, R. M., Roffwarg, H. P., Kennedy, S. J., et al.: Sleep-wake disorders based on a polysomnographic diagnosis: A national cooperative study. *Journal of the American Medical Association*, 247:997-1003, 1982.

Coons, P. M.: Treatment progress in twenty patients with multiple personality disorder. *Journal of Nervous and Mental Disease*, 174(12):715-721, 1986a.

Coons, P. M.: Child abuse and multiple personality disorder: Review of the literature and suggestions for treatment. *Child Abuse and Neglect* (England), 10(4):455-462, 1986b.

Coppen, A., Abou-Saleh, M. T., Nilln, P., et al.: Lithium continuation therapy following electroconvulsive therapy. *British Journal of Psychiatry*, 139:284-287, 1981.

Coppen, A., Chaudhry, S., & Swade, C.: Folic acid enhances lithium prophylaxis. *Journal of Affective Disorders*, 10(1):9-13, 1986.

Cordingley, G. J., Dean, B. C., & Hallett, C.: A multi-centre, double-blind parallel trial of bromazepam (lexotan) and lorazepam to compare the acute benefit-risk ratio in the treatment of patients with anxiety. *Current Medical Research and Opinion*, 9(7):505-510, 1985.

Coryell, W., Lavori, T., Endicott, J., et al.: Outcome in schizoaffective, psychotic, and non-psychotic depression. Course during a six-to-twenty-four-month follow-up. *Archives of General Psychiatry*, 41(8):787-791, 1984.

Cotten-Huston, A. L., & Wheeler, K. A.: Preorgasmic group treatment: Assertiveness marital adjustment and sexual function in women. *Journal of Sex & Marital Therapy*, 9(4):296-302, 1983.

Cottraux, J. A., Bouvard, M., Claustrat, B., et al.: Abnormal dexamethasone suppression test in primary obsessive-compulsive patients: A confirmatory report. *Psychiatry Research*, 13(2):159-165, 1984.

Covi, L., Lipman, R. S., Roth, D., et al.: Cognitive group psychotherapy in depression: A pilot study. *American Journal of Psychiatry*, in press.

Critchley, M.: Periodic hypersomnia and megaphagia in adolescent males. *Brain*, 85:628-656, 1962.

Croughan, J. L., Saghir, M., Cohen, R., et al.: A comparison of treated and untreated male cross-dressers. *Archives of Sexual Behavior*, 10(6):515-528, 1981.

Csanalosi, I., Schweizer, E., Case, W. G., et al.: Gepirone in anxiety: A pilot study. *Journal of Clinical Psychopharmacology*, 7(1):31-33, 1987.

Cytrynbaum, S., & Ken, K.: The Connecticut wilderness program: A preliminary report. State of Connecticut, Council on Human Services, Hartford, Connecticut, 1975.

Daghestani, A. N.: Impotence associated with compulsive gambling. *Journal of Clinical Psychiatry*, 48(3):115-116, 1987.

Dalton, R., Haslett, N., & Baul, G.: Alternative therapy with a recalcitrant firesetter. *Journal of the American Academy of Child Psychiatry*, 25(5):715-717, 1986.

D'Angelo, D. J., & Wolowitz, H. M.: Defensive constellation and styles of recovery from schizophrenic episodes. *Hillside Journal of Clinical Psychiatry*, 8(1):3-14, 1986.

de la Fuente, J. R., Verlanga, C., & Leon-Andrade, C.: Mania induced by tricyclic MAOI combination therapy in bipolar treatment-resistant disorder: Case reports. *Journal of Clinical Psychiatry*, 47(1):40-41, 1986.

De Luca, R. V., & Holborn, S. W.: A comparison of relaxation training and competing response training to eliminate hair-pulling and nailbiting. *Journal of Behavioral Therapy and Experimental Psychiatry*, 15(1):67-70, 1984.

Del Zompo, M., Bocchetta, A., Piccardi, M. P., et al.: Dopamine agonists in the treatment of schizophrenia. *Progress in Brain Research*, 65:41-48, 1986.

den Boer, J. A., Verhoeven, W. M., & Westenberg, H. G.: Remoxipride in schizophrenia. A preliminary report. *Acta Psychiatrica Scandanavica*, 74(4):409-414, 1986.

DePaulo, J. R., Jr., Correa, E. I., & Sapir, D. G.: Renal function and lithium: A longitudinal study. *American Journal of Psychiatry*, 143(7):892–895, 1986.

Dickey, B., Cannon, N. L., McGuire, T. G., et al.: The quarterway house: A two-year cost study of an experimental residential program. *Hospital and Community Psychiatry*, 37(11):1136–1143, 1986.

Dietzel, M., Saletu, B., Lesch, O. M., et al.: Light treatment in depressive illness. Polysomnographic psychometric and neuroendocrinological findings. *European Neurology*, 25(Supplement 2):93–103, 1986.

Doane, J. A., Goldstein, M. J., Miklowitz, D. J., et al.: The impact of individual and family treatment on the affective climate of the families of schizophrenics. *British Journal of Psychiatry*, 148:279–287, 1986.

Dominguez, R. A., Goldstein, B. J., Jacobson, A. F., et al.: Comparative efficacy of estazolam, flurazepam and placebo in outpatients with insomnia. *Journal of Clinical Psychiatry*, 47:362–365, 1986.

Donlon, P. T., Hopkin, J. T., Tupin, J. P., et al.: Haloperidol for acute schizophrenic patients: An evaluation of three oral regimens. *Archives of General Psychiatry*, 37(6):691–695, 1980.

Dossing, M., & Andreasen, B.: Drug-induced liver disease in Denmark: An analysis of 572 cases of hepatotoxicity reported to the Danish Board of Adverse Reactions to Drugs. *Scandinavian Journal of Gastroenterology*, 17:205–211, 1982.

Dowd, E. T., & Swoboda, J. S.: Paradoxical interventions in behavior therapy. *Journal of Behavioral Therapy and Experimental Psychiatry*, 15(3):229–234, 1984.

Drake, R. E., Gates, C., & Cotton, E. G.: Suicide among schizophrenics: A comparison of attemptors and completed suicides. *British Journal of Psychiatry*, 149:784–787, 1986.

Drake, R. E., & Sederer, L. I.: Inpatient psychosocial treatment of chronic schizophrenia: Negative effects and current guidelines. *Hospital and Community Psychiatry*, 37(9):897–901, 1986a.

Drake, R. E., & Sederer, L. I.: The adverse effects of intensive treatment of chronic schizophrenia. *Comprehensive Psychiatry*, 27(4):313–326, 1986b.

Dubovsky, S. L., Franks, R. D., Allen, S., et al.: Calcium antagonists in mania: A double blind study of verapamil. *Psychiatry Research*, 18(4):309–320, 1986.

Dunbar, G. C., Naarala, M., & Hiltumen, H.: A double-blind group comparison of mianserin and clomipramine in the treatment of mildly depressed psychiatric outpatients. *Acta Psychiatrica Scandinavica*, 320 (Supplements):60–66, 1985.

Dunner, D. L., Ishiki, D., Avery, D. H., et al.: Effect of alprazolam and diazepam on anxiety and panic attacks in panic disorder: A controlled study. *Journal of Clinical Psychiatry*, 47(9):458–460, 1986.

Earle, J. R., Jr., & Folks, D. G.: Factitious disorder and coexisting depression: A report of successful psychiatric consultation and case management. *General Hospital Psychiatry*, 8(6):448–450, 1986.

el-Bayoumi, M., el-Sherbini, O., & Mostafa, M.: Impotence in diabetics: Organic vs psychogenic factors. *Urology*, 24(5):459–463, 1984.

Elliott, F. A.: Neurological aspects of antisocial behavior. In W. H. Reid (Ed.), *The Psychopath: A Comprehensive Study of Antisocial Disorders and Behaviors*. New York: Brunner/Mazel, 1978.

Emrich, H. M., Dose, M., & von Zerssen, D.: The use of sodium valproate, carbamazepine, and oxcarbazepine in patients with affective disorders. *Journal of Affective Disorders*, 8(3):243–250, 1985.

Essa, M.: Grief as a crisis: Psychotherapeutic interventions with elderly bereaved. *American Journal of Psychotherapy*, 40(2):243–251, 1986.

Evans, D. L., Davidson, J., & Raft, D.: Early and late side effects of phenelzine. *Journal of Clinical Psychopharmacology*, 2:208–210, 1982.

Evans, D. L., Strawn, S. K., Haggerty, J. J., Jr., et al.: Appearance of mania in drug-resistant bipolar depressed patients after treatment with L-triiodothyromine. *Journal of Clinical Psychiatry*, 47(10):521–522, 1986.

Everaerd, W., & Dekker, J.: Treatment of male sexual dysfunction: Sex therapy compared to the systematic desensitization and rational emotive therapy. *Behaviour Research and Therapy*, 23(1):13–25, 1985.

Falcon, S., Ryan, C., Chamberlain, K., et al.: Tricyclics: Possible treatment for posttraumatic stress disorder. *Journal of Clinical Psychiatry*, 46(9):385–388, 1985.

Faraone, S. V., Brown, W. A., & Laughren, T. P.: Serum neuroleptic levels, prolactin levels, and relapse: A two year study of schizophrenic outpatients. *Journal of Clinical Psychiatry*, 48(4):151–154, 1987.

Faraone, S. V., Curran, J. P., Laughren, T., et al.: Neuroleptic bioavailability, psychosocial factors, and clinical status: A one year study of schizophrenic outpatients after dose reduction. *Psychiatry Research* (Ireland), 19(4):311–322, 1986.

Fenves, A. Z., Emmett, M., & White, M. G.: Lithium intoxications associated with acute renal failure. *Southern Medical Journal*, 77(11):1472–1474, 1984.

Fichten, C. S., Libman, E., & Brender, W.: Methodological issues in the study of sex therapy: Effective components in the treatment of secondary orgasmic dysfunction. *Journal of Sex & Marital Therapy*, 9(3):191–202, 1983.

Finkel, M. J.: Phenytoin revisited. *Clinical Therapeutics*, 6(5):577–591, 1984.

Fogelson, D. L., Marder, S. R., & van Putten, T.: Dialysis for schizophrenia: Review of clinical trials and implications for further research. *American Journal of Psychiatry*, 137(5):605–607, 1980.

Folks, D. G., & Freeman, A. M., III: Munchausen syndrome and other factitious illness. *Psychiatric Clinics of North America*, 8(2):263–278, 1985.

Fontaine, R., & Chouinard, G.: An open clinical trial of fluoxetine in the treatment of obsessive-compulsive disorder. *Journal of Clinical Psychopharmacology*, 6(2):98–101, 1986.

Fontaine, R., Mercier, T., Veaudry, T., et al.: Bromazepam and lorazepam in generalized anxiety: A placebo-controlled study with measurement of blood plasma concentrations. *Acta Psychiatrica Scandinavica*, 74(5):451–458, 1986.

Frances, A., & Carpenter, W. T., Jr.: A schizophrenic patient who resists phenythiazines. *Hospital and Community Psychiatry*, 34(2):115–116, 1983.

Frances, A., & Wise, T. N.: Treating a man who wears women's clothes. *Hospital and Community Psychiatry*, 38(3):233–234, 1987.

Freund, K.: Therapeutic sex drive reduction. *Acta Psychiatrica Scandinavica*, 287(Supplement):5–38, 1980.

Freund, K., & Blanchard, R.: The concept of courtship disorder. *Journal of Sex & Marital Therapy*, 12(2):79–92, 1986.

Freund, K., Scher, H., & Hucker, S.: The courtship disorders: A further investigation. *Archives of Sexual Behavior*, 13(2):133–139, 1984.

Frosch, J. P.: The treatment of antisocial and borderline personality disorders. *Hospital and Community Psychiatry*, 34(3):243–248, 1983.

Gagne, P.: Treatment of sex offenders with medroxyprogesterone acetate. *American Journal of Psychiatry*, 138(5):644–646, 1981.

Galatzer-Levy, R. M.: The opening phase of psychotherapy of hypochondriacal states. *International Journal of Psychoanalytic Psychotherapy*, 9:389–413, 1982.

Ganzarain, R.: Some key issues in the group psychotherapy of narcissistic and borderline patients: Introduction. *International Journal of Group Psychotherapy*, 32(1):3–7, 1982.

Garbutt, J. C., & Loosen, P. T.: A dramatic behavioral response to thyrotropin-releasing hormone following low-dose neuroleptics. *Psychoneuroendocrinology*, 9(3):311–314, 1984.

Gardner, B. L., & Cowdry, R. W.: Positive effects of carbamazepine on behavioral dyscontrol in borderline personality disorder. *American Journal of Psychiatry*, 143(4):519–522, 1986.

Gardos, G., & Casey, B.: *Tardive Dyskinesia and Affective Disorders*. Washington, D.C.: American Psychiatric Press, 1984.

Gelenberg, A. J., & Gibson, C. J.: Tyrosine for the treatment of depression. *Nutrition and Health*, 3(3):163–173, 1984.

Gerner, R. H.: Present status of drug therapy of depression in late life. *Journal of Affective Disorders*, 1(Supplement):S23–S31, 1985.

Getto, C. J.: V Codes for conditions not attributable to a mental disorder that are a focus of treatment. In J. H. Greist, J. W. Jefferson, & R. L. Spitzer (Eds.), *Treatment of Mental Disorders*. New York: Oxford University Press, 1982.

Getto, C. J., & Ochitill, H.: Psychogenic pain disorder. In J. H. Griest, J. W. Jefferson, & R. L. Spitzer (Eds.), *Treatment of Mental Disorders*. New York: Oxford University Press, 1982.

Ghadirian, A. M., & Lalinec-Michaud, M.: Report of a patient with lithium-related alopecia and psoriasis. *Journal of Clinical Psychiatry*, 47(4):212–213, 1986.

Glick, I. D., Fleming, L., DeChillo, N., et al.: A controlled study of transitional daycare for non-chronically-ill patients. *American Journal of Psychiatry*, 143(12):1551–1556, 1986.

Glover, J. H.: A case of kleptomania treated by covert sensitization. *British Journal of Clinical Psychology*, 24(Part 3):213–214, 1985.

Goldberg, H. L., Rickels, K., & Finnerty, R.: Treatment of neurotic depression with a new antidepressant. *Journal of Clinicial Psychopharamacology*, 1(6, Supplement):35S–38S, 1981.

Goldberg, M. A.: The treatment of Kleine-Levine syndrome with lithium. *Canadian Journal of Psychiatry*, 28:491–493, 1983.

Goldberg, S. C., Schulz, S. C., Schulz, P. M., et al.: Borderline and schizotypal personality disorders treated with low-dose thiothixene vs placebo. *Archives of General Psychiatry*, 43(7):680–686, 1986.

Goldman, H. W., Cooper, I. S., Simpson, G. M., et al.: Reversal of severe tardive dyskinesia and dystonia following bilateral CT-guided stereotactic thalatomy (abstract). *Fourth World Congress of Biological Psychiatry*. Philadelphia, Pa., 1985.

Goodnick, P. J., Fieve, R. R., Schlagel, A., et al.: Predictors of interepisode symptoms and relapse in affective disorder patients treated with lithium carbonate. *American Journal of Psychiatry*, 144(3):367–369, 1987.

Goodwin, F. K., Prange, A., Post, R., et al.: Potentiation of antidepressant effects by L-triiodothyronine in tricyclic non-responders. *American Journal of Psychiatry*, 139:34–38, 1982.

Graber, B. G.: Demystifying "sex therapy." *American Journal of Psychotherapy*, 35(4):481–488, 1981.

Graber, B. G.: *Circumvaginal musculature and sexual function*. Basel, Switzerland: S. Karger, 1982.

Gralnick, A.: The future of the chronic schizophrenic patient: Prediction and recommendations. *American Journal of Psychotherapy*, 40(3):419–429, 1986.

Granier, F., Girard, M., Schmitt, L., et al.: Depression and anxiety: Mianserin and nomifensime compared in a double-blind multicentre trial. *Acta Psychiatrica Scandinavica*, 320(Supplement):67–74, 1985.

Greben, S. E.: The multi-dimensional inpatient treatment of severe character disorders. *Canadian Journal of Psychiatry*, 28(2):97–101, 1983.

Greenblatt, D. J., Harmatz, G. S., Zinny, M. A., et al.: Effect of gradual withdrawal on the rebound sleep disorder after discontinuation of triazolam. *New England Journal of Medicine*, 317:722–728, 1987.

Greil, W., Stoltzenburg, M. C., Mairhofer, M. L., et al.: Lithium dosage in the elderly. A study with matched age groups. *Journal of Affective Disorders*, 9(1):1-4, 1985.

Grigsby, J. T.: Use of imagery in the treatment of posttraumatic stress disorder. *Journal of Nervous and Mental Disease*, 175(1):55-59, 1987.

Gross, G., & Huber, G.: Classification and prognosis schizophrenic disorders in light of the Bonn follow-up studies. *Psychopathology*, 19(1-2):50-59, 1986.

Guilleminault, C., Carskadon, M., & Dement, W. C.: On the treatment of rapid eye movement narcolepsy. *Archives of Neurology*, 30:90-93, 1974.

Guilleminault, C., & Flagg, W.: Effects of baclofen on sleep-related periodic leg movements. *Annals of Neurology*, 15:234-239, 1984.

Guilleminault, C., Nino-Murcia, G., Heldt, G., et al.: Alternative treatment to tracheostomy in obstructive sleep apnea syndrome: Nasal continuous positive airway pressure in young children. *Pediatrics*, 78:797-802, 1986.

Guilleminault, C., Quera-Salva, M. A., Nino-Murcia, G., et al.: Central sleep apnea and partial obstruction of the airway. *Annals of Neurology*, 21:465-469, 1987.

Haggerty, J., Jr., & Jackson, R.: Mania following change from trazodone to imipramine. *Journal of Clinical Psychopharmacology*, 5(6):342-343, 1985.

Handwerker, J. V., Jr., & Palmer, R. F.: Clonidine and the treatment of "restless leg" syndrome. *New England Journal of Medicine*, 313:1228-1229, 1985.

Harrison, W. M., Rabkin, J. G., Ehrhardt, A. A., et al.: Effects of antidepressant medication on sexual functions: A controlled study. *Journal of Clinical Psychopharmacology*, 6(3):144-149, 1986.

Hartman, L. M.: Effects of sex and marital therapy on sexual interaction and marital happiness. *Journal of Sex & Marital Therapy*, 9(2):137-151, 1983a.

Hartman, L. M.: Resistance in directive sex therapy: Recognition and management. *Journal of Sex & Marital Therapy*, 9(4):283-295, 1983b.

Hauri, P. J.: *The Sleep Disorders*. Kalamazoo, MI: Upjohn, 1977, pp. 1-76.

Hauri, P. J.: *The Sleep Disorders: Current Concepts*. Kalamazoo, MI: Upjohn Scope Publications, 1982, p. 54.

Hauri, P. J.: Primary sleep disorders and insomnia. In T. L. Riley (Ed.), *Clinical Aspects of Sleep Disturbance*. London: Butterworths 5:98-100, 1985.

Hawton, K., & Catalan, J.: Prognostic factors in sex therapy. *Behaviour Research and Therapy Journal*, 24(4):377-385, 1986.

Heiman, J. R., & LoPiccolo, J.: Clinical outcome of sex therapy. Effects of daily vs weekly treatment. *Archives of General Psychiatry*, 40(4):443-449, 1983.

Hening, W. A., Walters, A., Kavey, N., et al.: Dyskinesias while awake and periodic movements in sleep in restless syndrome: Treatment with opioids. *Neurology*, 36:1363-1366, 1986.

Herrmann, W. M., & Beach, R. C.: Pharmacotherapy for sexual offenders: Review of the actions of antiandrogens with special references to their psychic effects. *Modern Problems in Pharmacopsychiatry*, 15:182-194, 1980.

Hirschfeld, R. M., Klerman, G. L., Keller, M. B., et al.: Personality of recovered patients with bipolar affective disorder. *Journal of Affective Disorders*, 11(1):81-89, 1986.

Hogarty, G. E., Anderson, C. M., Reiss, D. J., et al.: Family psychoeducation, social skills training and maintenance chemotherapy in the aftercare treatment of schizophrenia. I. One-year effects of a controlled study on relapse and expressed emotion. *Archives of General Psychiatry*, 43(7):633-642, 1986.

Holcomb, W. R.: Stress inoculation therapy with anxiety and stress disorders of acute psychiatric patients. *Journal of Clinical Psychology*, 42(6):864-872, 1986.

Hollister, L. E.: Pharmacotherapeutic considerations in anxiety disorders. *Journal of Clinical Psychiatry*, 47(June Supplement):33-36, 1986.

Holman, S. L.: A group program for borderline mothers and their toddlers. *International Journal of Group Psychotherapy*, 35(1):79-93, 1985.

Hoon, P. W.: Physiologic assessment of sexual response in women: The unfulfilled promise. *Clinical Obstetrics and Gynecology*, 27(3):767–780, 1984.

Horne, D. J., McCormack, H. M., Collins, J. P., et al.: Psychological treatment of phobic anxiety associated with adjuvant chemotherapy. *Medical Journal of Australia*, 145(7):346–348, 1986.

Horowitz, M. J.: Stress-response syndromes: A review of posttraumatic and adjustment disorders. *Hospital and Community Psychiatry*, 37(3):241–249, 1986.

Horowitz, M. J., Marmar, C., Weiss, D. S., et al.: Brief psychotherapy of bereavement reactions. The relationship of process to outcome. *Archives of General Psychiatry*, 41(5):438–448, 1984.

Horwitz, L.: Divergent views on the treatment of borderline patients. *Bulletin of the Menninger Clinic*, 49(6):525–545, 1985.

Hyler, S. B., & Sussman, N.: Chronic factitious disorder with physical symptoms (The Munchausen Syndrome). *Psychiatric Clinics of North America*, 4(2):365–377, 1981.

Hymowitz, P., Frances, A., Jacobsberg, L. B., et al.: Neuroleptic treatment of schizotypal personality disorder. *Comprehensive Psychiatry*, 27(4):267–271, 1986.

Inoue, K., Nakajima, T., & Kato, N.: A longitudinal study of schizophrenia in adolescents. In the one-to-three-year outcome. *Japanese Journal of Psychiatry and Neurology*, 40(2):143–151, 1986.

Insel, T. R., Mueller, E. A. III, Gillin, J. C., et al.: Biological markers in obsessive-compulsive and affective disorders. *Journal of Psychiatric Research*, 18(4):407–423, 1984.

Insel, T. R., Mueller, E. A., Gillin, J. C., et al.: Tricyclic response in obsessive-compulsive disorder. *Progress in Neuropsychopharmacological and Biological Psychiatry*, 9(1):25031, 1985.

Insel, T. R., Murphy, D. L., Cohen, R. M., et al.: Obsessive-compulsive disorder. *Archives of General Psychiatry*, 40:605–612, 1983.

International Drug Therapy Newsletter. New hope for tricyclic refractory unipolar depressives? 16(7):25–27, 1981.

International Drug Therapy Newsletter: Buspirone: A new generation anxiolytic. 19:1–4, 1984.

Jaeger, A., Sauder, P., Kopfreschmitt, J., et al.: Toxicokinetics of lithium intoxication treated by hemodialysis. *Journal of Toxicology and Clinical Toxicology*, 23(7–8):501–517, 1985.

Jann, M. W., Saklad, S. R., Ereshefsky, L., et al.: Effects of smoking on haloperidol and reduced haloperidol plasma concentrations and haloperidol clearance. *Psychopharmacology* (Berlin), 19(4):468–470, 1986.

Jansson, L., Jerremalm, A., & Ost, L. G.: Follow-up of agoraphobic patients treated with exposure in vivo or applied relaxation. *British Journal of Psychiatry*, 149: 486–490, 1986.

Jarrett, R. B., & Rush, A. J.: Psychotherapeutic approaches for depression. In N. R. Michaels, J. O. Cavenar, Jr., et al. (Eds.), *Psychiatry, Volume 1*. Philadelphia: J. B. Lippincott, 1986.

Jefferson, J. W., Greist, J. H., & Ackerman, D. L.: *Lithium Encyclopedia for Clinical Practice*. Washington, D.C.: American Psychiatric Press, 1983.

Jelinek, J. M., & Williams, T.: Post-traumatic stress disorder and substance abuse in Vietnam combat veterans: Treatment problems, strategies and recommendations. *Journal of Substance Abuse Treatment*, 1(2):87–97, 1984.

Jenkins, S. C., & Maruta, T.: Therapeutic use of propranolol for Intermittent Explosive Disorder. *Mayo Clinic Proceedings*, 62(3):204–214, 1987.

Jensen, S. B.: Sexual dysfunction in younger insulin-treated diabetic females: A comparative study. *Diabete et Metabolisme*, 11(5):278–282, 1985.

Joffe, R. T., & Brown, P.: Clinical and biological correlates of sleep deprivation in depression. *Canadian Journal of Psychiatry*, 29(6):530–536, 1984.

Johansen, K. H.: The impact of patients with chronic character pathology on a hospital inpatient unit. *Hospital and Community Psychiatry*, 34(9):842–846, 1983.

Johnson, B., Geller, J., Gordon, J., et al.: Group psychotherapy with schizophrenic patients: Pairing group. *International Journal of Group Psychotherapy*, 36(1):75–96, 1986.
Johnson, C., Shenoy, R. S., & Langer, S.: Relaxation therapy for somatoform disorders. *Hospital and Community Psychiatry*, 32(6):423–424, 1981.
Johnson, S. B., Alvarez, W. A., & Freinhar, J. P.: A case of massive rhabdomyolysis following molindone administration. *Journal of Clinical Psychiatry*, 47(12):607–608, 1986.
Joint Commission on Accreditation of Hospitals: *Accreditation Manual for Hospitals.* Chicago, 1988.
Jorgensen, P.: Long-term course of acute reactive paranoid psychosis. A follow-up study. *Acta Psychiatrica Scandanavica*, 71(1):30–37, 1985.
Jorgensen, P., & Munk-Jorgensen, P.: Paranoid psychosis in the elderly. A follow-up study. *Acta Psychiatrica Scandinavica*, 72(4):358–363, 1985.
Kales, A., & Kales, J. D.: *Evaluation and Treatment of Insomnia.* New York: Oxford University Press, 1984.
Kales, A., Soldatos, C. R., Bixler, E. O., et al.: Narcolepsy-cataplexy. II. Psychosocial consequences and associated psychopathology. *Archives of Neurology*, 39:169–171, 1982.
Kales, A., Soldatos, C. R., Cadieux, R., et al.: Propranolol in the treatment of narcolepsy. *Annals of Internal Medicine*, 91:742–743, 1979.
Kane, J. M., & Smith, J. M.: Tardive dyskinesia: Prevalence and risk factors. *Archives of General Psychiatry*, 39:473–481, 1982.
Kane, J. M., Woerner, M., Weinhold, P., et al.: Incidence of tardive dyskinesia: Five year data from the prospective study. *Psychopharmacology Bulletin*, 20:387–389, 1984.
Kaplan, C. A.: The challenge of working with patients diagnosed as having a borderline personality disorder. *Nursing Clinics of North America*, 21(3):429–438, 1986.
Kaplan, H. S.: *The New Sex Therapy.* New York: Brunner/Mazel, 1974.
Kaplan, H. S.: *Disorders of Sexual Desire.* New York: Brunner/Mazel, 1979.
Kaplan, H. S.: Psychosexual dysfunctions. In R. M. Michaels & J. O. Cavenar (Eds.), *Psychiatry, Volume 1.* Philadelphia: J. B. Lippincott, 1986.
Karacan, I., Moore, C. A., & Williams, R. L.: The narcoleptic syndrome. *Psychiatric Annals*, 9(7):377–381, 1979.
Karacan, I., Thornby, J., Anch, M., et al.: Prevalence of sleep disturbance in a primarily urban Florida county. *Social Science and Medicine*, 10:239–244, 1976.
Karasu, T. D.: Psychotherapy of the psychosomatic patient. *American Journal of Psychotherapy*, 33(3):354–364, 1979.
Kartman, L. L.: Music hath charms. . . . *Journal of Gerontological Nursing*, 10(6):20–24, 1984.
Katz, R. J.: Effects of zometapine, a structurally novel antidepressant, in an animal model of depression. *Pharmacology and Biochemical Behavior*, 21(4):487–490, 1984.
Kaufman, K. R., & Okeya, V. L.: Lithium in pregnancy—Avoidance of toxicity. A case report. *Biological Research in Pregnancy and Perinatology*, 6(2):55–58, 1985.
Kazi, H. A.: An open clinical trial with the long-acting neuroleptic zuclopenthixol decanoate in the maintenance treatment of schizophrenia. *Pharmatherapeutica*, 4(9):555–560, 1986.
Keller, M. V., Lavori, P. W., Coryell, W., et al.: Differential outcome of pure manic, mixed/cycling and pure depressive episodes in patients with bipolar illness. *Journal of the American Medical Association*, 255(22):3138–3142, 1986.
Kellner, R.: Psychotherapy in psychosomatic disorders: A survey of controlled studies. *Archives of General Psychiatry*, 32:1021–1030, 1975.
Kellner, R.: Psychotherapeutic strategies in hypochondriasis: A clinical study. *American Journal of Psychotherapy*, 36(2):146–157, 1982a.
Kellner, R.: Disorders of impulse control. In J. H. Greist, J. W. Jefferson, & R. L. Spitzer (Eds.), *Treatment of Mental Disorders.* New York: Oxford University Press, 1982b.

Kellner, R.: Prognosis of treated hypochrondriasis. A clinical study. *Acta Psychiatrica Scandinavica*, 67(2):69-79, 1983.
Kellner, R.: Functional somatic symptoms and hypochondriasis. A survey of empirical studies. *Archives of General Psychiatry*, 42(8):821-833, 1985.
Kentsmith, D. K., & Eaton, M. T.: *Treating Sexual Problems in Medical Practice*. New York: Arco, 1979.
Kernberg, O. F.: Narcissistic personality disorder. In R. M. Michaels & J. O. Cavenar (Eds.), *Psychiatry, Volume I*. Philadelphia: J. B. Lippincott, 1986a.
Kernberg, O. F.: Hysterical and histrionic personality disorders. In R. Michaels & J. O. Cavenar, Jr. (Eds.), *Psychiatry, Volume 1*. Philadelphia: J. B. Lippincott, 1986b.
Khan, A., Jaffe, J. H., Nelson, W. H., et al.: Resolution of neuroleptic malignant syndrome with dantrolene sodium: Case report. *Journal of Clinical Psychiatry*, 46(6):244-246, 1985.
Khuri, R., & Gehi, M.: Psychogenic amenorrhea: An integrated review. *Psychosomatics*, 22(10):883-893, 1981.
Kiev, A.: Cluster analysis profiles of suicide attempts. *American Journal of Psychiatry*, 133(2):150-153, 1976.
Kilmann, P. R., Boland, J. C., Norton, S. P., et al.: Perspectives of sex therapy outcome: A survey of AASECT providers. *Journal of Sex & Marital Therapy*, 12(2):116-138, 1986.
Kimball, C. T.: *The Biopsychosocial Approach to the Patient*. Baltimore: Williams & Wilkins, 1981.
Kimball, R. O.: Wilderness experience program: Final evaluation report. Santa Fe, New Mexico, Health and Environment Department, 1979.
Kinney, J. L.: Nomifensine malleate: A new second-generation antidepressant. *Clinical Pharmacology*, 4(6):625-636, 1984.
Kitchner, I., & Greenstein, R.: Low dose lithium carbonate in the treatment of posttraumatic stress disorder: Brief communication. *Military Medicine*, 150(7):378-381, 1985.
Klar, H.: The setting for psychiatric treatment. In R. E. Hales & A. J. Frances (Eds.), *Psychiatry Update, Annual Review, Volume 6*. Washington, D.C.: American Psychiatric Press, 1987, pp. 336-352.
Klonoff, E. A., Youngner, S. J., Moore, E. J., et al.: Chronic factitious illness: A behavioral approach. *International Journal of Psychiatry and Medicine*, 13(3):173-183, 1983.
Kluft, R. P.: An update on multiple personality disorder. *Hospital and Community Psychiatry*, 38(4):363-373, 1987.
Knobler, H. Y., Itzchaky, S., Emanuel, D., et al.: Trazodone-induced mania. *British Journal of Psychiatry*, 149: 787-789, 1986.
Koehler, K., & Sauer, H.: First rank symptoms as predictors of ECT response in schizophrenia. *British Journal of Psychiatry*, 142:280, 1983.
Koenigsberg, H. W.: Indications for hospitalization in the treatment of borderline patients. *Psychiatric Quarterly*, 56(4):247-258, 1984.
Koles, M. R., & Jenson, W. R.: Comprehensive treatment of chronic firesetting in a severely disordered boy. *Journal of Behavioral Therapy and Experimental Psychiatry*, 16(1):81-85, 1985.
Kolko, D. J.: Multicomponent parental treatment of firesetting in a six-year-old boy. *Journal of Behavioral Therapy and Experimental Psychiatry*, 14(4):349-353, 1983.
Kravitz, H. M., Sabelli, H. C., & Fawcett, J.: Dietary supplements of phenylalanine and other amino acid precursors of brain neuroamines in the treatment of depressive disorders. *Journal of the American Osteopathic Association*, 84(Supplement):119-123, 1984.
Kretsch, R., Goren, Y., & Wasserman, A.: Change patterns of borderline patients in individual and group therapy. *International Journal of Group Therapy*, 37(1):95-112, 1987.

Krishnan, R. R., Davidson, J., & Miller, R.: MAO inhibitor therapy in trichotillomania associated with depression: Case report. *Journal of Clinical Psychiatry*, 45(6):267-268, 1984.

Kuch, K., Swinson, R. P., & Kirby, M.: Post-traumatic stress disorder after car accident. *Canadian Journal of Psychiatry*, 30(6):426-427, 1985.

Lamontagne, Y., & Lesage, A.: Private exposure and covert sensitization in the treatment of exhibitionists. *Journal of Behavioral Therapy and Experimental Psychiatry*, 17(3):197-201, 1986.

Lanza, U.: The contribution of acupuncture to clinical psychotherapy by means of biofeedback (EMG-BME) training. *Acupuncture & Electrotherapeutics Research*, 11(1):53-57, 1986.

Laws, D. R.: Sexual fantasy alteration: Procedural considerations. *Journal of Behavioral Therapy and Experimental Psychiatry*, 16(1):39-44, 1985.

Lawy, A. J., Sack, R. L., Fredrickson, R. H., et al.: The use of bright light in the treatment of chronobiologic sleep and mood disorders: The phase-response curve. *Psychopharmacology Bulletin*, 19(3):523-525, 1983.

Lawy, A. J., Sack, R. L., & Singer, C. M.: Treating phase-typed chronobiologic sleep and mood disorders using appropriately timed bright artificial light. *Psychopharmacology Bulletin*, 21:368-372, 1985.

Lazara, A.: Conversion symptoms. *New England Journal of Medicine*, 305(13):745-748, 1981.

Lazarus, J. H., McGregor, A. M., Ludgate, M., et al.: Effect of lithium carbonate therapy on thyroid immune status in manic depressive patients: A prospective study. *Journal of Affective Disorders* (Netherlands), 11(2):155-169, 1986.

Lazarus, L. W., Davis, J. M., & Dysken, M. W.: Geriatric depression: A guide to successful therapy. *Geriatrics*, 40(6):43-48, 52-53, 1985.

Ledermann, R.: Narcissistic disorder and its treatment. *Journal of Analytical Psychology*, 27:303-321, 1982.

Lehman, C. R., Ereshefsky, L., Saklad, S. R., & Mings, T. E.: Very high dose loxapine in refractory schizophrenic patients. *American Journal of Psychiatry*, 138:1212-1214, 1981.

Lelliott, P. T., & Monteiro, W. O.: Drug treatment of obsessive-compulsive disorder. *Drugs*, 31(1):75-80, 1986.

Lenox, R. H., Modell, J. G., & Weiner, S.: Acute treatment of manic agitation with lorazepam. *Psychosomatics*, 21(1, Supplement):28-32, 1986.

Lerer, B.: Alternative therapies for biopolar disorder. *Journal of Clinical Psychiatry*, 46(8):309-316, 1985.

Lerer, B., Moore, N., Meyendorff, E., et al.: Carbamazepine vs. lithium in mania: A double-blind study. *Journal of Clinical Psychiatry*, 48(3):89-93, 1987.

Lesser, M. S., Cahan, M., Brenner, R., & Nayak, D.: Dantrolene sodium as a possible prophylactic agent against NMS. *Hillside Journal of Clinical Psychiatry*, 8(1):34-37, 1986.

Levinson, D., & Simpson, G.: EPS with fever: Heterogeneity of the neuroleptic malignant syndrome. *Archives of General Psychiatry*, 43:839-848, 1986.

Levinson, D., & Simpson, G.: Antipsychotic drug side effects. In R. E. Hales & A. J. Frances (Eds.), *Psychiatry Update, Annual Review, Volume 6.* Washington, D.C.: American Psychiatric Press, 1987, pp. 704-723.

Lewis, D. A., & Nasrallah, H. A.: Mania associated with electroconvulsive therapy. *Journal of Clinical Psychiatry*, 47(7):366-367, 1986.

Lewis, J. L., & Winokur, G.: The induction of mania, a natural history study with controls. *Archives of General Psychiatry*, 39: 303-306, 1982.

Lewy, A. J., Sack, R. L., Miller, L. S., et al.: Antidepressants and circadian phase-shifting effects of light. *Science*, 235(4786):352-354, 1987.

Lewy, A. J., Sack, R. L., & Singer, C. M.: Melatonin, light and chronobiological disorders. *Ciba Foundation Symposia*, 117:231-252, 1985.

Libman, E., Fichten, C. S., Brinder, W., et al.: A comparison of three therapeutic formats in the treatment of secondary orgasmic dysfunction. *Journal of Sex & Marital Therapy,* 10(3):147–159, 1984.
Lichstein, T. R.: Caring for the patient with multiple somatic complaints. *Southern Medical Journal,* 79(3):310–314, 1986.
Liebowitz, M. R.: Imipramine in the treatment of panic disorder and its complications. *Psychiatric Clinics of North America,* 8(1):37–47, 1985.
Lindberg, F. H., & Distad, L. J.: Post-traumatic stress disorders in women who experienced childhood incest. *Child Abuse and Neglect,* 9(3):329–334, 1985.
Lindsay, W. R., Gansu, C. V., McLaughlin, E., et al.: A controlled trial of treatments for generalized anxiety. *British Journal of Clinical Psychology,* 26(part 1):3–15, 1987.
Lion, J. R.: Countertransference and other psychotherapy issues. In W. H. Reid (Ed.), *The Treatment of Antisocial Syndromes.* New York: Van Nostrand Reinhold, 1981.
Lisansky, J., Fava, G. A., Buckman, M. T., et al.: Prolactin, amitriptyline, and recovery from depression. *Psychopharmacology* (Berlin), 84(3):331–335, 1984.
LoPiccolo, J., Heiman, J. R., Hogan, D. R., et al.: Effectiveness of single therapist vs. cotherapy teams in sex therapy. *Journal of Consulting and Clinical Psychology,* 53(3):287–294, 1985.
Louie, A. K., & Meltzer, H. Y.: Lithium potentiation of antidepressant treatment. *Journal of Clinical Psychopharmacology,* 4(6):316–321, 1984.
Lowe, M. R., & Batchelor, D. H.: Depot neuroleptics and manic-depressive psychosis. *International Clinical Psychopharmacology* (England), 1(Supplement 1):53–62, 1986.
Lukoff, D., Wallace, C. J., Liberman, R. P., et al.: A holistic program for chronic schizophrenic patients. *Schizophrenia Bulletin,* 12(2):274–282, 1986.
Lybiard, R. B.: Obsessive-compulsive disorder successfully treated with trazodone. *Psychosomatics,* 27(12):858–859, 1986.
Macaskill, N. D.: Therapeutic factors in group therapy with borderline patients. *International Journal of Group Psychotherapy,* 32(1):61–73, 1982.
MacHovec, F. J.: Hypnosis to facilitate recall in psychogen amnesia and fugue states: Treatment variables. *American Journal of Clinical Hypnosis,* 24(1):7–13, 1981.
Mahapatra, R. K., Paul, S. K., Mahapatra, D., et al.: Cardiovascular effects of polycyclic antidepressants. *Angiology,* 37(10):709–717, 1986.
Mahgoub, O. M.: A remarkable response of chronic severe obsessive-compulsive neurosis to phenelzine. *Acta Psychiatrica Scandinavica,* 75(2):222–223, 1987.
Maj, M., Starace, F., Nolfe, G., et al.: Minimum plasma lithium levels required for effective prophylaxis in DSM-III bipolar disorder: A prospective study. *Pharmacopsychiatry* (West Germany), 19(6):420–423, 1986.
Majid, I.: A double-blind comparison of one-daily flupenthixol and mianserin in depressed hospital outpatients. *Pharmatherapeutica,* 4(7):405–410, 1986.
Maletzky, V. M.: *Multiple-monitored Electroconvulsive Therapy.* Boca Raton, FL: CRC, 1981.
Malinow, K. L.: Dependent personality. In J. R. Lion (Ed.), *Personality Disorders: Diagnosis and Management* (Second Edition). Baltimore: Williams & Wilkins, 1981.
Mamelak, M., & Webster, P.: Treatment of narcolepsy and sleep apnea with gamma-hydroxybutyrate: A clinical and polysomnographic case study. *Sleep,* 4:105–111, 1981.
Manchanda, R., & Hirsch, S. R.: Does propranolol have an antipsychotic effect? A placebo-controlled study in acute schizophrenia. *British Journal of Psychiatry,* 148: 701–707, 1986.
Mander, A. J.: Clinical prediction of the outcome of lithium response in bipolar affective disorder. *Journal of Affective Disorders,* 11(1):35–41, 1986.
Marder, S. R., van Putten, T., Mintz, J., et al.: Maintenance therapy in schizophrenia: New findings. In J. M. Kane (Ed.), *Drug Maintenance Strategies in Schizophrenia.* Washington, D.C.: American Psychiatric Press, 1984.
Marks, I. M.: Review of behavioral psychotherapy. I. Obsessive-compulsive disorders. *American Journal of Psychiatry,* 138(5):584–592, 1981a.

Marks, I. M.: Review of behavioral psychotherapy. II: Sexual disorders. *American Journal of Psychiatry*, 138(6):750-756, 1981b.
Marks, I. M.: Behavioral psychotherapy for anxiety disorders. *Psychiatric Clinics of North America*, 8(1):25-35, 1985.
Marmor, J.: The psychodynamic approach in the treatment of sexual problems. In M. R. Zales (Ed.), *Eating, Sleeping, and Sexuality: Treatment of Disorders in Basic Life Functions*. New York: Brunner/Mazel, 1982.
Martin, B. A.: Electroconvulsive therapy: Contemporary standards of practice. *Canadian Journal of Psychiatry*, 31:759-771, 1986.
Martin, W. R., Sloan, J. W., Sapira, J. D., et al.: Physiologic, subjective and behavioral effects of amphetamine, methamphetamine, ephedrine, phenmetrazine and methylphenidate in man. *Clinical Pharmacology & Therapeutics*, 12:245-258, 1971.
Masters, W., & Johnson, V.: *Human Sexual Inadequacy*. Boston: Little, Brown, 1970.
Mattes, J. A.: Metoprolol for intermittent explosive disorder. *American Journal of Psychiatry*, 142(9):1108-1109, 1985.
Mavissakalian, M. M., & Michelson, L.: Agoraphobia: Behavioral and pharmacological treatments. *Psychopharmacology Bulletin*, 18: 91-103, 1982.
Mavissakalian, M., & Michelson, L.: Agoraphobia: Relative and combined effectiveness of therapist-assisted in vivo exposure and imipramine. *Journal of Clinical Psychiatry*, 47(3):117-122, 1986a.
Mavissakalian, M., & Michelson, L.: Two-year follow-up of exposure and imipramine treatment of agoraphobia. *American Journal of Psychiatry*, 143(9):1106-1112, 1986b.
Mawson, B., Marks, I., Ramm, E., et al.: Guided mourning for morbid grief: A controlled study. *British Journal of Psychiatry*, 138: 185-193, 1981.
May, P. R. A., van Putten, T., Jenden, D. J., et al.: Chlorpromazine levels and the outcome of treatment in schizophrenic patients. *Archives of General Psychiatry*, 38: 202-207, 1981.
McCabe, B., & Tsuang, M. T.: Dietary considerations in MAO inhibitor regimens. *Journal of Clinical Psychiatry*, 43:178-181, 1982.
McCann, I. L., & Holmes, D. S.: Influence of aerobic exercise on depression. *Journal of Personality and Social Psychology*, 46(5):1142-1147, 1984.
McConaghy, N., Armstrong, M. S., Blaszczynski, A., et al.: Controlled comparison of aversive therapy and imaginal desensitization in compulsive gambling. *British Journal of Psychiatry*, 142:366-372, 1983.
McCormick, R. A., Russo, A. M., Ramirez, L. F., et al.: Affective disorders among pathological gamblers seeking treatment. *American Journal of Psychiatry*, 141(2):215-218, 1984.
McCreadie, R., Mackie, M., Morrison, D., et al.: Once weekly pimozide vs. fluphenazine decanoate and maintenance therapy in chronic schizophrenia. *British Journal of Psychiatry*, 140:280-286, 1982.
McEvoy, J. P., & Lohr, J. B.: Diazepam for catatonia. *American Journal of Psychiatry*, 141(2):284-285, 1984.
McEvoy, R. D., & Thornton, A. T.: Treatment of obstructive sleep apnea syndrome with nasal continuous positive airway pressure. *Sleep*, 7(4):313-325, 1984.
McGlashan, T. H.: Intensive individual psychotherapy of schizophrenia. A review of techniques. *Archives of General Psychiatry*, 40(8):909-920, 1983.
McGlashan, T. H.: Schizotypal personality disorder. Chestnut Lodge follow-up study: VI. Long-term follow-up perspectives. *Archives of General Psychiatry*, 43(4):329-334, 1986.
McMillan, D. E., Fody, E. P., Couch, L., et al.: Drug holidays and serum haloperidol levels in schizophrenic patients. *General Clinical Psychiatry*, 47(7):373-374, 1986.
McNair, D. M., Kahn, R. J., Frankenthaler, L. M., et al.: Amoxapine and amitriptyline. I. Relative speed of antidepressant action. *Psychopharmacology* (Berlin), 83(2):129-133, 1984a.

McNair, D. M., Kahn, R. J., Frankenthaler, L. M., et al.: Amoxapine and amitriptyline. II. Specificity of cognitive effects during brief treatment of depression. *Psychopharmacology* (Berlin), 83(2):134–139, 1984b.

Meadow, R.: Fictitious epilepsy. *Lancet*, 2(8393):25–28, 1984.

Mellion, M. B.: Exercise therapy for anxiety and depression. 1. Does the evidence justify its recommendation? *Postgraduate Medicine*, 77(3):59–66, 1985.

Meltzer, H. Y., Sommers, A. A., & Luchins, D. J.: The effect of neuroleptics and other psychotropic drugs on negative symptoms in schizophrenia. *Journal of Clinical Psychopharmacology*, 6(6):329–338, 1986.

Mendlewicz, J., Hubain, T. P., & Koumakis, C.: Further investigation of the dexamethasone suppression test in affective illnesses: Relationship to clinical diagnosis and therapeutic response. *Neuropsychobiology*, 12(1):23–26, 1984.

Michelson, L., & Ascher, L. M.: Paradoxical intention in the treatment of agoraphobia and other anxiety disorders. *Journal of Behavioral Therapy and Experimental Psychiatry*, 15(3):215–220, 1984.

Micheroli, R., & Battegay, R.: Ambulantate behandlung von sexualdelinquenten mit cyproteronacetat (Androcur) eime katannestiche untersuchung. *Schweiz Arch. Neurol. Psychiatr.*, 136(5):37–58, 1985.

Mitchell, J. D., & Poplin, M. K.: Antidepressant drug therapy and sexual dysfunction in men: A review. *General Clinical Psychopharmacology*, 3:76–79, 1983.

Mitler, M. M., Browman, C. P., Menn, S. J., et al.: Nocturnal myoclonus: Treatment efficacy of clonazepam and temazepam. *Sleep*, 9(3):385–392, 1986.

Modell, J. G., Lenox, R. H., & Weiner, S.: Inpatient clinical trials of lorazepam for the management of manic agitation. *Journal of Clinical Psychopharmacology*, 5:109–113, 1985.

Moldofsky, H., & Lue, F. A.: The relationship of alpha and delta EEG frequencies to pain and mode in fibrositis patients treated with chlorpromazine and L-tryptophan. *Electroencephalography & Clinical Neurophysiology*, 50:71–80, 1980.

Moldofsky, H., Musisi, S., & Phillipson, E. A.: Treatment of a case of advanced sleep-phase syndrome by phase advance chronotherapy. *Sleep* 9(1):61–65, 1986.

Monroe, R. R.: The problem of impulsivity in personality disturbances. In J. R. Lion (Ed.), *Personality Disorders: Diagnosis and Management* (Second Edition). Baltimore: Williams & Wilkins, 1981.

Montplaisir, J., Godbout, R., Boghen, D., et al.: Familial restless legs with periodic movements in sleep: Electrophysiologic biochemical and pharmacological study. *Neurology*, 35:130–134, 1985.

Mosher, L. R., & Keith, S. J.: Research on the psychosocial treatment of schizophrenia: A summary report. *American Journal of Psychiatry*, 137(5):623–631, 1979.

Moss, E., & Garb, R.: Integrated psychotherapeutic treatment of somatoform and other psychophysiological disorders. *Psychotherapy and Psychosomatics*, 25(2):105–112, 1986.

Mukherjee, S., Rosen, A. M., Caracci, G., et al.: Persistent tardive dyskinesia in bipolar patients. *Archives of General Psychiatry*, 43(4):342–346, 1986.

Muller, Y. L.: Depersonalisation—Symptoms, meaning, therapy. *Acta Psychiatrica Scandinavica*, 66(6):451–458, 1982.

Murphy, E.: General management of depression in late life. *Journal of Affective Disorders*, (Supplement 1):S7–S10, 1985.

Murphy, G. E., Simons, A. D., Wetzle, R. D., et al.: Cognitive therapy and pharmacotherapy: Singly and together in the treatment of depression. *Archives of General Psychiatry*, 41:33, 1984.

Murphy, M. F., & Davis, K. L.: Biological perspectives in chronic pain, depression, and organic mental disorders. *Psychiatric Clinics of North America*, 4(2):223–237, 1981.

Murray, J. B.: Successful treatment of obsessive-compulsive disorders. *Genetic, Social, & General Psychology Monographs*, 112(2):173–199, 1986.

Mutter, C. B.: A hypno-therapeutic approach to exhibitionism: Outpatient therapeutic strategy. *Journal of Forensic Sciences*, 26(1):129–133, 1981.

Myall, R. W., Collins, F. J., Ross, A., et al.: Chronic factitious illness: Recognition and management of deception. *Journal of Oral and Maxillofacial Surgery*, 42(2):97–100, 1984.

Myers, E. D., & Calvert, E. J.: Information, compliance and side effects: A study of patients on antidepressant medication. *British Journal of Clinical Pharmacology*, 17(1):21–25, 1984.

Naylor, G. J., & Martin, B.: A double-blind out-patient trial of indalpine vs. mianserin. *British Journal of Psychiatry*, 147: 306–309, 1985.

Neborsky, R., Janowsky, D., Munson, E., et al.: Rapid treatment of acute psychotic symptoms with high- and low-dose haloperidol: Behavioral considerations. *Archives of General Psychiatry*, 38: 195–199, 1981.

Neidigh, L., & Kinder, B. N.: The use of audiovisual materials in sex therapy: A critical overview. *Journal of Sex & Marital Therapy*, 13(1):64–72, 1987.

Nemiah, J. C.: Dissociative disorders (hysterical neurosis, dissociative type). In H. I. Kaplan, A. M. Freedman, & B. J. Sadock (Eds.), *Comprehensive Textbook of Psychiatry*, 3rd ed., vol. 2. Baltimore, MD: Williams & Wilkins, 1980.

Nestoros, J. N., Suranyl-Cadotte, B. E., Spees, R. C., et al.: Diazepam in high doses is effective in schizophrenia. *Progress in Neuro-Psychopharmacology and Biological Psychiatry*, 6(4–6):513–516, 1982.

Newton, R. E., Marunycz, J. D., Alderdice, M. T., et al.: Review of the side-effect profile of buspirone. *American Journal of Medicine*, 80(3b):17–21, 1986.

Noyes, R., Jr., Chaudry, D. R., & Domingo, D. V.: Pharmacologic treatment of phobic disorders. *Journal of Clinical Psychiatry*, 47(9):445–452, 1986.

Nurnberg, H. G.: Survey of psychotherapeutic approaches to narcissistic personality disorder. *Hillside Journal of Clinical Psychiatry*, 6(2):204–220, 1984.

Nurnberg, H. G., & Feldman, A.: Hospital management of borderline patients. In J. H. Masserman (Ed.), *Current Psychiatric Therapies, Volume 22*. New York: Grune & Stratton, 1983, pp. 221–229.

Nurnberg, H. G., & Levine, P. E.: Schizophrenia and antipsychotic drugs. *Comprehensive Therapeutics*, 12(10):42–52, 1986.

O'Connell, R. A., Mayo, J. A., Eng, L. K., et al.: Social support and long-term lithium outcome. *British Journal of Psychiatry*, 147:272–275, 1985.

O'Regan, J. B.: Hypersomnia and MAOI antidepressants. *Canadian Medical Association Journal*, 111:213, 1974.

Orne, M. T.: The use and misuse of hypnosis in court. *International Journal of Clinical and Experimental Hypnosis*, 27(4):311–341, 1979.

Osborne, M., Crayton, J. W., Javaid, J., et al.: Lack of effect of a gluten-free diet on neuroleptic blood levels in schizophrenic patients. *Biological Psychiatry*, 17(5):627–629, 1982.

Oswald, I.: Symptoms that depress the doctor: Insomnia. *British Journal of Sleep Medicine*, 31:219–224, 1984.

Pare, C. M.: The present status of monoamine oxidase inhibitors. *British Journal of Psychiatry*, 146:576–584, 1985.

Parkes, J. D.: Daytime drowsiness. *Lancet*, 2:1213–1218, 1981.

Parsons, C. L.: Group reminiscence therapy and levels of depression in the elderly. *Nurse Practitioner*, 11(3):68–76, 1986.

Pathy, M. S. J., Bayer, A. J., & Stoker, M. J.: A double-blind comparison of chloramathiazole and temazepam in elderly patients with sleep disturbance. *Acta Psychiatrica Scandinavica*, 73(329):99–103, 1986.

Pecknold, J. C., & Fleury, D.: Alprazolam-induced manic episode in two patients with panic disorder. *American Journal of Psychiatry*, 143(5):652–653, 1986.

Perenyi, A., Szuchs, R., & Frecska, E.: Tardive dyskinesia in patients receiving lithium maintenance therapy. *Biological Psychiatry*, 19(11):1573-1578, 1984.

Perry, J. C., & Flannery, R. B.: Passive-aggressive personality disorder. Treatment implications of a clinical typology. *Journal of Nervous and Mental Disease*, 170(3):164-173, 1982.

Peteet, J. R., & Gutheil, T. G.: The hospital and the borderline patient: Management guidelines for the community mental health center. *Psychiatric Quarterly*, 51(2):106-118, 1979.

Petrie, W. M., Van, T. A., Berney, S., et al.: Loxapine in psychogeriatrics: A placebo and standard controlled clinical investigation. *Journal of Clinical Psychopharmacology*, 2:122-126, 1982.

Pickar, D., Wolkowitz, O. M., Doran, A. R., et al.: Clinical and biochemical effects of verapamil administration to schizophrenic patients. *Archives of General Psychiatry*, 44(2):113-118, 1987.

Pickard Bartanian, F., Bunney, W. E., Maier, H. P., et al.: Short-term naloxone administration in schizophrenic and traumatic patients: A world health organization collaborative study. *Archives of General Psychiatry*, 39:313-318, 1982.

Plakun, E. M., Burkhardt, T. E., & Muller, J. T.: Fourteen-year follow-up of borderline and schizotypal personality disorders. *Comprehensive Psychiatry*, 26(5):448-455, 1985.

Pollack, M. H., Tesar, G. E., Rosenbaum, J. F., et al.: Clonazepam in the treatment of panic disorder and agoraphobia: A one-year follow-up. *Journal of Clinical Psychopharmacology*, 6(5):302-304, 1986.

Potkin, S. G., Weinberger, D., Kleinman, J., et al.: Wheat gluten challenge in schizophrenic patients. *American Journal of Psychiatry*, 138(9):1208-1211, 1981.

Pottash, A. L. C., Gold, M. S., & Extein, I.: The use of the clinical laboratory. In L. I. Sederer (Ed.), *Inpatient Psychiatry: Diagnosis and Treatment* (2nd Edition). Baltimore: Williams & Wilkins, 1986, pp. 197-218.

Prasad, A.: Efficacy of trazodone as an anti-obsessional agent. *Neuropsychobiology*, 15(Supplement 1):19-21, 1986.

Preskorn, S. H., & Othmer, S. C.: Evaluation of buproprion hydrochloride: The first of a new class of atypical antidepressants. *Pharmacotherapy*, 4:20-34, 1984.

Price, W. A., & Giannini, A. J.: Neurotoxicity caused by lithium-verapamil synergism. *Journal of Clinical Pharmacology*, 26(8):717-719, 1986.

Prien, R. F., Kupfer, D. J., Mansky, P. A., et al.: Drug therapy and the prevention of recurrence in unipolar and bipolar affective disorders. Report of the NIMH collaborative study group comparing lithium carbonate, imipramine, and a lithium carbonate-imipramine combination. *Archives of General Psychiatry*, 41(11):1096-1104, 1984.

Puzynski, S., & Klosiewicz, L.: Valproic acid amide in the treatment of affective and schizoaffective disorders. *Journal of Affective Disorders*, 6(1):115-121, 1984.

Quality Assurance Project: Treatment outlines for the management of anxiety states. *Australia and New Zealand Journal of Psychiatry*, 19(2):138-151, 1985a.

Quality Assurance Project: Treatment outlines for the management of obsessive-compulsive disorders. *Australia and New Zealand Journal of Psychiatry*, 19(3):240-253, 1985b.

Rabiner, C. J., Wegner, J. T., & Kane, J. M.: Outcome study of first-episode psychosis. I: Relapse rates after one year. *American Journal of Psychiatry*, 143(9):1155-1158, 1986.

Ragheb, M.: Ibuprofen can increase serum lithium level in lithium-treated patients. *Journal of Clinical Psychiatry*, 48(4):161-163, 1987.

Rajagopal, K. R., Abbrecht, P. H., & Jabbari, B.: Effects of medroxyprogesterone acetate in obstructive sleep apnea. *Chest*, 90(6):815-821, 1986.

Ramirez, L. F., McCormick, R. A., Russo, A. M., et al.: Patterns of substance abuse in pathological gamblers undergoing treatment. *Addictive Behaviors*, 8(4):425-428, 1983.

Rampertaap, M. P.: Neuroleptic malignant syndrome. *Southern Medical Journal*, 79(3):331-336, 1986.

Rankin, H.: Control rather than abstinence as a goal in the treatment of excessive gambling. *Behaviour Research and Therapy*, 20(2):185-187, 1982.

Rasmussen, S. A.: Lithium and tryptophan augmentation in clomipramine-resistant obsessive-compulsive disorder. *American Journal of Psychiatry*, 141(10):1283-1285, 1984.

Ratey, J. J., Sands, S., & O'Driscoll, G.: The phenomenology of recovery in the chronic schizophrenic. *Psychiatry*, 49(4):277-289, 1986.

Reich, J.: The relationship between antisocial behavior and affective illness. *Comprehensive Psychiatry*, 26(3):296-303, 1985.

Reich, P., & Gottfried, L. A.: Factitious disorders in a teaching hospital. *Annals of Internal Medicine*, 99(2):240-247, 1983.

Reid, W. H.: Treatment of somnambulism in military trainees. *American Journal of Psychotherapy*, 29(1):101-106, 1975.

Reid, W. H.: Antisocial personality and related syndromes. In J. R. Lion (Ed.), *Personality Disorders: Diagnosis and Management*. Baltimore: Williams & Wilkins, 1981a.

Reid, W. H. (Ed.):*The Treatment of Antisocial Syndromes*. New York: Van Nostrand Reinhold, 1981b.

Reid, W. H.: *Treatment of the DSM-III Psychiatric Disorders*. New York: Brunner/Mazel, 1983.

Reid, W. H.: The antisocial personality: A review. *Hospital and Community Psychiatry*, 36(8):831-837, 1985.

Reid, W. H.: Antisocial personality. In R. M. Michels & J. O. Cavenar, Jr. (Eds.), *Psychiatry*. Philadelphia: J. B. Lippincott, 1986.

Reid, W. H., Ahmed, I., & Levie, C. A.: Treatment of sleepwalking: A controlled study. *American Journal of Psychotherapy*, 35(1):27-37, 1981.

Reid, W. H., Blouin, P., & Schermer, M.: A review of psychotropic medications and the glaucomas. *International Pharmacopsychiatry*, 11(3):163-174, 1976.

Reid, W. H., & Gutnik, B. D.: Organic treatment of chronically violent patients. *Psychiatric Annals*, 12(5):526-542, 1982.

Reid, W. H., Haffke, E. A., & Chu, C. C.: Diazepam in treatment of intractable sleepwalking. *Hillside Journal of Clinical Psychiatry*, 6(1):49-55, 1984.

Reid, W. H., & Matthews, W.: A wilderness experience treatment program for antisocial offenders. *International Journal of Offender Therapy and Comparative Criminology*, 24(2):171-178, 1980.

Reid, W. H., & Solomon, G. H.: Community-based offender programs. In W. H. Reid (Ed.), *The Treatment of Antisocial Syndromes*. New York: Van Nostrand Reinhold, 1981.

Richardson, G. S., Carskadon, M. A., Flagg, W., et al.: Excessive daytime sleepiness in man: Multiple sleep latency measurement in narcoleptic and controlled subjects. *Electroencephalography & Clinical Neurophysiology*, 45:621-627, 1978.

Richelson, E.: Schizophrenia: Treatment. In R. Michaels & J. O. Cavenar, Jr., et al. (Eds.), *Psychiatry, Volume 1*. New York: J. B. Lippincott, 1986.

Rickels, K., Morris, R. J., Mauriello, R., et al.: Brotizolam, a triazolothiendodiazepine in insomnia. *Clinical Pharmacology and Therapy*, 40:293-299, 1986.

Ries, R. K., Bokan, J. A., Katon, W. J., et al.: The medical care abuser: Differential diagnosis and management. *Journal of Family Practice*, 13(2):257-265, 1981.

Rifkin, A., Quitkin, F., Carillo, C., et al.: Lithium treatment in emotionally unstable character disorders. *Archives of General Psychiatry*, 27:519-523, 1972.

Rifkin, A., & Siris, S. G.: Panic disorder: Response to sodium lactate and treatment with antidepressants. *Progress in Neuro-Psychopharmacology and Biological Psychiatry*, 9(1):33-38, 1985.

Rihmer, Z., Arato, M., Gyorgy, S., et al.: Dexamethasone suppression test as an aid for selection of specific antidepressant drugs in patient with endogenous depression. *Pharmacopsychiatry*, 18(5):306-308, 1985.

Ritzler, B. A.: Paranoia—Prognosis and treatment: A review. *Schizophrenia Bulletin*, 7(4) 710-728, 1981.

Robey, A.: Personal communication, 1981.
Robinson, A. D., & McCreadie, R. G.: The nithsdale schizophrenia survey. V. Follow-up of tardive dyskinesia at 3½ years. *British General Psychiatry*, 149:621-623, 1986.
Roselaar, S. E., Langdon, N., Lock, C. B., et al.: Selegiline in narcolepsy. *Sleep*, 10(5):491-495, 1987.
Rosenbaum, M. B.: Sex therapy today. *Bulletin of the Menninger Clinic*, 49(3):270-279, 1985.
Rosenbaum, M. S.: Treating hair-pulling in a seven-year-old male: Modified habit reversal for use in pediatric settings. *Journal of Development and Behavioral Pediatrics*, 3(4):241-242, 1982.
Rosenbluth, M.: The inpatient treatment of the borderline personality disorder: A critical review and discussion of aftercare implications. *Canadian Journal of Psychiatry*, 32(3):228-237, 1987.
Rosenthal, M. S.: Therapeutic communities: A treatment alternative for many but not all. *Journal of Substance Abuse Treatment*, 1(1):55-58, 1984.
Ross, W. P., Schultz, J. R., & Edelstein, P.: The biopsychosocial approach: Clinical examples from a consultation-liaison service. *Psychosomatics*, 23(2):141-151, 1982.
Roth, T., Zorick, F., Wittig, R., et al.: Pharmacological and medical considerations in hypnotic use. *Sleep*, 5:S46-S52, 1982.
Rowlands, D.: Therapeutic touch: Its effects on the depressed elderly. *Australian Nurses Journal*, 13(11):45-52, 1984.
Ruedrich, S. L., Chu, C. C., & Wadle, C. V.: The amytal interview in the treatment of psychogenic amnesia. *Hospital and Community Psychiatry*, 26(10):1045-1046, 1985.
Rush, A. J.: Diagnosis of affective disorders. In A. J. Rush & K. Z. Altshuler (Eds.), *Depression: Basic Mechanisms, Diagnosis, and Treatment*. New York: Guilford Press, 1986, pp. 1-31.
Rush, A. J., Beck, A. T., Kovacs, M., et al.: Comparative efficacy of cognitive therapy and pharmacotherapy in the treatment of depressed outpatients. *Cognitive Therapy and Research*, 1:17, 1977.
Rush, A. J., Beck, A. T., Kovacs, M., et al.: Comparison of the effects of cognitive therapy and pharmacotherapy on hopelessness and self-concept. *American Journal of Psychiatry*, 139:862-866, 1982.
Russo, A. M., Taber, J. I., McCormick, R. A., et al.: An outcome study of an inpatient treatment program for pathological gamblers. *Hospital and Community Psychiatry*, 35(8):823-827, 1984.
Sachs, C., Persson, H. E., & Hagenfeldt, K.: Menstruation-related periodic hypersomnia: A case study with successful treatment. *Neurology*, 32(12):1376-1379, 1982.
Salzman, C.: The use of ECT in the treatment schizophrenia. *American Journal of Psychiatry*, 137: 1032, 1980.
Salzman, C., Green, A. I., Rodriguez-Villa, F., et al.: Benzodiazepines combined with neuroleptics for acute and severe disruptive behavior. *Psychosomatics*, 27 (Supplement):17-21, 1987.
Salzman, L.: Psychotherapeutic management of obsessive-compulsive patients. *American Journal of Psychotherapy*, 39(3):323-330, 1985.
Saul, T., Jones, B. P., Edwards, K. G., et al.: Randomized comparison of atenolol and placebo in the treatment of anxiety: A double-blind study. *European Journal of Clinical Pharmacology*, 28(Supplement):109-110, 1985.
Scarzella, L., Scarzella, R., Mailland, F., et al.: Amineptine in the management of the depressive syndromes. *Progress in Neuro-Psychopharmacology and Biological Psychiatry*, 9(4):429-439, 1985.
Schmidt, K.: Pipothiazine palmitate: A versatile, sustained-action neuroleptic in the psychiatric practice. *Current Medical Research and Opinion* (England), 10(5):326-329, 1986.
Schneider-Helmert, D.: DSIP in sleep disturbances. *European Neurology*, 25(2):154-157, 1986.

Schneider-Helmert, D., & Spinweber, C. L.: Evaluation of L-tryptophan for treatment of insomnia: A review. *Psychopharmacology* (Berlin), 89:1–7, 1986.

Schnitt, J. M., & Nocks, J. J.: Alcoholism treatment of Vietnam veterans with post-traumatic stress disorder. *Journal of Substance Abuse Treatment*, 1(3):179–189, 1984.

Schover, L. R., & vonEschenbach, A. C.: Sex therapy and the penile prosthesis: A synthesis. *Journal of Sex & Marital Therapy*, 11(1):57–66, 1985.

Schover, L. R., vonEschenbach, A. C., Smith, D. B., et al.: Sexual rehabilitation of urologic cancer patients. A practical approach. *CA*, 34(2):66–74, 1984.

Schreter, R. K.: Treating the untreatable: A group experience with somaticizing borderline patients. *International Journal of Psychiatry and Medicine*, 10(3):205–215, 1980.

Schwartz, L. S., Robinson, M. V., Flaherty, J. A., et al.: A supportive care clinic: Maintaining the chronic psychiatric patient. *Hillside Journal of Clinical Psychiatry*, 8(2):202–208, 1986.

Sederer, L. I., & Thorbeck, J.: First do no harm: Short-term inpatient psychotherapy of the borderline patient. *Hospital and Community Psychiatry*, 37(7):692–697, 1986.

Seidel, W. F., Cohen, S. A., Bliwise, N. G., et al.: Dose-related effects of triazolam and flurazepam on a circadian rhythm insomnia. *Clinical Pharmacology and Therapeutics*, 40:31420, 1986.

Serban, G., & Siegel, S.: Response of borderline and schizotypal patients to small doses of thiothixene and haloperidol. *American Journal of Psychiatry*, 141(11):1455–1458, 1984.

Shah, J. H., DeLeon-Jones, F. A., Schickler, R., et al.: Symptomatic reactive hypoglycemia during glucose tolerance tests in lithium-treated patients. *Metabolism*, 35(7):634–639, 1986.

Shalev, A., & Munitz, H.: Conversion without hysteria: A case report and review of literature. *British Journal of Psychiatry*, 148:198–203, 1986.

Shapira, B., Oppenheim, G., Zohar, J., et al.: Lack of efficacy of estrogen supplementation to imipramine in resistant female depressives. *Biological Psychiatry*, 20(5):576–579, 1985.

Shapiro, W. R.: Treatment of cataplexy with clomipramine. *Archives of Neurology*, 32:653–656, 1975.

Sheline, Y. I., & Miller, M. B.: Catatonia relieved by oral diazepam in a patient with a pituitary microadenoma. *Psychosomatics*, 27(12):860–862, 1986.

Shively, D., & Petrich, J.: Correctional mental health. *Psychiatric Clinics of North America*, 8(3):537–550, 1985.

Shukla, S., Cook, B. L., & Miller, M. G.: Lithium-carbamazepine vs lithium-neuroleptic prophylaxis in bipolar illness. *Journal of Affective Disorders*, 9(3):219–222, 1985.

Siebel, M. M., Freeman, M. G., & Graves, W. L.: Carcinoma of the cervix and sexual functioning. *Obstetrics and Gynecology*, 55(4):484–487, 1980.

Sifneos, P. E.: Short-term dynamic psychotherapy for patients with physical symptomatology. *Psychotherapy and Psychosomatics*, 42(1–4):48–51, 1984.

Sifneos, P. E.: Short-term dynamic psychotherapy of phobic and mildly obsessive-compulsive patients. *American Journal of Psychotherapy*, 39(3):314–322, 1985.

Silver, D.: Psychotherapy of the characterologically difficult patient. *Canadian Journal of Psychiatry*, 28(7):513–521, 1983.

Silver, D.: Psychodynamics and psychotherapeutic management of the self-destructive character-disordered patient. *Psychiatric Clinics of North America*, 8(2):357–375, 1985.

Simmons, D. A., Daamen, M. J., Harrison, J. W., et al.: Hospital management of a patient with factitial dermatitis. *General Hospital Psychiatry*, 9(2):147–150, 1987.

Simon, J. I.: Day hospital treatment for borderline adolescents. *Adolescence*, 21(83):561–572, 1986.

Simons, A. D., Levine, J. L., Lustman, P. J., et al.: Patient attrition in a comparative outcome study of depression: A follow-up report. *Journal of Affective Disorders*, 6:163, 1984.

Simpson, G. M., Pi, E. H., & Sramek, J. J., Jr.: Neuroleptics and antipsychotics. In N. B. Blackwell (Ed.), *Meyler's Side Effects of Drugs* (Tenth Edition). New York: Elsevier, 1984.
Smith, P. L., Haponik, E. F., Allen, R. P., et al.: The effects of protriptylene in sleep-disordered breathing. *American Review of Respiratory Diseases*, 127(1):8–13, 1983.
Smith, P. L., Haponik, E. F., & Bleeker, E. R.: The effects of oxygen in patients with sleep apnea. *American Review of Respiratory Diseases*, 130:985–963, 1984.
Smith, R. C.: A clinical approach to the somatizing patient. *Journal of Family Practice*, 21(4):294–301, 1985.
Smith, R. C., Veroulis, G., Shvartsburd, A., et al.: RBC and plasma levels of haloperidol and clinical response in schizophrenia. *American Journal of Psychiatry*, 139:1054, 1982.
Snaith, R. P., & Collins, S. A.: Five exhibitionists and a method of treatment. *British Journal of Psychiatry*, 138: 126–130, 1981.
Snyder, D. K., & Berg, P.: Predicting couples' response to brief directive sex therapy. *Journal of Sex & Marital Therapy*, 9(2):114–120, 1983.
Snyder, S.: Trichotillomania treated with amitriptyline. *Journal of Nervous and Mental Disease*, 168(8):505–507, 1980.
Socarides, C. W.: Some problems encountered in psychoanalytic treatment of overt male homosexuality. *American Journal of Psychotherapy*, 33(4):506–520, 1979.
Soloff, P. H., George, A., Nathan, R. S., et al.: Progress in pharmacotherapy of borderline disorders. A double-blind study of amitriptyline, haloperidol, and placebo. *Archives of General Psychiatry*, 43(7):691–697, 1986a.
Soloff, P. H., George, A., Nathan, S., et al.: Amitriptyline and haloperidol in unstable and schizotypal borderline disorders. *Psychopharmacology Bulletin*, 22(1):177–182, 1986b.
Soloff, P. H., George, A., Nathan, R. S., et al.: Paradoxical effects of amitriptyline on borderline patients. *American Journal of Psychiatry*, 143(12):1603–1605, 1986c.
Solomon, L., & Williamson, P.: Verapamil in bipolar illness. *Canadian Journal of Psychiatry*, 31(5):442–444, 1986.
Spencer, J.: Maximization of biofeedback following cognitive stress preselection in generalized anxiety. *Perceptual and Motor Skills*, 63(1):239–242, 1986.
Spiegel, D.: Multiple personality of a post-traumatic stress disorder. *Psychiatric Clinics of North America*, 7(1):101–110, 1984.
Spielman, A. J., Saskin, P., & Thorpy, M. J.: Treatment of chronic insomnia by restriction of time in bed. *Sleep*, 10(1):45–56, 1987.
Spiker, B. G., Hanin, I., Cofsky, J., et al.: Pharmacological treatment of delusional depressives. *Psychopharmacology Bulletin*, 17:201–202, 1981.
Squire, L. R., & Slater, P. C.: Electroconvulsive therapy and complaints of memory dysfunction: A prospective three-year follow-up study. *British Journal of Psychiatry*, 142: 1, 1983.
Sranek, J. J., Simpson, G. N., Morrison, R. L., et al.: A prospective study of anticholinergic agents for prophylaxis of neuroleptic-induced dystonic reactions. *Journal of Psychiatry*, 47:305–309, 1986.
Stern, B. A., Fromm, M. G., & Sacksteder, J. L.: From coercion to collaboration: Two weeks in the life of a therapeutic community. *Psychiatry*, 49(1):18–32, 1986.
Stevens, M. J.: Behavioral treatment of trichotillomania. *Psychological Reports*, 55:987–990, 1984.
Stewart, J. W., Harrison, W., Quitkin, F., et al.: Phenelzine-induced pyridoxine deficiency. *Journal of Clinical Psychopharmacology*, 4:225–226, 1984.
Sticher, M., Abramovits, W., & Newcomer, V. V.: Trichotillomania in adults. *Cutis*, 26(1):90, 97–101, 1980.
Stone, J. L., McDaniel, K. D., Hughes, J. R., et al.: Episodic dyscontrol disorder and paroxysmal EEG abnormalities: Successful treatment with carbamazepine. *Biological Psychiatry*, 21(2):208–212, 1986.

Stone, M. H.: Schizotypal personality: Psychotherapeutic aspects. *Schizophrenia Bulletin*, 11(4):576–589, 1985a.
Stone, M. H.: Analytically oriented psychotherapy in schizotypal and borderline patients: At the border of treatability. *Yale Journal of Biological Medicine*, 58(3):275–288, 1985b.
Stone, M. H.: Borderline personality disorder. In R. Michels, J. O. Cavenar, Jr., et al. (Eds.), *Psychiatry, Volume I*. Philadelphia: J. B. Lippincott, 1986.
Stone, M. H.: Psychotherapy of borderline patients in light of long-term follow-up. *Bulletin of the Menninger Clinic*, 51(3):231–347, 1987.
Storms, L. H., Clopton, J. M., & Wright, C.: Effects of gluten on schizophrenics. *Archives of General Psychiatry*, 39(3):323–327, 1982.
Strain, J. J.: Diagnostic considerations in the medical setting. *Psychiatric Clinics of North America*, 4(2):287–300, 1981.
Strider, F. D., & Menolascino, F. J.: Treatment of antisocial syndromes in the mentally retarded. In W. H. Reid (Ed.), *The Treatment of Antisocial Syndromes*. New York: Van Nostrand Reinhold, 1981.
Stringer, A. Y., & Josef, N. C.: Methylphenidate in the treatment of aggression in two patients with antisocial personality disorder. *American Journal of Psychiatry*, 140(10):1365–1366, 1983.
Stromgren, L. S., & Boller, S.: Carbamazepine in treatment and prophylaxis of manic-depressive disorder. *Psychiat. Dev.*, 3(4):349–367, 1985.
Stürup, G. K., & Reid, W. H.: Herstedvester: An historical overview of institutional treatment. In W. H. Reid (Ed.), *The Treatment of Antisocial Syndromes*. New York: Van Nostrand Reinhold, 1981.
Szapocznik, J., Kurtines, W. M., Santisteban, D., et al.: Ethnic and cultural variations in the care of the aged. New directions in the treatment of depression in the elderly: A life enhancement counseling approach. *Journal of Geriatric Psychiatry*, 15(2):257–281, 1982.
Szasz, G., Paty, D., & Maurice, W. L.: Sexual dysfunctions in multiple sclerosis. *Annals of the New York Academy of Sciences*, 436:443–452, 1984.
Szymanski, H. V., Simon, J. C., & Gutterman, N.: Recovery from schizophrenic psychosis. *American Journal of Psychiatry*, 140(3):335–338, 1983.
Taber, J. I., McCormick, R. A., Russo, A. M., et al.: Follow-up of pathological gamblers after treatment. *American Journal of Psychiatry*, 144(6):757–761, 1987.
Takeda, M., Tanino, S., Nishinuma, K., et al.: A case of hypophyseal prolactinoma with treatable delusions of dermatozoiasis. *Acta Psychiatrica Scandinavica*, 72(5):470–475, 1985.
Talbott, J. A.: Chronic mental illness. *Audio Digest Psychiatry*, 11(2), January 1982.
Talley, J.: Geriatric depression: Avoiding the pitfalls of primary care. *Geriatrics*, 42(4):53–60, 65–66, 1987.
Tanney, B.: Electroconvulsive therapy and suicide. *Suicide and Life-Threatening Behavior*, 16(2):116–140, 1986.
Tarachow, S.: *An Introduction to Psychotherapy*. New York: International Universities Press, 1963.
Tarrier, N., & Main, C. J.: Applied relaxation training for generalised anxiety and panic attacks: The efficacy of a learnt coping strategy on subjective reports. *British Journal of Psychiatry*, 149:330–336, 1986.
Taylor, P., & Fleminger, J. J.: ECT for schizophrenia. *Lancet*, i: 1380, 1980.
Taylor, R. E.: Imagery for the treatment of obsessional behavior: A case study. *American Journal of Clinical Hypnosis*, 27(3):175–179, 1985.
Tearnan, B. H., Goetsch, V., & Adams, H. E.: Modification of disease phobia using a multi-faceted exposure program. *Journal of Behavior Therapy and Experimental Psychiatry*, 16(1):57–61, 1985.
Tesar, G. E., & Rosenbaum, J. F.: Successful use of clonazepam in patients with treatment-resistant panic disorder. *Journal of Nervous and Mental Disease*, 174(8):477–482, 1986.

Theorell, T.: Life events and manifestations of ischemic heart disease: Epidemiological and psychophysiological aspects. *Psychotherapy and Psychosomatics,* 34:135–148, 1980.

Thigpen, C. H., & Cleckley, H. M.: *The Three Faces of Eve.* New York: McGraw-Hill, 1957.

Thompson, C. J., & Baylis, P. H.: Asymptomatic Graves' disease during lithium therapy. *Postgraduate Medical Journal,* 62(726):295–296, 1986.

Thyer, B. A.: Audio-taped exposure therapy in the case of obsessional neurosis. *Journal of Behavioral Therapy and Experimental Psychiatry,* 16(3):271–273, 1985.

Tollefson, G.: Alprazolam in the treatment of obsessive symptoms. *Journal of Clinical Psychopharmacology,* 5(1):39–42, 1985.

Tolpin, T. H.: A change in the self: The development and transformation of an idealizing transference. *International Journal of Psychoanalysis,* 64(part 4):461–483, 1983.

Trabert, W., von Blohm, G., & Gawlitza, M.: Schwere Hypermatrianie Imrahmeneiner Katatomen Schizophrenie. *Fortschr. Neurol. Psychiatr.,* 54(6):196–198, 1986.

Tune, L. E., Creese, I., DePaulo, J. R., et al.: Clinical state and serum neuroleptic levels measured by radioreceptor assay in schizophrenia. *American Journal of Psychiatry,* 137: 187, 1980.

Tupin, J. P., Smith, D. B., Clannon, T. L., et al.: The long-term use of lithium in aggressive prisoners. *Comprehensive Psychiatry,* 13:209–214, 1972.

Vaamonde, C. A., Millian, N. E., Magrinat, G. S., et al.: Longitudinal evaluation of glomerular filtration rate during long-term lithium therapy. *American Journal of Kidney Diseases,* 7(3):213–216, 1986.

Van den Hoed, T., Kraemer, H., Guilleminault, C., et al.: Disorders of excessive daytime somnolence: Polygraphic and clinical data for 100 patients. *Sleep,* 4:23–37, 1981.

van Ree, J. M., Verhoeven, W. M., Claas, F. H., et al.: Antipsychotic action of gamma-type endorphins: Animal and human studies. *Progress in Brain Research,* 65: 221–235, 1986.

Varner, R. V., & Gaitz, C. M.: Schizophrenic and paranoid disorders in the aged. *Psychiatric Clinics of North America,* 5(1):107–118, 1982.

Vasile, R. G., Samson, J. A., Bemporad, J., et al.: A biopsychosocial approach to treating patients with affective disorders. *American Journal of Psychiatry,* 144(3):341–344, 1987.

Vestergaard, P., & Schou, M.: The effect of age on lithium dosage requirements. *Pharmacopsychiatry,* 17(6)199–201, 1984.

Vidalis, A. A., & Baker, G. H.: Factors influencing effectiveness of day hospital treatment. *International Journal of Social Psychiatry* (England), 32(3):3–8, 1986.

Videka-Sherman, L., & Lieberman, M.: The effects of self-help and psychotherapy intervention on child loss: The limits of recovery. *American Journal of Orthopsychiatry,* 55(1):70–82, 1985.

Viner, J.: Milieu concepts for short-term hospital treatment of borderline patients. *Psychiatric Quarterly,* 57(2):127–133, 1986.

Virkkunen, M.: Reactive hypoglycemic tendency among arsonists. *Acta Psychiatrica Scandinavica,* 69(5):445–452, 1984.

Vital-Herne, J., Gerbino, L., Kay, S. R., et al.: Mesoridazine and thioridazine: Clinical effects and blood levels in refractory schizophrenics. *Journal of Clinical Psychiatry,* 47(7):375–379, 1986.

Vlissides, D. N., Venulet, A., & Jenner, F. A.: A double-blind gluten-free/gluten-load controls trial in a secure ward population. *British Journal of Psychiatry,* 148:447–452, 1986.

Volavka, J., & Cooper, T. V.: Review of haloperidol blood level and clinical response: Looking through the window. *Journal of Clinical Psychopharmacology,* 7(1):25–30, 1987.

Volavka, J., Meziroglu, F., & Yaryura-Tobias, J. A.: Clomipramine and imipramine in obsessive-compulsive disorder. *Psychiatry Research*, 14(1):85–93, 1985.
Waldinger, R. J.: Intensive psychodynamic therapy with borderline patients: An overview. *American Journal of Psychiatry*, 144(3):267–274, 1987.
Waldinger, R. J., & Gunderson, J. G.: Completed psychotherapies with borderline patients. *American Journal of Psychotherapy*, 38(2):190–202, 1984.
Warnes, H.: The termination phase of psychoanalysis in a narcissistic personality. *International Journal of Psychoanalysis and Psychotherapy*, 10: 159–171, 1984.
Watkins, J. G., & Watkins, H. H.: Hazards to the therapist in treatment of multiple personalities. *Psychiatric Clinics of North America*, 7(1):111–119, 1984.
Watson, C. G., & Buranen, C.: The frequency and identification of false positive conversion reactions. *Journal of Nervous and Mental Disease*, 167:234, 1979.
Watters, W. W.: Supra-biological factors in the assessment of males seeking penile prostheses. *Canadian Journal of Psychiatry*, 31(1):25–31, 1986.
Watts, C. A.: A long-term follow-up of schizophrenic patients: 1946–1983. *Journal of Clinicial Psychiatry*, 46(6):210–216, 1985.
Waynik, M.: Paranoia as a cultural phenomenon: Treatment of an Indian physician. *American Journal of Psychotherapy*, 39(4):587–592, 1985.
Weeke, A., & Vaeth, M.: Excess mortality of bipolar and unipolar manic-depressive patients. *Journal of Affective Disorders* (Netherlands), 11(3):227–234, 1986.
Wehr, T. A., Rosenthal, N. E., Sack, D. A., et al.: Antidepressant effects of sleep deprivation in bright and dim light. *Acta Psychiatrica Scandinavica*, 72(2):161–165, 1985.
Weiner, R. D.: ECT and the physically ill. *Journal of Psychiatric Treatment and Evaluation*, 5:457–462, 1983.
Weiner, R. D., Rogers, H. J., Davidson, J., et al.: Evaluation of the central nervous system risks of ECT. *Psychopharmacology Bulletin*, 18:29–31, 1982.
Weisman, G. K.: Crisis-oriented residential treatment as an alternative to hospitalization. *Hospital and Community Psychiatry*, 36(12):1302–1305, 1985.
Weitzman, E. D., Czeisler, C. A., Coleman, R. M., et al.: Delayed sleep-phase syndrome: A chronobiological disorder associated with sleep-onset insomnia. *Archives of General Psychiatry*, 38:737–746, 1981.
Weizsacker, M., Woller, W., & Tegeler, J.: Lithium in der behandlung periodisch auftretender katatoner erregungszustande bel schizophrenen. *Nervenarzt*, 55(7):382–384, 1984.
White, K., Razani, J., Cadow, B., et al.: Tranylcypromine vs nortriptyline vs placebo in depressed outpatients: A controlled trial. *Psychopharmacology* (Berlin), 82(3):258–262, 1984.
Wik, G., Wiesel, F. A., Eneroth, P., et al.: Dexamethasone suppression test in schizophrenic patients before and during neuroleptic treatment. *Acta Psychiatrica Scandanavica*, 74(2):161–167, 1986.
Williams, W.: Anesthetic ejaculation. *Journal of Sex & Marital Therapy*, 11(1):19–29 (Spring), 1985.
Williams, R. L., Karacan, I., & Hursch, C. J.: *Electroencephalography (EEG) of Human Sleep: Clinical Applications*. New York: John Wiley & Sons, 1974.
Willner, A., & Radiner, C. J.: Reluctance to readmit psychiatric patients. *Hillside Journal of Clinical Psychiatry*, 5(2):203–209, 1983.
Wilson, P. H., Goldin, J. C., & Charbonneau-Powis, M.: Comparative effects on behavioral and cognitive treatments of depression. *Cognitive Therapy Research*, 7:111, 1983.
Wincze, J. T., Bansai, S., & Malamud, M.: Effects of medroxyprogesterone acetate on subjective arousal, arousal through erotic stimulation, and nocturnal penile tumescence in male sex offenders. *Archives of Sexual Behavior*, 15(4):293–305, 1986.
Wise, T. N.: Psychotherapy of an aging transvestite. *Journal of Sex and Marital Therapy*, 5(4):368–373, 1979.

Wise, T. N.: Fetishism—Etiology and treatment: A review from multiple perspectives. *Comprehensive Psychiatry*, 26(3):249–257, 1985.

Wistedt, B.: A comparative trial of haloperidol deconoate and fluphenazine decanoate in chronic schizophrenic patients. *International Clinical Psychopharmacology*, 1(Supplement 1):1523, 1986.

Wolff, R.: Satiation in the treatment of inappropriate firesetting. *Journal of Behavioral Therapy and Experimental Psychiatry*, 15(4):337–340, 1984.

Wolpe, J.: Behavior therapy for psychosomatic disorders. *Psychosomatics*, 21(5):379–385, 1980.

Wolpe, J.: Carbon dioxide inhalation treatments of neurotic anxiety: An overview. *Journal of Nervous and Mental Disease*, 175(3):129–133, 1987.

Woods, S. W., Tesar, G. E., Murray, G. B., et al.: Psychostimulant treatment of depressive disorders secondary to medical illness. *Journal of Clinical Psychiatry*, 47(1):12–15, 1986.

Woody, G. E., McLellan, A. T., Luborsky, L., et al.: Sociopathy and psychotherapy outcome. *Archives of General Psychiatry*, 42(11):1081–1086, 1985.

Woollcott, T., Jr.: Prognostic indicators in the psychotherapy of borderline patients. *American Journal of Psychotherapy*, 39(1):17–29, 1985.

Wyler, A. R., Wilkins, R. J., & Trupin, A. S.: Methysergide in the treatment of narcolepsy. *Archives of Neurology*, 32:265–268, 1975.

Young, W. C.: Restraints in the treatment of a patient with multiple personality. *American Journal of Psychotherapy*, 40(4):601–606, 1986.

Zetin, M., Garber, D., DeAntonio, M., et al.: Prediction of lithium dose: A mathematical alternative to the test dose method. *Journal of Clinical Psychiatry*, 47(4):175–178, 1986.

Zisook, S., Braff, D. L., & Click, M. A.: Monoamine oxidase inhibitors in the treatment of atypical depression. *Journal of Clinical Psychopharmacology*, 5(3):131–137, 1985.

Zoccolillo, M. S., & Cloninger, C. R.: Excess medical care of women with somatization disorder. *Southern Medical Journal*, 79(5):532–535, 1986.

Zucker, D. K., Livingston, R. L., Makra, R., et al.: B-12 deficiency and psychiatric disorders: Case report and literature review. *Biological Psychiatry*, 16(2):197–205, 1981.

Zung, W. W.: Effect of chlorazepate on depressed mood in anxious patients. *Journal of Clinical Psychiatry*, 48(1):13–14, 1987.

Appendix A

DRUG-DRUG INTERACTIONS*
(**Boldface** indicates known clinically significant interaction)

NEUROLEPTICS interacting with

Anticholinergics	**Increase anticholinergia**
	Delay neuroleptic effect
	? Alter neuroleptic level
	? Increase risk of hyperthermia
Antacids, cholestyramine activated charcoal, kaolin, pectin	Delay oral absorption of neuroleptic
Lithium	? **Increase CNS toxicity**
	? Decrease neuroleptic level
Phenytoin	? Increase phenytoin toxicity
	Decrease neuroleptic level
Narcotics	**Increase sedation**
	Augment analgesia
	Augment hypotension
	Increase respiratory depression
	Augment anticholinergia
Benzodiazepines	**Increase sedation**
	Decrease akathisia
Cyclic antidepressants	**Increase sedation**
	Increase hypotension
	Increase anticholinergia
	? Increase neuroleptic effect
	? Increase seizure risk

*Adapted with permission from Tables 1–6 Glassman, R., & Salzman, C.: *Hospital and Community Psychiatry*, 38(3):236–242, 1987.

L-dopa	**May exacerbate psychosis** **Decreased antiparkinson effect**
Amphetamines	**Possibly psychotogenic**
Caffeine	Decrease sedation ? Delay neuroleptic effect
Hypnotics, barbiturates	**Increase sedation** **Decrease neuroleptic effect**
Insulin, other hypoglycemics	Neuroleptic increase blood glucose
Iproniazid	**Hepatotoxicity, encephalopathy** **Decrease neuroleptic effect**
Reserpine, clonidine, guanethidine, bethanidine, debrisoquine	Decrease antihypertensive effect
Ammonium chloride	Decrease neuroleptic effect
Phenylpropanolamine	Ventricular arrhythmias with thioridazine May increase sedation
Propranolol	Increase neurotoxicity Increase neuroleptic effect Seizure/cardiopulmonary arrest (one case report)
Dichloralphenazone, rifampin, dioxyline, griseofulvin, phenylbutazone, carbamazepine	May decrease neuroleptic effect
Chloramphenicol, disulfiram, MAO inhibitors, oral contraceptives, acetaminophen	May increase neuroleptic effect
Epinephrine	**Augment hypotension**
Coumarin, phenindione	May increase bleeding (*but* haloperidol may decrease bleeding)
Methyldopa	Dementia with haloperidol Increase sexual desire with chlorpromazine
Hydralazine, minoxidil	Increase hypotensive effect
Succinylcholine	May prolong ECT apnea
Enflurane, Isoflurane, anesthetics	**Profound hypotension with phenothiazines**
Indomethacin	? Severe sedation with haloperidol
Bromocriptine	Neuroleptics antagonize bromocriptine effects

* *

CYCLIC ANTIDEPRESSANTS *interacting with*

Cimetidine, methylphenidate, acetaminophen, isoniazid, oral contraceptives, MAO inhibitors, chloramphenicol	**Increase antidepressant level & toxicity**

Disulfiram	Increase antidepressant level Possible psychosis, confusion
Guanethidine, debrisoquine, bethanidine	**Decrease antihypertensive effect** Decrease antidepressant effect
Clonidine	Decrease antihypertensive effect Decrease antidepressant effect ? Hypertensive crisis (case report with imipramine)
Thiazide diuretics, acetazolamide	Increased hypotension
Quinidine, procainamide	**Prolong cardiac conduction**
Methyldopa	Increase agitation, tremor, tachycardia
Propranolol	Decrease antidepressant effect
Coumarin anticoagulants	**Increase bleeding**
Neuroleptics	? Increase neuroleptic level
Phenytoin, barbiturates, other hypnotics, rifampin, dichloralphenazone, doxycycline, griseofulvin, carbamazepine, phenylbutazone	**Decrease antidepressant effect**
Anticholinergic drugs	Increase anticholinergia
Lithium, triiodothyronine (T3, liothyronine)	May increase antidepressant effect
Activated charcoal, kaolin	Decrease antidepressant absorption (e.g., in TCA overdose)
Estrogen	? Decrease imipramine effect Lethargy, headache, hypotension Akathisia
Testosterone	Paranoid psychosis, aggression
Halothane, enflurane, anesthetics	Tachycardia with imipramine
Phenytoin, phenylbutazone, aspirin, aminopyrine, scopolamine	Increase antidepressant effect
Epinephrine-containing drugs	**Increase hypotension** **Increase nasal surgery bleeding**
Benzodiazepines	**Increase sedation, confusion** **Decrease motor function** Increase suicide risk
Phenothiazines	Increase tricyclic levels Possible ventricular arrhythmia with thioridazine combinations
L-dopa	Possibly increase rigidity, tremor, agitation Decrease antidepressant level
Alcohol	Increase sedation

MAO INHIBITORS interacting with

Amphetamines, ephedrine, metaraminol, levarterenol methylphenidate, L-dopa, phenylephrine, dopamine, pseudoephedrine, epinephrine-containing drugs/anesthetics, mephentermine, chlorpheniramine	...**Increase blood pressure, possible hypertensive crisis**
Cyclic antidepressants	...**Possible toxicity, hyperpyrexia, rigidity, seizures, coma if improperly used** Increase antidepressant effect Weight gain
Meperidine	...**Excitation, sweating, hypotension (possibly severe)**
Succinylcholine	...Phenelzine may prolong ECT apnea
General anesthetics, sedative-hypnotics, anticholinergics, antihistamines, benzodiazepines	...Increase CNS depression
Insulin, sulfonylurea, phenformin	...Increase hypotension
Thiazide diuretics, reserpine, hydralazine, phenothiazines	...Increase hypotension
Guanethidine	...Decreases antihypotensive effect
Methyldopa	...Excitation, possible visual hallucinations with pargyline
Alcohol	...Decreases MAO inhibition CNS depression

* *

LITHIUM interacting with

Indomethacin, piroxicam, sulindac, ibuprofen, phenylbutazone, naproxen, zomepirac, thiazide diuretics, spironolactone, triamterene, amiloride, tetracycline, spectinomycin	...**Increase lithium effect & toxicity**
Neuroleptics	...**Decrease neuroleptic levels** **Decrease lithium nausea** Possibly increase neurotoxicity
Phenytoin	...Possibly increase neurotoxicity of both drugs
Theophylline, acetazolamide, aminophylline	...**Decrease lithium effect**

Succinylcholine, pancuronium, ...**Prolong ECT apnea**
decamethonium
Amphetamines.....................May increase amphetamine effect
Benzodiazepines ....Hypothermia with diazepam
(case report)
Potassium iodide..................May precipitate hypothyroidism
NaCl, Sodium bicarbonate, ...**Decrease lithium effect**
urea, mannitol
Carbamazepine ....Increase neurotoxicity of both
lithium and carbamazepine
Increase polyuria, ataxia
Cyclic antidepressants ....May increase lithium
neurotoxicity & tremor
Ketamine ....**Increases lithium toxicity**
Digitalis ....Possible cardiac arrhythmias
Furosemide ....**Increase lithium toxicity**
Insulin ....Lithium alters glucose tolerance
Mazindol ....**Increase lithium toxicity**
Norepinephrine ....Decrease pressor response

BENZODIAZEPINE interacting with

Cimetidine, isoniazid, ...Increases benzodiazepine toxicity
disulfiram, oral contraceptives
Phenytoin, rifampin ....Decrease benzodiazepine effect
Antacids, anticholinergics............Delay benzodiazepine absorption
Digoxin..........................Increases digoxin level
Alcohol, sedative-hypnotics, ...**Increases sedation/CNS depression**
neuroleptics, narcotics,
antihistamines
Cyclic antidepressants ....Increases sedation/CNS depression
Increases tricyclic level
L-dopa ....May decrease L-dopa effect

* *

CARBAMAZEPINE interacting with

Lithium..........................**May increase ataxia, dizziness,
feelings of unreality**
Neurotoxicity even with normal
levels of both
Inhibits polyuria & diuresis
associated with lithium
Haloperidol ....May decrease levels of both
Cimetidine, erythromycin, ...**May produce somnolence, nausea,
isoniazid lethargy, nystagmus, dizziness**
Increases carbamazepine level
Propoxyphene ....**Increases carbamazepine level**
Possible headache, nausea, ataxia,
dizziness

Clonazepam	Decreases clonazepam level
Activated charcoal	Binds carbamazepine in gut (e.g., treatment of overdose)
Phenytoin	Decreases carbamazepine level
Phenobarbital, primidone	Decreases carbamazepine level
Corticosteroids, coumarin anticoagulants, doxycycline, oral contraceptives	Decreases carbamazepine effect
Verapamil	Increases carbamazepine toxicity (especially neurotoxicity)

Appendix B

GENERIC AND TRADE NAMES OF MEDICATIONS
("In" means that the generic product is part of a brand-name combination. Suffixes [e.g., HCL, maleate, decanoate] have been omitted.)

GENERIC NAME	TRADE NAME®

Neuroleptics
Acetophenazine	Tindal
Chlorpromazine	Thorazine
Chlorprothixene	Taractan
Fluphenazine	Prolixin, Permitil
Haloperidol	Haldol
Loxapine	Loxitane
Mesoridazine	Serentil
Molindone	Moban
Perphenazine	Trilafon; in Triavil, Etrafon, others
Pimozide	Orap
Piperacetazine	Quide
Promazine	Sparine
Thioridazine	Mellaril, others
Trifluoperazine	Stelazine, others
Triflupromazine	Vesprin

Antidepressants
Amitriptyline	Elavil, Endep, others; in Triavil, Etrafon, Limbitrol, others
Amoxapine	Asendin
Buproprion	Wellbutryn
Clomipramine	Anafranil
Desipramine	Norpramin, Pertofrane
Doxepin	Adapin, Sinequan

Fluoxetine	Prozac
Imipramine	Tofranil, SK-Pramine, Janimine, others
Isocarboxazid	Marplan
Maprotiline	Ludiomil
Mianserin	Bolvidon
Nomafensine	Merital
Nortriptyline	Pamelor
Pargyline	Eutonyl
Phenelzine	Nardil
Protriptyline	Vivactil
Tranylcypromine	Parnate
Trazodone	Desyrel
Trimipramine	Surmontil

Anxiolytics

Alprazolam	Xanax
Chlordiazepoxide	Librium, SK-Lygen, others; in Limbitrol, Menrium, Librax
Clorazepate	Tranxene
Diazepam	Valium, T-Quil, others
Halazepam	Paxipam
Hydroxyzine	Atarax, Vistaril, Durrax, Neucalm, others
Lorazepam	Ativan, others
Meprobamate	Miltown, Equanil, SK-Bamate, others; in Deprol, Equagesic, Pathibamate, PMB
Oxazepam	Serax, others
Prazepam	Centrax

Other

Lithium	Eskalith, Lithane, Lithobid, Cibalith-S, others
Amantadine	Symmetrel
Benztropine	Cogentin, others
Biperiden	Akineton
Diphenhydramine	Benadryl, Allerdryl, others
Procyclidine	Kemadrin
Trihexyphenidyl	Artane, others
Chloral Hydrate	Chloral Hydrate
Flurazepam	Dalmane, others
Glutethimide	Doriden, other
Secobarbital	Seconal, others; in Tuinal
Temazepam	Restoril, others
Triazolam	Halcion
Carbamazepine	Tegretol
Clonazepam	Klonopin

Phenobarbital	Luminal, others
Phenytoin	Dilantin, others
Primidone	Mysoline, others
Valproic acid	Depakene
Benzphetamine	Didrex
Dextroamphetamine	Dexedrine
Methamphetamine	Desoxyn
Methylphenidate	Ritalin
Pemoline	Cylert
Amobarital	Amytal, in Tuinal
Atenolol	Tenormin
Bromocriptine	Parlodel
Cyproterone	Androcur
Dantrolene	Dantrium
Dexamethasone	Decadron, Hexadrol, others
Disulfiram	Antabuse, others
L-tryptophan	Trofan, Tryptacin, others; in Tryptoplex
Medroxyprogesterone IM	Depo-Provera
Methadone	Dolophine, others
Methohexital	Brevital
Naltrexone	Trexan
Physostigmine	Antilirium
Propranolol	Inderal, others
Succinylcholine	Anectine, others
Thiamine	Various
Triiodothyronine, Liothyronine, T_3	Cytomel, in Thyrolar
Verapamil	Calan, Isoptin, others

Name Index

Abbrecht, P. H., 306
Abel, G. G., 275, 280
Abou-Saleh, M. T., 212
Abrahms, J. L., 140
Abramovits, W., 319
Abrams, R., 107
Ackerman, D. L., 183, 208
Adams, H. E., 261
Adams, R. D., 73, 74, 89–90, 114
Adelman, S. A., 345
Adler, G., 343, 347
Afchoff, J., 307
Aguglia, D., 190
Ahmed, I., 272, 309
Akiskal, H. S., 197
Alderdice, M. T., 257
Alexander, B., 87
Alexander, D. D., 246
Alexander, F., 330
Alexander, P. E., 246
Allen, C. B., 168, 175
Allen, R. E., 98, 126
Allen, R. M., 106
Allen, R. P., 306
Allen, S., 211
Allsopp, L. F., 251
Althof, S. E., 34
Alvarez, E., 252
Alvarez, W. A., 183

Amdurski, S., 75
Ames, D., 218
Amrung, S. A., 23
Ananth, J., 252
Anch, M., 301
Anderson, C. M., 186
Anderson, E., 84
Anderson, G., 75
Anderson, J. W., 102
Anderson, W., 142
Andreasen, B., 178
Andrews, E., 261
Aniline, O., 98, 126
Anker, A. L., 143
Ansseau, M., 257
Appel, G., 333
Arana, G. W., 197
Arato, M., 218
Arieti, S., 194
Arky, R. A., 115
Armstrong, M. S., 318
Ascher, L. M., 250
Astrup, C., 198
Atsmon, A., 96
Ausabel, D. P., 138–139
Avery, D. H., 256
Ayde, F. J., 64

Babiker, I. E., 188
Baizerman, M., 319
Baker, G. H., 186, 193

Baldessarini, R. J., 128–129, 197
Balis, G. U., 60, 68, 93, 99–100, 102, 108, 110, 126, 142
Ban, T. A., 79, 85–86, 238
Bancroft, J., 286, 288
Bansai, S., 279
Barnes, R., 85
Barry, M. J., 107
Bastani, J. B., 276
Batchelor, D. H., 211
Battegay, R., 279, 347
Baul, G., 319
Baum, N., 290
Bayer, A. J., 299
Bayer, E. M., 299
Baylis, P. H., 207
Bayne, J. R. D., 72
Beach, R. C., 279
Bear, D., 99
Beck, A. T., 240–241
Beck, L., 21
Becker, J. V., 275, 280
Behemns, M. M., 96
Bellard, J., 261
Bemporad, J., 240
Benedek, E. T., 337
Benson, D. F., 76, 83, 89, 91

393

Benson, D. M., 185
Benvenuto, J. A., 121, 124
Beresin, E., 339
Berg, P., 289
Berger, P. A., 93–95, 98, 120, 124–125, 128, 138, 142
Bergman, B., 286
Berkovic, S. F., 75
Berlant, J., 106, 190
Berlin, F. S., 279
Berman, E., 210
Berney, S., 85, 176
Bertrand, S., 100, 102, 143
Bespalec, D. A., 144
Bianchi, G., 144
Biehl, H., 193
Bigger, J. T., 79
Bill, W., 140
Billiard, M., 304
Bisette, G., 9
Bixler, E. O., 301, 302
Black, F. W., 100, 102
Black, J. L., 87, 107
Blackwell, B., 223, 231
Blaine, J. D., 138
Blanchard, R., 277
Blaszczynski, A., 318
Bleeker, E. R., 305
Bliss, E. L., 267
Blitt, C. D., 70
Bliwise, N. G., 307
Bloodworth, R., 106
Blouin, P., 178, 231
Blue, F. R., 271
Blum, I., 96
Blumenthal, M. D., 81
Blumer, D., 99, 111
Bocchetta, A., 172
Boettger, M. L., 75
Boghen, D., 304
Bokan, J. A., 262
Boland, J. C., 289–291, 293
Boller, S., 211
Bootzin, R. R., 301
Bouvard, M., 252
Braconnier, M. A., 85–86
Bradford, J. M., 279
Brady, J. P., 136
Braff, D. L., 223
Branbilla, F., 190
Branchy, L. B., 196

Branchy, M. H., 196
Brantley, J. T., 283
Braunstein, G. D., 290
Brautigan, W., 330
Brender, W., 289–291
Brenner, R., 183
Bridge, T. P., 197
Bridges, C. K., 108
Brinder, W., 291
Brix, R. J., 319
Brizer, D. A., 185
Brocker, N., 90
Brodsky, L., 100, 102
Brook, C. G. D., 31
Brott, T., 75
Browman, C. P., 305
Brown, J., 90
Brown, L. S., 287
Brown, M., 90
Brown, P., 239
Brown, W. A., 174, 189
Brownell, L. G., 306
Bruun, R. D., 36
Bucci, L., 190
Buckman, M. T., 219
Buigues, J., 246
Bumpas, E. R., 319
Bunney, W. E., 183
Buranen, C., 262
Burck, H. D., 251
Burest, J. C. M., 96
Burkhardt, T. E., 335
Burrows, G., 218
Butler, R. W., 79
Byck, R., 143

Cade, J. F. J., 115
Cadieux, R., 303
Cadow, B., 223
Cahan, M., 183
Caine, E. D., 76
Calvert, E. J., 229
Cami, J., 119
Campbell, M., 43
Cannon, N. L., 194
Cape, R. D. T., 72
Capponi, R., 226
Caracci, G., 208
Carbaat, P. A. T., 75
Carney, F., 336
Carpenter, W. T., 185, 189, 194
Carr, J., 8–9
Carskadon, M., 302–303
Casas, M., 252

Case, W. G., 257
Casenas, E. R., 100, 102
Casey, B., 180
Casley-Smith, J. R., 190
Cassem, N. H., 75
Catalan, J., 285
Chamberlain, K., 254
Chandler, G. M., 251
Charbonneau-Powis, M., 242
Charney, D. S., 119, 246, 248
Chaudhry, S., 211, 227
Chaudry, D. R., 251
Chen, H. C., 258
Chessick, R. D., 342
Childress, A. R., 136
Chodoff, P., 346
Chouinard, G., 252
Christie, J. E., 84
Chu, C. C., 270
Cierpka, M., 316
Claas, F. H., 172
Clannon, T. L., 315, 337
Clark, B. G., 299
Claustrat, B., 252
Clay, T. H., 20
Cleckley, H., 266, 338
Clement, W. R., 93
Click, M. A., 223
Climo, L. H., 166
Cloninger, C. R., 262
Clopton, J. M., 184
Cobble, J. C., 137
Coccaro, E. F., 233
Cofsky, J., 228
Cohen, I. L., 43
Cohen, L. J., 262
Cohen, M. R., 107
Cohen, R., 283
Cohen, S. I., 331
Cohens, S. A., 307
Cohn, C. K., 107
Cole, J. O., 85–86, 345
Cole, M., 285
Coleman, R. M., 304, 307
Collins, F. J., 312
Collins, G. H., 74, 89–90
Collins, J. P., 251
Collins, S. A., 275–276
Conn, D. K., 107
Cook, B. L., 211
Coons, D. J., 75
Coons, P. M., 267–268
Cooper, D. S., 106

Name Index 395

Cooper, I. S., 179
Cooper, T. V., 174, 189
Coppen, A., 211, 212, 227
Cordingley, G. J., 256
Correau, E. I., 208
Coryell, W., 210, 240
Cotten-Huston, A. L., 291
Cotton, E. G., 186
Cottraux, J. A., 252
Covi, L., 242
Cowdry, R. W., 345
Coyle, P. K., 102
Crayton, J. W., 184
Creese, I., 174
Critchley, M., 304
Croughan, J. L., 283
Crout, J. R., 105
Crowley, T. J., 143
Csanalosi, I., 257
Cullen, J. W., 144
Cullen, M. R., 106–107
Cummings, J. L., 76, 83, 99, 107
Cunningham-Rather, J., 275, 280
Curran, J. P., 174
Cytrynbaum, S., 353
Czechowicz, D., 112–113, 115–116, 120–121, 124–125
Czeisler, C. A., 307

D'Angelo, D. J., 194
Dackis, C. A., 106, 119, 143
Daghestani, A. N., 318
Dalton, R., 319
Damber, J. E., 286
Davidson, D. W., 288
Davidson, J., 232, 237, 319
Davie, J. W., 81
Davies, B., 218
Davies, P., 84
Davies, R. K., 79
Davis, B. M., 84, 168, 175
Davis, J. M., 84, 121, 124–125, 225
Davis, K. L., 168, 175, 264
Dawson, G. W., 299
de la Fuente, J. R., 230
Dean, B. C., 256

DeAntonio, M., 206
DeChillo, N., 186
Deering, R. B., 251
Degan, R. O., 117
Dekker, J., 291
Del Zompo, M., 172
Delahunt, J., 100–101
DeLeon, G., 140
DeLeon-Jones, F. A., 207
DeLuca, R. V., 319
Dement, W. C., 303, 304
den Boer, J. A., 172
DePaulo, J. R., 174, 208
Dermer, S. W., 108, 110–111
DeVaul, R. A., 107
Dhib-Jalbut, S., 75
Diaz-Cabal, R., 106
Dickey, B., 194
Dietzel, M., 217, 239
Dimascio, A., 140
Dische, S., 40
Distad, L. J., 254
Doane, J. A., 186
Dole, V. P., 138
Domingo, D. V., 251
Dominguez, R. A., 299
Donlon, P. J., 164
Doran, A. R., 172
Dose, M., 211
Dossing, M., 178
Douglas, J., 70
Douglas, V., 20
Doumont, A., 257
Dowd, E. T., 250
Drake, R. E., 186, 191, 195
Druley, D. A., 141
Dubovsky, S. L., 64, 66, 71, 211
Dunbar, G. C., 226
Dundee, J. W., 90
Dunner, D. L., 256
Durack, D. T., 74
Duro, T., 252
Dysken, M. W., 225

Eames, P., 109, 111
Earle, J. R., 312
Eaton, M. T., 275
Edelstein, P., 329
Edwards, K. G., 257
Ehrhardt, A. A., 286
Eisendrath, S. J., 70
Eisenman, A. J., 116

el-Bayoumi, M., 287
el-Sherbini, O., 287
Ellinwood, E. H., 120, 125
Elliott, F. A., 108, 314–315
Elliott, F. P., 110
Emanuel, D., 230
Emmett, M., 208
Emrich, H. M., 211
Emrick, C. D., 137
Emshoff, B., 319
Endicott, J., 240
Eng, L. K., 212
Engelaar, H. F. W. J., 85
Epstein, L. J., 138
Ereshefsky, L., 189
Essa, M., 324
Estabrook, W., 79
Evans, B. D., 139
Evans, D. L., 103, 213, 230, 232
Evans, L. E. J., 105, 139
Evans, R. W., 20
Everaerd, W., 291
Extein, I., 106, 218

Fagerstrom, K., 144
Fairburn, C. G., 31
Falcon, S., 254
Falk, W. E., 103, 105
Faraone, S. V., 174, 189
Farebrother, M., 144
Fava, G. A., 219
Fawcett, J., 227
Feibel, J. H., 107
Feldman, A., 341
Fenves, A. Z., 208
Ferguson, J., 84
Fermaglich, J., 75
Ferris, S. H., 85
Fichten, C. S., 289–291
Fieve, R. R., 210
Finkel, M. J., 315
Finlayson, D. C., 71
Finnerty, R., 243
Fisher, C. M., 73
Flagg, W., 302, 305
Flaherty, J. A., 186
Flannery, R. B., 351
Fleming, L., 186
Fleminger, J. J., 167
Fleury, D., 247
Fllewellen, E. H., 74
Flynn, D. D., 84

Fogelson, D. L., 185
Folks, D. G., 312
Fontaine, R., 252, 256
Forrest, C., 139
Forrest, D. V., 107
Forsyth, A. B., 144
Foulks, E. T., 136
Frances, A., 185, 283, 334
Francis, F. J., 86
Frankenthaler, L. M., 224–225
Franklin, J. E., 86
Franks, R. D., 211
Fraser, J. F., 116
Frecska, E., 208
Fredrickson, R. H., 307
Freeman, A. M., 312
Freeman, M. G., 286
Freeman, R., 99
Freinhar, J. P., 183
Freinkel, N., 115
Freund, K., 277, 279
Fricchione, G. L., 75
Fromm, M. G., 341
Frosch, J. P., 344
Fry, R. V., 141
Fundudis, T., 42

Gagne, P., 279
Gaitz, C. M., 86, 197
Galatzer-Levy, R. M., 260
Gansu, C. V., 255
Ganzarain, R., 347
Garb, R., 263
Garber, D., 206
Gardner, B. L., 345
Gardos, G., 180
Gates, C., 186
Gauthier, S., 100, 102, 143
Gawin, F. H., 143
Gawlitza, M., 166
Gehi, M., 329
Gelenberg, A. J., 227
Geller, J., 195
Gelmers, H. J., 104
George, A., 334, 345
Gerard, D. L., 136
Gerbino, L., 190
Gerner, R., 79, 225
Gershon, S., 85, 94
Getto, C. J., 264, 354
Ghadirian, A. M., 100, 102, 207

Giannini, A. J., 211
Giannini, A. M., 143
Giardina, E. V., 79, 144
Gibson, C. J., 227
Gillespie, L., 105
Gillin, J. C., 252
Girard, M., 226
Glaser, G. H., 105
Glassman, A. H., 79, 144
Glazer, W., 140
Glick, I. D., 186
Glover, J. H., 316
Godbout, R., 304
Godwin, C. D., 70
Goekoop, J. G., 75
Goetsch, V., 261
Goggans, F. C., 106
Gold, M. S., 106, 119, 143, 218
Goldberg, H. L., 243
Goldberg, M. A., 304
Goldberg, S. C., 334, 344
Goldfrank, L., 128–129
Goldin, J. C., 242
Goldman, B., 70
Goldman, H. W., 179
Goldstein, A., 119, 138
Goldstein, B. J., 299
Goldstein, M. J., 186
Goodnick, P. J., 210
Goodwin, E. W., 137
Goodwin, F. K., 227
Gordon, C., 339
Gordon, J., 195
Goren, Y., 344
Gottfried, L. A., 312
Gounan, J., 108, 110
Graber, B. G., 284, 291
Gralnick, A., 193
Granacher, R. P., 128–129
Granato, J. E., 75
Granier, F., 226
Graves, W. L., 286
Greben, S. E., 340
Greden, J. F., 127
Green, A. I., 138, 165
Green, R., 33
Greenberg, R. D., 106
Greenblatt, D. J., 93–94, 114, 299
Greenfield, H., 140
Greenhill, L. L., 20
Greenstein, R., 139, 254
Greil, W., 207

Greist, J. H., 183, 208
Grigsby, J. T., 254
Gritz, E. R., 144
Gross, G., 193
Gross, M. D., 5
Gualtieri, C. T., 20
Guilleminault, C., 303–306
Gunderson, J., 345
Gutheil, T. G., 341
Gutnik, B. D., 315
Gutterman, N., 186
Guy, W., 238
Gyorgy, S., 218

Hagenfeldt, K., 304
Haggerty, J. J., 213, 230
Hales, R. H., 107
Hall, R. W., 106
Hall, S. M., 144
Hallett, C., 256
Halpern, R., 106
Hamilton, L. D., 80
Hamilton, S. H., 42
Handelsman, L., 143
Handwerker, J. V., 304
Hanin, I., 228
Hanlon, T. E., 194
Haponik, E. F., 305, 306
Hargreaves, A., 119
Harmatz, G. S., 299
Harmon, R. L., 106
Harrison, W., 232
Harrison, W. M., 286
Harrow, M., 79
Hartman, L. M., 289
Hartman, N., 185
Haskett, R. F., 106
Haslett, N., 319
Hass, W. K., 73, 86
Hauri, P. J., 296, 306
Hawkins, N., 42
Hawton, K., 285
Healey, M., 90
Heiman, J. R., 285, 290–291
Heinrichs, D. W., 189, 194
Heizer, J. R., 63, 70, 128
Heldt, G., 306
Hening, W. A., 304
Heninger, G. R., 246
Henry, J. F., 79
Henschke, P. J., 72
Hermann, W. M., 279

Name Index

Hermans, N. B. M., 85
Hernandez, J. M., 23
Hershey, S. C., 107
Hersov, L., 12, 28
Hesselbrock, R., 75
Heston, L. L., 84
Hill, D., 105
Hillman, F. J., 75
Hiltumen, H., 226
Hirsch, S. R., 172
Hirschfeld, R. M., 212
Hirt, M., 140
Hjalmarson, A. I. M., 144
Hoffman, K., 307
Hoffman, R. S., 87
Hogan, D. R., 291
Hogarty, G. E., 186
Holborn, S. W., 319
Holcomb, W. R., 258
Holi, T. C., 109, 111
Hollister, L. E., 85, 117, 246, 251
Hollon, S. V., 241
Holman, S. L., 344
Holmes, D. S., 241
Hoon, P. W., 289
Hopkin, J. T., 164
Hoppe, S. K., 23
Hormazabal, L., 226
Horne, D. J., 251
Horowitz, M. J., 321, 323
Horwitz, L., 343
Hrdina, P. D., 79
Hsie, M. T., 258
Huber, G., 193
Hucker, S., 277
Hughes, J. R., 314
Huitson, A., 251
Hunt, W. A., 144
Hursch, C. J., 296
Hyler, S. B., 311
Hymowitz, P., 334

Ifabumuyi, O. L., 95
Inoue, K., 193
Insel, T. R., 252
Inturrisi, C. E., 119
Isbell, H., 116
Ishiki, D., 256
Itzchaky, S., 230

Jabbari, B., 306
Jackson, R., 230
Jacobsberg, L. B., 334
Jacobson, A. F., 299

Jaeger, A., 208
Jaffe, J. H., 75, 144
Jamieson, R. C., 107
Jampala, V. C., 107
Jann, M. W., 189
Janowsky, D., 84, 125, 164
Jansson, L., 248
Jarrett, R. B., 242
Jarvik, M. E., 144
Jasinski, D. R., 119
Javaid, J., 184
Jefferson, J. W., 183, 208
Jeffries, J. J., 95
Jelinek, J. M., 255
Jenden, D. J., 172
Jenike, M. A., 80, 106
Jenkins, S. C., 315
Jenner, F. A., 184
Jensen, S. B., 286
Jenson, M. R., 319
Jerremalm, A., 248
Jessee, S., 75
Joffe, R. T., 239
Johansen, K. H., 340
Johns, C. A., 84
Johnson, A. F., 190
Johnson, B., 195
Johnson, C., 263
Johnson, R. E., 119
Johnson, R. W., 144
Johnson, S. B., 183
Johnson, V., 284, 288
Johnston, A. W., 105
Jones, B. P., 257
Jorgensen, P., 185, 197
Josef, N. C., 337
Judson, B. A., 119, 138
Jue, S. G., 299

Kahn, A., 75
Kahn, R. J., 224-225
Kalant, H., 114
Kales, A., 298, 302-303
Kales, J. D., 298, 301
Kane, J. M., 99, 180, 185
Kantor, S. J., 79
Kaplan, C. A., 340
Kaplan, H. S., 287-288, 291
Karacan, I., 296, 301
Karasu, T. D., 263, 330
Karoff, S. N., 74, 75
Kartman, L. L., 238
Kathol, R. G., 100-101

Kato, N., 193
Katon, W. J., 262
Katz, N. W., 144
Katz, R. J., 226
Kaufman, E., 137
Kaufman, K. R., 207
Kavey, N., 304
Kawecki, A., 106
Kay, S. R., 190
Kazi, H. A., 188
Keck, P. E., 104
Keith, S. J., 195
Keller, A. C., 34
Keller, M. B., 212
Keller, M. V., 210
Kellner, R., 85, 259-260, 263, 317-318
Ken, K., 353
Kentsmith, D. K., 275, 276
Kernberg, O. F., 346-347
Keutzer, C., 42
Khantzian, E. J., 117, 141
Khoska, N., 90
Khuri, R., 329
Kiev, A., 349
Kilmann, P. R., 289-291, 293
Kimball, C. T., 331
Kimball, R. O., 353
Kinder, B. N., 288
Kinney, J. L., 226
Kirby, M., 254
Kissin, B., 138
Kitchner, I., 254
Klar, H., 171
Kleber, H. D., 119, 141, 143
Klein, J. M., 140
Kleinman, J., 184
Kleist, K., 74
Klempner, M. S., 105
Klerman, G. L., 103, 140, 212
Klonoff, E. A., 312
Klosiewicz, L., 226
Kluft, R. P., 267
Knobler, H. Y., 230
Kocher, T. R., 119
Koehler, K., 167
Koenigsberg, H. W., 340
Koles, M. R., 319
Kolko, D. J., 319
Kolvin, I., 42
Kopfreschmitt, J., 208

Kovacs, M., 240–241
Kraemer, H., 306
Krahn, D., 106
Kramer, S. I., 106
Krauthammer, C., 103
Kravitz, H. M., 227
Kretsch, R., 344
Krishnan, R. R., 319
Kuch, K., 254
Kuhn, R., 108, 111
Kupfer, D. J., 210, 213, 221
Kurtines, W. M., 238
Kwentus, J. A., 89, 104

Lalinec-Michaud, M., 207
Lamontagne, Y., 275
Lang, P. J., 32
Langdon, N., 303
Langer, S., 263
Langfold, W., 21
Lanza, U., 258
Lapierre, Y. D., 107
Laughren, T. P., 174, 189
Lavori, P. W., 210
Lavori, T., 240
Laws, D. R., 280
Lawy, A. J., 307
Lazara, A., 262
Lazare, A., 142
Lazarus, J. H., 208
Lazarus, L. W., 225
Ledermann, R., 347
Lehman, H. E., 85–86
Leigh, D., 109
Leigh, H. S., 106
Lelliott, P. T., 252
Lennard, H. L., 138
Lenox, R. H., 165, 211
Leon-Andrade, C., 230
Lerer, B., 211
Lesage, A., 275
Lesch, O. M., 217, 239
Lesser, M. S., 183
LeVann, L. J., 43
Levenson, J. L., 74, 75
Levi, A., 75
Levie, C. A., 272, 309
Levin, H. S., 89
Levine, D. J., 144
Levine, J. L., 241, 312
Levine, P. E., 173
Levinson, D., 177, 182
Lewis, D. A., 230

Lewis, D. C., 71, 98, 124, 126, 128
Lewis, J. L., 212
Lewis, V., 90
Lewy, A. J., 239
Lezak, M. D., 89, 109
Libman, E., 289–291
Lichstein, T. R., 263
Lieberman, M., 323
Liebowitz, M. R., 246
Lindberg, F. H., 254
Lindsay, W. R., 255
Ling, M. H. M., 98, 105
Ling, W., 138
Lion, J. R., 336
Lipman, R. S., 242
Lipowski, Z. J., 64–65, 71–72, 91, 95, 99, 106
Lipsey, J. R., 107
Lipton, M. A., 9
Lisansky, J., 219
Liskow, B., 142
Liston, E. H., 72
Littbrand, B., 286
Livingston, R. L., 198
Lock, C. B., 303
Lockshin, M. D., 105
Lohr, J. B., 166
LoPiccolo, J., 285, 290–291
Lothstein, L. M., 34, 35
Louie, A. K., 227
LoVerme, S., 76, 83
Lowe, M. R., 211
Lowinson, J. H., 138
Luborsky, L., 140–141, 338
Lucas, M. J., 81, 85
Luchins, D. J., 173
Ludgate, M., 208
Lue, F. A., 301
Lustman, P. J., 241, 312
Lybiard, R. B., 252

Macaskill, M. D., 344
Macedo, C. A., 23
MacHovec, F. J., 270
MacIndoe, J. H., 87
Mack, J. E., 141
MacKay, M., 21
MacKenzie, T. B., 99
Mackie, M., 188
Magrinat, G. S., 207–208
Mahapatra, D., 225, 230

Mahapatra, R. K., 225, 230
Mahgoub, O. M., 252
Mahnke, M. W., 103, 105
Maier, H. P., 183
Mailland, F., 226
Main, C. J., 258
Mair, R. G., 90
Mairhofer, M. L., 207
Maj, M., 210
Majid, I., 226
Majovski, L. V., 84
Makra, R., 198
Malamud, M., 279
Maletsky, V. M., 237
Malinow, K. L., 349
Maloney, A. J. F., 84
Mamelak, M., 303
Manchanda, R., 172
Mander, A. J., 210
Mann, L. S., 144
Mansky, P. A., 210, 213, 221
Marder, S. R., 185, 189
Marini, J. L., 108
Marks, I. M., 250, 280, 295, 323
Marmar, C., 323
Marmor, J., 284
Marsden, D. C., 91
Marsh, G. M., 84
Marshall, R. W., 75
Martin, B., 226
Martin, B. A., 184, 234, 237
Martin, M. J., 87, 107
Martin, W. R., 303
Marunycz, J. D., 257
Maruta, T., 315
Mash, D. C., 84
Massironi, R., 190
Masters, W., 284, 288
Mastri, A. R., 84
Mathew, R. J., 91
Mattes, J. A., 110, 315
Matthews, W., 353
Maurer, J. I., 93–94
Maurer, K., 193
Maurice, W. L., 287
Mauriello, R., 299
Mavissakalian, M., 249
Mawson, B., 323
May, D. C., 75
May, P. R. A., 172
Mayo, J. A., 212

Name Index 399

McAllister, T. W., 76
McCabe, B., 224
McCann, I. L., 241
McCarron, M. M., 75
McConaghy, N., 318
McCord, J., 22
McCormack, H. M., 251
McCormick, R. A., 317–318
McCreadie, R., 180, 188
McDaniel, K. D., 314
McElroy, S. L., 104
McEntee, 90
McEvoy, J. P., 91, 166
McGahan, J. A.., 141
McGlashan, T. H., 195, 335
McGregor, A. M., 208
McGuire, T. G., 194
McKay, A. C., 90
McKenna, G. J., 117
McKenna, P. J., 99
McLaughlin, E., 255
McLellan, A. T., 139–141, 338
McMahon, T., 105
McNair, D. M., 224–225
McNeal, S. A., 42
McNeilly, A., 286
McNutt, B. A., 5
Meadow, R., 312
Meadows, J. C., 91
Mees, H. L., 42
Mehl, R., 108, 110
Mehr, J. J., 109, 111
Meisch, R., 90
Melamed, B. G., 32
Meliek, M., 128–129
Mellion, M. B., 241
Mello, N., 115
Meltzer, H. Y., 173, 227
Mendelson, J., 115
Mendez, M. F., 107
Menn, S. J., 305
Menolascine, F. J., 353
Mercier, T., 256
Messner, E., 128–129
Meyer, J. S., 91
Meyer, R. E., 138, 140
Meziroglu, F., 252
Michelson, L., 249–250
Micheroli, R., 279
Mienecke, C. F., 279
Mikkelsen, E. J., 40
Miklowitz, D. J., 186

Miller, L. S., 239
Miller, M. B., 166
Miller, M. G., 211
Miller, R., 319
Miller, S. I., 140
Millian, N. E., 207–208
Millman, R. B., 138
Minde, K., 20
Mintz, J., 189
Mirin, S. M., 138, 140
Mitchell, J. D., 231
Mitler, M. M., 305
Modell, J. G., 165, 211
Mogelnicki, S. R., 71
Mohr, J. P., 73
Mohs, R. C., 84
Moldofsky, H., 301, 307
Money, J., 144
Monroe, R. R., 108, 314
Monteiro, W. O., 252
Montplaisir, J., 304
Montzenbecker, R. P., 117
Moore, D. P., 65
Moore, E. J., 312
Morril, R., 108, 110
Morris, R. J., 299
Morris, S. W., 75
Morrison, D., 188
Morrison, R. L., 177
Mosher, L. R., 195
Moss, E., 263
Mostafa, M., 287
Mueller, E. A., 252
Mueller, P. S., 75
Mukherjee, S., 208
Muller, J. T., 335
Muller, Y. L., 271
Munitz, H., 262
Munk-Jorgensen, P., 197
Munson, E., 164
Murphy, E., 238
Murphy, G. E., 241
Murphy, M. F., 264
Murray, G. B., 107, 228
Murray, J. B., 252
Musisi, S., 307
Myall, R. W., 312
Myers, E. D., 229

Naarala, M., 226
Naeser, M. A., 185
Nakajima, T., 193
Nasrallah, H. A., 230
Nathan, R. S., 334, 345

Nayak, D., 183
Naylor, G. J., 226
Neborsky, R., 164
Neidigh, L., 288
Nelson, T. E., 74
Nelson, W. H., 75
Nemeroff, C. B., 9, 103
Nemeth, E., 20
Nemiah, J. C., 270
Nestoros, J. N., 165
Neubauer, H., 94
Newcomer, V. V., 319
Newton, R. E., 257
Nicassio, P. N., 301
Nichols, S. E., 87, 106
Nilln, P., 212
Nino-Murcia, G., 306
Nishinuma, K., 259
Niska, R. W., 107
Nixon, R. A., 105
Nocks, J. J., 255
Nolfe, G., 210
Norton, S. P., 289–291, 293
Noyes, R., 251
Nurcombe, B., 144
Nurnberg, H. G., 173, 341, 347
Nyswander, M., 138

O'Brien, B. P., 141
O'Carroll, R., 286
O'Connell, R. A., 212
O'Donnell, J. A., 138
O'Driscoll, G., 192
O'Malley, J. E., 142
O'Regan, J. B., 302
Oates, J. A., 105
Ochitill, H., 264
Ogata, M., 115
Okada, F., 105
Okeya, V. L., 207
Okimoto, J., 85
Oppenheim, G., 227
Orleans, C. T., 144
Orne, M. T., 269
Osborne, M., 184
Ost, L. G., 248
Ostrow, D. G., 87, 106
Othmer, S. C., 233
Overall, J. E., 86
Oxenburg, G., 108, 110
Oyewumi, L. K., 107

Palmer, R. F., 304

Palmer, T. B., 22
Pare, C. M., 223
Parish, K., 99
Parkes, J. D., 302
Parsons, C. L., 238
Pathy, M. S. J., 299
Patten, B. M., 89
Pattison, E. M., 137
Paty, D., 287
Paul, S. K., 225, 230
Pearce, S., 144
Pearlman, C., 106
Pearlman, M., 77, 79, 81
Pearsal, H., 106
Peck, J. J., 75
Pecknold, J. C., 247
Perel, J. M., 79, 144
Perenyi, A., 208
Perlson, G. D., 107
Perry, J. C., 351
Perry, P. J., 98, 105
Perry, S., 69, 84, 97
Persson, H. E., 304
Pertshuk, M., 136
Pescor, F. T., 116
Peteet, J. R., 341
Peters, B. H., 89
Peterson, P., 108
Petrich, J., 338
Petrie, W. M., 85, 176
Petty, W. C., 70
Phelps, R. E., 42
Phillips, L. R. F., 72
Phillipson, E. A., 307
Pi, E. H., 178
Piccardi, M. P., 172
Pickar, D., 172
Pickard Bartanian, F., 183
Pickens, R., 90
Pitts, F. N., 98, 126
Plakun, E. M., 335
Plutzky, M., 81
Pohl, H., 307
Pollack, M. H., 247-248
Pope, H. G., 75, 104
Popkin, G. D., 99
Poplin, M. K., 231
Poskanzer, D. C., 103, 105
Post, R., 227
Potkin, S. G., 184
Pottash, A. C., 106
Pottash, A. L. C., 119, 218
Potter, L. T., 84

Potter, W. K., 42
Prange, A., 9, 227
Prasad, A., 252
Preskorn, S. H., 70, 233
Preston, B., 319
Price, D. L., 84
Price, T. R., 76, 107
Price, W. A., 211
Prichard, B. N. C., 105
Prien, R. F., 210, 213, 221
Puente, R. M., 108
Puzynski, S., 226

Quinn, P. O., 5
Quitkin, F., 232

Rabiner, C. J., 185
Rabkin, J. G., 286
Rada, R., 85
Radiner, C. J., 337
Radwan, M., 75
Raft, D., 232
Ragheb, M., 207
Rajagopal, K. R., 306
Ramirez, L. F., 318
Ramm, E., 323
Rankin, H., 317
Rapoport, J. L., 5, 40
Raskind, M. A., 81, 85
Rasmussen, S. A., 252
Ratey, J. J., 108, 110, 192
Razani, J., 223
Redmond, D. E., 119
Reich, P., 312
Reid, J. B., 42
Reid, K. M., 42
Reid, W. H., 178, 231, 256, 272, 309, 315, 335-337, 353
Reisberg, B., 84, 85
Reisman, J., 28
Reiss, D. J., 186
Resnick, R. B., 119, 139-140
Reus, V. I., 106
Richardson, G. S., 302
Richardson, M. A., 196
Richelson, E., 167
Rickels, K., 141, 243, 299
Rieder, R., 20
Ries, R. K., 262
Rifkin, A., 246, 315
Rihmer, Z., 218
Ringel, A., 75

Riordan, C. E., 119
Risse, S. C., 81, 85
Ritzler, B. A., 193, 199
Robey, A., 317
Robinson, A. D., 180
Robinson, D. S., 79
Robinson, M. V., 186
Robinson, R. G., 107
Rodriguez-Villa, F., 165
Rogeness, G. A., 23
Rogers, H. J., 237
Rollinson, R. D., 91
Romand, A., 139
Roose, S., 79
Rose, R. M., 106
Roselaar, S. E., 303
Rosen, A. M., 208
Rosen, W., 84
Rosenbaum, A. H., 107
Rosenbaum, J. F., 247-248
Rosenbaum, M. B., 285
Rosenbaum, M. S., 319
Rosenthal, M. S., 138, 338
Rosenthal, N. E., 239
Ross, A., 312
Ross, W. P., 329
Roth, D., 242
Roth, T., 298
Rothstein, E., 137
Rounsaville, B. J., 140-141
Rovei, V., 79
Rowlands, D., 238
Ruedrich, S. L., 270
Rugg, D., 144
Rundall, J. R., 106
Rush, A. J., 239-242
Russell, G. F. M., 31
Russo, A. M., 317-318
Rutter, M., 12, 28
Ryan, C., 254

Sabelli, H. C., 227
Sachs, C., 304
Sack, D. A., 239
Sack, R. L., 239, 307
Sacksteder, J. L., 341
Saenger, G., 136
Saghir, M., 283
Sahpira, B., 227
Saklad, S. R., 189
Sakles, C. J., 60
Saletu, B., 217, 239

Name Index

Salomon, M., 345
Salzman, C., 77–81, 85–86, 165, 184
Salzman, L., 253
Sampson, J. P., 251
Sampson, N., 137
Samson, J. A., 240
San, L., 119
Sands, S., 192
Santisteban, D., 238
Sapir, D. G., 208
Sapira, J. D., 303
Saskin, P., 298, 301
Sauder, P., 208
Sauer, H., 167
Saul, T., 257
Scarlett, J. D., 75
Scarzella, L., 226
Scarzella, R., 226
Scharf, M. D., 90, 301
Schatzberg, A. F., 141
Scher, H., 277
Schermer, M., 178, 231
Schickler, R., 207
Schiff, D., 99
Schlagel, A., 210
Schmid-Burgk, W., 226
Schmidt, K., 188, 190
Schmitt, L., 226
Schneider, N. G., 144
Schneider-Helmert, D., 299–300
Schnitt, J. M., 255
Schottenfeld, R. S., 106–107
Schou, M., 207
Schover, L. R., 287, 290
Schreier, H. A., 108, 110
Schreter, R. K., 263
Schubart, C., 193
Schultz, J. R., 329
Schulz, P. M., 334, 344
Schulz, S. C., 334, 344
Schuyton-Resnick, E. S., 139–140
Schwartz, L. S., 186
Schweizer, E., 257
Sederer, L. I., 191, 195, 342
Seidel, W. F., 307
Sekerke, J., 84, 125
Sellers, E. M., 114
Sells, S. B., 140–142
Selzer, M. L., 136

Senay, E. C., 71, 98, 124, 126, 128
Serban, G., 334, 344
Sergent, J. S., 105
Seymour, D. G., 72
Shader, R. I., 77, 79, 81, 93–94, 114, 138
Shah, J. H., 207
Shalev, A., 262
Shapiro, A. K., 36
Shapiro, E. S., 36
Shapiro, W. R., 303
Sharpless, N. S., 84
Shea, V., 107
Sheard, M. H., 108
Sheline, Y. I., 166
Shenoy, R. S., 263
Shering, A., 84
Shibuya, T. K., 258
Shipley, R. H., 144
Shively, D., 338
Shulkla, S., 211
Shvartsburd, A., 174
Siebel, M. M., 286
Siegel, S., 334, 344
Siever, L. J., 233
Sifneos, P. E., 251, 253, 263
Silver, D., 342–344
Silver, J., 90
Silverman, J. J., 89, 104
Simon, J. C., 186
Simon, J. I., 340
Simons, A. D., 241, 312
Simpson, D. D., 141–142
Simpson, F. O., 105
Simpson, G., 177, 182
Simpson, S., 70
Singer, C. M., 239, 307
Siris, S., 79, 246
Slater, P. C., 236
Sloan, J. W., 303
Sluping, J. R., 91
Small, A. M., 43
Smego, R. A., 74
Smith, D. B., 287, 315, 337
Smith, D. L., 116
Smith, J. M., 180
Smith, P. L., 305, 306
Smith, R. C., 174, 263
Snaith, R. P., 275–276
Snyder, D. K., 289
Snyder, S., 319
Socarides, C. W., 295

Soldatos, C. R., 302–303
Soloff, P. H., 334, 345
Solomon, G. H., 353
Solomon, L., 211
Solursh, L. P., 93
Sommers, A. A., 173
Sorensen, J. L., 119
Spees, R. C., 165
Spencer, J., 258
Spiegel, D., 267
Spielman, A. J., 298
Spiker, B. G., 228
Spinweber, C. L., 300
Sprague, M., 89, 104
Springer, C. J., 107
Squire, L. R., 236
Sramek, J. J., 178
Sranek, J. J., 177
Starace, F., 210
Steele, C., 81, 85
Stending-Lindberg, G., 115
Sterman, A. B., 102
Stern, B. A., 341
Stern, B. J., 75
Stern, M., 53
Sternberg, D. E., 119
Stevens, L., 90
Stevens, M. J., 319
Stever, J., 79
Stewart, J. W., 232
Stewart, R. M., 75
Sticher, M., 319
Stoker, M. J., 299
Stoltzenburg, M. C., 207
Stone, J. L., 314
Stone, M. H., 334, 343, 346
Storey, P. B., 108
Storms, L. H., 184
Stoudemire, A., 87
Strain, J. J., 331
Straughan, J. H., 42
Strawn, S. K., 213, 230
Strider, F. D., 353
Stringer, A. Y., 337
Stromgren, L. S., 211
Strub, R. L., 100, 102
Struble, R. G., 84
Sturup, G. K., 337
Stuss, D. T., 185
Stybel, L. J., 144
Summers, W. K., 84
Sundland, D. M., 94

Suranyl-Cadotte, B. E., 165
Sussman, N., 311
Swade, C., 211, 227
Sweatman, P., 306
Sweeney, D. R., 119
Sweeney, J., 185
Sweet, T. R. D., 36
Swinson, R. P., 254
Swoboda, J. S., 250
Szapocznik, J., 238
Szasz, G., 287
Szuchs, R., 208
Szymanski, H. V., 186

Taber, J. I., 317
Takeda, M., 259
Talbott, J. A., 190
Talley, J., 238
Tanino, S., 259
Tanney, B., 234, 237
Tarachow, S., 350
Targum, S. D., 106
Tarrier, N., 258
Tawlak, A., 279
Taylor, P., 167
Taylor, R. E., 252
Taylor, R. L., 93–94
Tearnan, B. H., 261
Tegeler, J., 166
Tennant, F. S., 142
Tesar, G. E., 228, 247–248
Thal, L. J., 84
Theorell, T., 329
Thigpen, C. H., 266
Thiry, D., 257
Thompson, C. J., 207
Thompson, T. L., 87
Thorbeck, J., 342
Thornby, J., 301
Thorpy, M. J., 298, 301
Thyer, B. A., 252
Tinklenberg, J. R., 85, 93–95, 98, 120, 124–125, 128, 138, 142
Tollefson, G., 252
Tolpin, T. H., 316
Toole, J. F., 91
Torres, S., 119
Trabert, W., 166
Troupin, A. S., 104, 108, 110
Trupin, A. S., 306

Tsuang, M. T., 98, 105, 224
Tucker, G. J., 79
Tune, L., 81, 85, 174
Tunks, E. R., 108, 110–111
Tunstall, C., 144
Tupin, J. P., 108, 164, 315, 337
Turner, P., 144
Turner, R., 100–101
Turpin, G., 37

Ursano, R. J., 106

Vaamonde, C. A., 207–208
Vaeth, M., 210
Vallejo, J., 246
Van den Hoed, T., 306
van Putten, T., 172, 185, 189
van Ree, J. M., 172
Van, T. A., 176
Varner, R. V., 86, 197
Varney, N. R., 87
Vasile, R. G., 240
Veaudry, T., 256
Veith, R., 85
Venulet, A., 184
Verhoeven, W. M., 172
Verlanga, C., 230
Veroulis, G., 174
Vester, J. W., 75
Vestergaard, P., 207
Victor, M., 74, 89–90, 114
Vidalis, A. A., 186, 193
Videka-Sherman, L., 323
Viner, J., 340
Virkkunen, M., 315
Vital-Herne, J., 190
Vlissides, D. N., 184
Vogt, T. M., 144
Volavka, J., 174, 189, 252
von Blohm, G., 166
von Eschenbach, A. C., 287, 290
von Frenckell, R., 257
von Loveren-Huyban, C. M. S., 85
von Zerssen, D., 211

Waal-Manning, H. J., 105
Wadle, C. V., 270

Waldinger, R. J., 343, 345
Waller, J. L., 71
Walter-Ryan, W. G., 261
Walters, A., 304
Warner, T., 288
Warnes, H., 348
Washton, A. M., 119, 139–140
Wasserman, A., 344
Watkins, H. H., 267
Watkins, J. G., 267
Watson, C. G., 262
Watters, W. W., 290
Watts, C. A., 193
Waynik, M., 198
Webster, P., 303
Weeke, A., 210
Wegner, J. T., 185
Wehr, T. A., 239
Weil, A. A., 100, 102
Weinberg, J. A., 119
Weinberger, D., 184
Weiner, R. D., 234, 237
Weiner, S., 165, 211
Weinhold, P., 180
Weisberg, M. P., 64, 66, 71
Weisman, G. K., 341
Weiss, D. S., 323
Weiss, G., 20
Weissman, M. M., 140, 141
Weitzman, E. D., 307
Weizsacker, W., 166
Wells, A. A., 105
Wells, C. E., 76, 107
Wender, P., 20
Werry, J., 20
Wesson, D. R., 116
West, L. J., 144
West, P., 306
Westenberg, H. G., 172
Westermeyer, J., 127, 143–144
Wetzle, R. D., 241
Wheeler, K. A., 291
White, K., 223
White, M. G., 208
White, N. J., 96
Whitehouse, P. J., 84
Whitlock, F. A., 105, 107, 139
Wikler, A., 116
Wilber, C. H., 140

Name Index

Wilbert, D. E., 63, 70, 128
Wilkins, R. J., 306
Willett, E. A., 140
Williams, C., 144
Williams, D., 108, 110
Williams, R. L., 296
Williams, T., 255
Williams, W., 292
Williamson, P., 211
Willner, A., 337
Wilson, P. H., 242
Wilson, W. H., 238
Wincze, J. T., 279
Winokur, G., 212
Wise, M. G., 106
Wise, T. N., 276, 283
Wistedt, B., 188
Wittig, R., 298
Woerner, M., 180
Wolanin, M. O., 72

Wolff, R., 319
Wolkowitz, O. M., 172
Woller, W., 166
Wolowitz, H. M., 194
Wolozin, B. L., 84
Wolpe, J., 258, 331
Wolpert, E. A., 210
Wood, L. L., 106
Wood, R., 109, 111
Woods, S. W., 228
Woody, G. E., 140–141, 338
Woollcott, T., 345
Wright, C., 184
Wright, J. R., 107
Wulff, M. H., 117
Wurmser, L., 137, 141
Wyatt, R. J., 197
Wyler, A. R., 306

Yaryura-Tobias, J. A., 252

Yesavage, J. A., 85
Young, J. E., 241
Young, W. C., 268
Youngner, S. J., 312
Yudofsky, S., 90, 108, 110
Yuke, W., 9

Zavardil, A., 40
Zetin, M., 206
Zimmerman, R., 75
Zinny, M. A., 299
Zisook, S., 223
Zoccolillo, M. S., 262
Zohar, J., 227
Zorick, R., 298
Zubenko, G., 75, 105
Zucker, D. K., 198
Zung, W. W., 256
Zuniga, J. S., 100, 102

Subject Index

Abnormal Involuntary Movement Scale, 181–182
Abstinence-oriented recovery models, 140
Academic inhibition, 326
Academic problems, 352
Academic skills disorders, 14
Acquired Immune Deficiency Syndrome, 141, 287
Adjustment disorders, 321–327
Adolescents, 42–44, *see also* Children
   Antisocial behavior and, 353–354
   Anxiety disorders and, 25–28
   Attention-deficit hyperactivity disorder and, 19
   drug treatment in, 4–6
   firesetting and, 318–319
   Gender identity disorders, 33–35
   Inhalant abuse and, 144
Agitation, 78
Agoraphobia, 246–249
Agranulocytosis, 179
Akathisia, 177
Alcohol, 23. *See also* Substance abuse; Withdrawal and withdrawal deliria
   abuse/dependence, 136–137
   Amnestic disorders and, 89–90
   Deliria and, 68
   Dementia and, 86
   Explosive type personality and, 110
   Intoxication, 123
   Wernicke's syndrome and, 73
Alcohol hallucinosis, 92–93

Alcohol withdrawal delirium, 114–115
Alprazolam, 26, 214–215, 226–227, 234, 334
   Anxiety disorders and, 246–248, 251–252, 256
Alzheimer's disease, 72, 76, 83–86, 105
Amantadine, 75, 143, 176, 179, 183
Amenorrhea, 329
Amineptine, 226
Amitriptyline, 300–301
Amnesia, 67, 237
   psychogenic, 269–270
Amnestic disorders, 76, 88–91
Amoxapine, 224–225, 232
Amphetamines
   abuse/dependence, 143
   Deliria and, 68–69
   Delusional disorders and, 96–97
   Intoxication, 125
   Major depression and, 228
   Organic anxiety disorders and, 101
   Sleep disorders and, 304
   withdrawal, 119–120
Anorexia nervosa, 29–31
Antiandrogenic medication, 275, 277, 279–283
Anticholinergic drugs, intoxication, 128–129
Anticoagulants, 72
Antidepressants, 219–227
   Bipolar disorders and, 213
   Dementia and, 79–80

Factitious disorders and, 312
monoamine oxidase inhibitors, *see*
  Monoamine oxidase inhibitors
Organic mood disorder and, 103, 105, 107
Personality disorders and, 334, 337, 345, 349
Schizoaffective disorder and, 202
side/adverse effects of, 228–234
Sleep disorders and, 302
tetracyclics, 224–225
tricyclic, 215–216, 219–224
  Anxiety disorders and, 246, 251, 254, 257
  side/adverse effects of, 229–231
  Somatoform disorders and, 265
withdrawal and, 120
Antihistamines, 78
Antihypertensive drugs, 105
Antiparkinsonism drugs, Schizophrenia and, 164–165, 176–177, 179
Antipsychotic medication, *see* Neuroleptics
Antisocial behavior
  adult, 352–353
  childhood/adolescent, 353–354
Antisocial personality disorder, 335–339, 353
Anxiety, 43
  Adjustment disorder with, 324
  Dementia and, 78
Anxiety disorders, 25–28, 245–258
  Agoraphobia, 246–249
  Generalized anxiety disorder, 255–258
  Obsessive compulsive disorder, 251–253
  Panic disorder, 246–247
  performance anxiety and, 250
  Post-traumatic stress disorder, 253–255
  Simple phobia, 250–251
  Social phobia, 249–250
Anxiety syndrome, 99–102
Anxiolytics, *see* Benzodiazepines
Arylcyclohexylamine, *see* Phencyclidine
Aspirin, 73, 86
Asthma, 330–331
Atenolol, 257
Atropine, 93
Attention-deficit disorder, undifferentiated, 44
Attention-deficit hyperactivity disorder, 16–22
  Conduct disorders and, 23
  lithium and, 6
  Oppositional defiant disorder and, 24
  Severe mental retardation and, 9

Speech disorders and, 41
Atypical psychosis, 203
Autistic disorder, 12–13
Aversive conditioning, 276, 280, 295, 317, 319
Avoidant disorders, 27
Avoidant personality disorder, 348

Baclofen, 305
Bad tripper, 93–94, 122
Barbiturates, 94, 124, 200, 203
  Bipolar disorder and, 205
  Dissociative disorders and, 270–271
  Schizophrenia and, 165
  withdrawal and, 116, 120
Behavior modification
  Alcohol abuse and, 137
  Anorexia nervosa and, 30
  Anxiety disorders and, 248, 252, 254, 258
  Attention-deficit hyperactivity disorder and, 18–19
  Depression and, 240
  Elective mutism and, 42
  Explosive personality type and, 111
  Factitious disorders and, 311–312
  Impulse control disorders and, 316–319
  Insomnia disorders and, 298
  Mental retardation and, 8–10
  Oppositional defiant disorder and, 24
  Overanxious disorder and, 28
  psychosomatic disorders and, 331
  Rumination disorder and, 32
  Sexual disorders and, 275–276, 280, 282, 287–288, 292–293
  Somatoform disorders and, 261, 263
  Stereotypy/habit disorder and, 44
Behavioral disorders, Mental retardation and, 8
Behavioral toxicity, 5
Benzodiazepines. *See also* Specific drug names
  abuse of, 141–142
  Alcohol abuse and, 137
  Alcohol hallucinosis and, 93
  Alcohol intoxication and, 123
  Alcohol withdrawal and, 114–115
  Amnestic disorders and, 90
  Anorexia nervosa and, 31
  Anxiety disorders and, 251, 255–256
  Avoidant disorder and, 27
  Brief reactive psychosis and, 200
  Deliria and, 64–65, 72
  Dementia and, 78

Benzodiazepines *(continued)*
  Dissociative disorders and, 271
  Explosive type personality and, 110
  Hallucinogen hallucinosis and, 94–95
  Identity disorders and, 43
  Intoxication and, 123–125
  Major depression and, 228, 239
  Organic anxiety syndrome and, 100–101
  Overanxious disorder and, 28
  Schizophrenia and, 164–165, 168, 177, 184
  Sleep disorders and, 298–299, 307–310
  withdrawal and, 116
Benzopyrones, 190
Benztropine, 177
Bereavement, 323, 356
Bethanechol, 228
Biperiden, 177
Bipolar disorders, 204–214
  in children, 6
  Cyclothymia, 213–214
  Depressed, 212–213
  Manic, 204–212
    maintenance treatment, 209–210
  Mixed, 213
Blood dyscrasias, 11
Body dysmorphic disorder, 259–261
Borderline intellectual functioning, 353
Borderline personality disorder, 339–346
Brain tumors, 102
Brief reactive psychosis, 187, 200–201
Bromocriptine, 75, 177, 183
Bulimia nervosa, 31
Buprenorphine, 139
Buproprion, 226, 233
Buspirone, 256–257
Butyrophenone, 172
  Autistic disorder and, 13

Caffeine, 101, 126–127, 300, 302
Cannabis, 93, 95
  abuse/dependence, 142
  Delusional disorders and, 97
  intoxication, 125–126
  Organic personality disorder and, 110
Carbamazepine, 99, 345
  Attention-deficit hyperactivity disorder and, 20
  Bipolar disorders and, 211, 213
  Conduct disorders and, 22
  Impulse control disorders and, 314
  Mental retardation and, 11
  Organic mood disorder and, 103

Organic personality disorder and, 108, 110
Carbon dioxide inhalation, 258
Cataplexy, 302–303
Catatonia, 74, 179
Catatonic schizophrenia, 166
Cathartics, 121
Child abuse, 43–44
Childhood-onset insomnia, 300
Children, 42–44, *see also* Adolescents
  adult disorders in, 6
  antisocial behavior and, 353–354
  Anxiety disorders and, 25–28
  Developmental disorders and, 7–15
  drug treatment in, 4–6
  Eating disorders in, 29–32
  Elimination disorders and, 38–40
  Factitious disorders and, 312
  firesetting and, 318–319
  Gender identity disorders, 33–35
  Multiple personality disorder and, 267
  parent-child problem, 355
  of a psychotic "primary," 203
Chloral hydrate, 5
Chlordiazepoxide, 114
Chlormethiazole, 299
Chloroquine, 68
Chlorpromazine, 301
  Bipolar disorder and, 204
  Schizophrenia and, 164–165, 172, 175, 178–179
Clomipramine, 246, 251–252
Clonazepam, 247, 305
Clonidine, 90, 247, 304
  Nicotine dependence and, 144
  Opioid withdrawal and, 118–119
  Tourette's disorder and, 36–37
Cluttering, 41
Cocaine
  abuse/dependence, 142–143
  Deliria and, 68–69
  Delusional disorders and, 96–97
  intoxication, 125
  Organic anxiety disorders and, 101
  withdrawal, 113, 120
Codeine, 68
Cognitive therapy, 31
  Depression and, 240, 242
Cognitive-behavioral approach, 255
  Sexual disorders and, 275
Conduct disorders, 14, 19, 22–23
Consultation-liaison approach, 329–330
Conversion disorder, 261–262
Countertransference, 267, 273, 284, 325, 330, 356

Personality disorders and, 332, 334, 336, 343, 351
Covert sensitization, 280-281
Cross-dressing, 34-35
Cushing's syndrome, 102
Cyclothymia, 213-214
Cyproterone acetate, 279

Dantrolene, 75
Decompensation, 203, 312, 333-334
Dehydration, 115
Delinquents, 22-23, 353-354
Deliria, 59-76
  Amphetamine or similarly acting sympathomimetic, 69
  anticholinegic substances and, 70-71
  associated with Axis III physical disorders, 73-76
  cocaine-induced, 68-69
  complicating dementias of the senium and presenium, 71-72
  Dementia and, 78
  dose-related, 68
  drugs capable of causing, 61-62
  etiologic treatment, 60, 62
  general therapeutic principles, 59-60
  idiosyncratic, 68
  multi-infarct dementia with, 72-73
  patient management, 65-67
  Phencyclidine or similarly acting arylcyclohexylamine, 69-70
  Psychoactive substance-induced, 68
  other psychoactive substances, 70
  symptomatic treatment, 63-65
  withdrawal and, 112-120
Delirium tremens, 114
Delta-sleep-inducing peptide, 299
Delusional (paranoid) disorder, 197-199
Delusions, 96-99
Dementia, 76-87
  arising in the senium and presenium, 83-86
  associated with Axis III physical disorders, 87
  Deliria and, 71-73
  delusions and, 99
  Depression and, 105-106
  etiologic treatment, 76-77
  Multi-infarct, 86
  patient management, 81-82
  Psychoactive substance-induced, 86-87
  symptomatic treatment, 77-81
Dependence syndromes, 133-145
  therapeutic principles, 134-136
Dependent personality disorders, 349

Depersonalization disorder, 270-271
Depot-injected medications, 188-189
Depression, *see also* Antidepressants
  Adjustment disorder and, 324
  Dementia and, 79-80, 105-106
  Dysthymia, 241-244
  in the elderly, 238
  Kleptomania and, 316
  Major, 214-241
    Conduct disorders and, 22
    psychotherapy and, 240-243
  maternal, 24-26
  neurological disorders associated with, 107
  opiate addicts and, 141
  Personality disorder and, 335-337, 345
  post-stroke, 107
  Post-traumatic stress disorder and, 255
  sexual dysfunction and, 285
  sexual masochism and, 281
  sleep and, 238-239
  subclinical hypothyroidism and, 106
Desensitization, 25-26, 248, 250, 252, 258
  Sexual disorders and, 289, 291-294
Desipramine
  Anxiety disorders and, 246
  Attention-deficit hyperactivity disorder, 20
  cocaine and, 143
  Conduct disorders and, 23
  Dementia and, 79
Detoxification, 113-114, 116-120, 134, 136-137, 139, 141
Developmental disorders, 7-15
Dexamethasone suppression test, 174, 217-219
Dexedrine, 20
Dextroamphetamine, 303
Diabetes, 286
Diazepam
  Alcohol withdrawal and, 114-115
  Deliria and, 64-65, 68-70
  Delusional disorders and, 98
  Dementia and, 78
  hallucinations and, 92
  intoxication and, 126-128
  Schizophrenia and, 165-166
Diazoxide, 70
Diclofesine, 226
Diethylpropion, deliria and, 69
Diethylstilbestrol, 283
Diphenhydramine, 5-6, 177
Disruptive behavior disorders, 16-24
Dissociative disorders, 266-272
Disulfiram, 135-136

Diuretics, 207
Divorce, 354
Doctor-patient relationship, 82
Dopamine beta hydroxylase, 23
Doxepin, 79, 141
Dream anxiety disorder, 308
Drug abuse, *see* Substance abuse
Drugs, *see* Psychopharmacology
Dyspareunia, 293
Dysphoria, 202, 282
Dyssomnias, 297–298
Dysthymia, 241–244
Dysthymic disorder, Speech disorders and, 41
Dystonia, 165, 177, 205

Eating disorders, 29–32, 261
Educational setting, 17–18
EEG, 22
Ego-dystonic homosexuality, 294–295
Elective mutism, 42
Electroconvulsive therapy, 80, 166–167, 184, 202
   Bipolar disorder and, 205, 210, 212
   Major depression and, 215–217, 234–237
   Organic mood disorder and, 103–107
   side/adverse effects of, 237
Elimination disorders, 38–40
Encopresis, 10, 13
   primary, 38
   secondary, 39
Enuresis, 10, 13
   Functional, 39–40
Epilepsy, 11
   Amnestic disorders and, 91
   delusions and, 95–96, 99
   Organic anxiety disorders and, 102
   Organic mood disorder and, 103–104
Episodic dyscontrol syndrome, 107
Estrogen, 227
Ethinyl estradiol, 31
Exhibitionism, 275–276
Explosive type personality, 100–111, 107
Exposure therapy, 248, 252, 254, 261
Extrapyramidal symptoms, 164–165, 182, 207

Factitious disorders, 311–313
Fading, 280, 295
Family therapy, 4, 355
   Alcohol abuse and, 137
   Anorexia nervosa and, 30
   Attention-deficit hyperactivity disorder and, 17

   Avoidant disorder and, 27
   Oppositional defiant disorder and, 24
   Organic personality disorder and, 108
Feingold diet, 20
Female sexual arousal disorder, 289–290
Fenfluramine, 12
Fetishism, 276–277
Firesetting, juvenile, 318–319
Flashbacks, 95, 98
Flooding, 248
Fluoxetine, 80, 226, 234, 251–252
Fluphenazine, 164, 173, 188, 211
Folic acid supplements, 210
Frotteurism, 277

Gambling, pathological, 317–318
Ganser's syndrome, 200, 313
Gender identity disorders, 33–35
Generic drugs, *see* Psychopharmacology
Gepirone, 257
Glaucoma, 178, 231
Glucose-naloxone test, 122
Gluten-free diets, 184–185
Glutethimide, 68, 124
Grand mal seizures, 112, 115–116
Graves' disease, 207
Grief, 323, 356
Group therapy
   Adjustment disorders and, 322
   opioid addicts and, 140
   Personality disorders and, 344, 348
   schizophrenics and, 195
   Sexual disorders and, 276, 280–281, 291
   Somatoform disorders and, 260
   Transsexualism and, 34
Growth retardation, 5
Guided mourning, 323

Hair-pulling, compulsive, 319
Hallucinations, 91–93, 96
Hallucinogen hallucinosis, 93–95
Hallucinogen mood disorder, 104
Hallucinogen abuse/dependence, 142
Haloperidol
   Attention-deficit hyperactivity disorder and, 20
   Atypical psychosis and, 203
   Bipolar disorders and, 211
   Deliria and, 63–65, 69–72
   Delusional disorders and, 98
   Dementia and, 81, 85
   Hypochondriasis and, 261
   Intoxication and, 125, 126

Mental retardation and, 10–11
Organic mood disorder and, 105
Personality disorders and, 334, 344
Schizophrenia and, 164–165, 173–174, 176, 188–189
Stereotypy/habit disorder and, 43
Tic disorders and, 36–37
Hemodialysis, 185
Heroin, 118–120, 124, 138–139
Histrionic personality disorder, 346–347
HIV, 141
Homosexual orientation, 33
Homosexuals, 287, 294–295
Hydrazine, 70
Hydroxyzine, 65, 257
Hyperactivity, 6. *See also* Attention-deficit hyperactivity disorder
Hypercortisolism, 102, 106–107
Hypersexuality, 110
Hypersomnia disorders, 301–308
Hypertension, 69–70, 86, 330–331
Hyperthermia, 69
Hyperthyroidism, 101
Hypnosis, 267–271, 275, 309, 319, 322, 324
Hypnotics
  abuse/dependence, 141–142
  intoxication, 123–124
  withdrawal, 116–117
Hypoactive sexual desire disorder, 288–289
Hypochondriasis, 259–261
Hypoglycemia, 59, 102, 115
Hypoparathyroidism, 101
Hypotension, 176
Hypothyroidism, 207
Hypothyroidism-induced depression, 106
Hypoxia, 59

Ibuprofen, 207
Identity disorder, 42–43
Imipramine
  Anorexia nervosa and, 29, 31
  Anxiety disorders and, 246–247, 249
  Attention-deficit hyperactivity disorder and, 20
  Avoidant disorder and, 27
  Conduct disorders and, 23
  Dementia and, 79–80
  Enuresis and, 40
  Mental retardation and, 10
  opiate addicts and, 141
  Oppositional defiant disorder and, 24
  Overanxious disorder and, 28
  Separation anxiety disorder and, 25–26
  Sleep disorders and, 309–310
Impulse control disorders, 314–320
Incest, 277, 281
Individual therapy, *see* Psychotherapy
Induced Psychotic Disorder, 202–203
Infants, 42–44
  Rumination disorder and, 32
Inhalants, 127, 143–144
Inhibited female orgasm, 291
Inhibited male orgasm, 292
Insomnia, 77–78, 296–301
  monoamine oxidase inhibitors and, 232
Intermittent explosive disorder, 314–316
Intoxication, 120–129
IQ level, 12
Irradiation, sexual dysfunction after, 286

Kleine-Levine Syndrome, 304
Kleptomania, 316–317

L-dopa, 173
L-tryptophan, *see* Tryptophan
La Posada program, 341
Language and speech disorders, 14
Lead poisoning, 31, 91, 127
Learning disorders, 17, 23
Levo-alpha-acetyl-methadol, 138
Liothyronine, 227
Lithium, 6
  antidepressants and, 227
  Anxiety disorders and, 252, 254
  Attention-deficit hyperactivity disorder and, 20
  Bipolar disorders and, 205–208, 212–214
  Dementia and, 87
  Impulse control disorders and, 315
  Mental retardation and, 11
  Neuroleptic malignant syndrome and, 74
  Organic mood disorder and, 103, 105, 107
  Organic personality syndrome and, 108
  patient instructions for, 208–209
  Personality disorder and, 337, 345
  Schizoaffective disorder and, 202
  Schizophrenia and, 166, 183
  side effects, 206–208
  Sleep disorders and, 304
  Stereotypy/habit disorder and, 44
Liver disorders, 11
Liver toxicity, 178
Lobeline sulfate, 144

Lorazepam
  Alcohol withdrawal and, 114
  Bipolar disorders and, 211
  Deliria and, 64–65, 69, 72, 75
  Delusional disorders and, 98
  Dementia and, 78
  Schizophrenia and, 165–166, 183
LSD, 93
  Organic personality disorder and, 110
Luekotomy, 185

Magnesium sulfate, 115
Male erectile disorder, 290–291
Malingering, 354
Mania, *see* Bipolar disorders, manic
Manic syndromes, 107
Maprotiline, 225, 233
Marital problems, 354–355
Masochism, sexual, 281–282
Masturbatory satiation, 280
MDT, 93
Medications, *see* Psychopharmacology
Medroxyprogesterone acetate, 279
Menstruation-associated hypersomnia, 303–304
Mental retardation, 7–11, 353
Meprobamate, 124, 257
Mescaline, 93
Methadone, 118–120, 124, 138–139, 141
Methadyl acetate, 119
Methaqualone, 124
Methylclonazepam, 257
Methylphenidate, 5
  Attention-deficit hyperactivity disorder and, 19–20
  Autistic disorder and, 13
  Deliria and, 69
  Major depression and, 228
  Personality disorders and, 337
  Sleep disorders and, 303
Metoprolol, 110, 315
Mianserin, 226, 233
Michigan Alcoholism Screening Test, 136
Molindone, 172, 181, 183
Monoamine oxidase inhibitors
  Anxiety disorders and, 246, 257
  Bipolar disorders and, 213
  Dementia and, 80
  Major depression and, 223–224
  Organic mood syndrome and, 103–105
  Personality disorders and, 334, 345
  Schizophrenia and, 190
  side effects of, 231–232
  Sleep disorders and, 302–303

Mood disorders, organic, 103–107
Morphine, 118–119
Motor skills disorders, 14
Multiple personality disorder, 266–268
Multiple Sleep Latency Test, 302
Multivitamins, 20

Naloxone, 118, 124, 139
  Schizophrenia and, 183
  Stereotypy/habit disorder and, 44
Naltrexone, 119, 139
  Stereotypy/habit disorder and, 44
Narcissistic personality disorder, 347–348
Narcolepsy, 302–303
Neuroleptic Malignant Syndrome, 74–76, 182–183
Neuroleptics, *see also* Specific drug names
  Alcohol abuse and, 137
  Alcohol withdrawal and, 114
  Amphetamine withdrawal and, 119–120
  Bipolar disorders and, 205, 208–209, 211
  Brief reactive psychosis and, 200
  Deliria and, 63–64, 70, 74–76
  Delusional (paranoid) disorder and, 197–198
  Delusional disorders and, 96–99
  Dementia and, 78, 80–81, 85
  equivalent doses of, 166
  Hallucinogen hallucinosis and, 94
  Intoxication and, 125
  lithium and, 206
  Mental retardation and, 11
  Organic mood disorder and, 103–107
  Personality disorders and, 333–334, 344–345
  rapid neuroleptization schedule, 163–166, 204
  Schizophrenia and, 172–175
  side and adverse effects of, 175–183
  Sleepwalking disorder and, 309
Nicotine, 120, 144
Nightmare disorder, 308
Nomifensine, 225–226, 233
Noncompliance, 355
Notriptyline, dementia and, 79

Object relations theory, 342
Obsessive compulsive
  disorder, 251–253
  personality disorder, 349–350
  symptoms, 31
Opioid
  abuse/dependence, 138–140
  intoxication, 124–125

withdrawal, 118
Oppositional defiant disorder, 23–24
Organic amnestic syndrome, 88–91
Organic anxiety syndrome, 99–102
Organic delusional syndrome, 96–99
Organic mental disorders
  causes of, 54–55
  definition, 52
  patient management, 53, 55–57
  treatment, 53
Organic Mental Syndrome
  definition, 52
  patient management and, 56–57
Organic mood syndrome, 103–107
Organic personality syndrome, 107–111
Orgasm disorders, 291–293
Overanxious disorder, 27–28
Oxazepam
  Deliria and, 64–65
  Dementia and, 78

Panic disorder, 246–247
Paradoxical intention, 250, 271
Paraldehyde, 65
Paranoid personality disorder, 333
Paranoid psychosis, 185, 193
Paraphilias, 343
Paraphrenia, 197
Parasomnias, 308–310
Parent-child problems, 355
Passive agressive personality disorder, 350–351
Patient noncompliance, 355
Pedophilia, 277–281
Pemoline, 20, 303
Penile plethysmography, 277
Pentobarbital, 117
Performance anxiety, 250
  Male erectile disorder and, 290
Pernicious anemia, 198
Personality disorders, 332–351
Pervasive developmental disorders, 11–14
Phencyclidine
  abuse/dependence, 142
  Deliria and, 68–70
  Delusional disorders and, 96–98
Phenelzine, 246, 252
Phenmetrazine, 303
Phenobarbital, 116–117, 120, 124
Phenothiazines, 172, 178–179, 193
  Anorexia nervosa and, 31
  Autistic disorder and, 13
  Mental retardation and, 11
  Overanxious disorder and, 28

Posthallucinogen perception disorder and, 95
Phenycyclidine
  intoxication, 126
  mood disorder and, 104
Phenylalanine, 227
Phenytoin, 110, 114–115
  Impulse control disorders and, 315
Pheochromocytoma, 102
Phobias, see Anxiety disorders
Physical condition, psychological factors affecting, 328–331
Physostigmine, 84, 176
  Amnestic disorders and, 89
  Deliria and, 63, 70
  intoxication and, 122, 128
Pica, 31–32
  Mental retardation and, 8
Pimozide, 188
  Tourette's disorder and, 36
Pipothiazine, 190
Piracetam, 85
Placebo effects, 4
Play therapy, 8, 10
Polysomnograms, 217
Post-traumatic stress disorder, 253–255, 266
  Sleep disorders and, 308
Postanesthetic malignant hyperthermia, 74
Posthallucinogen perception disorder, 95
Power struggle, 39
Pregnancy, 208, 231
Premature ejaculation, 292–293
Primary hypersomnia, 306
Primary insomnia, 301
Probationed Offender's Rehabilitation and his Treatment Program, 338
Prolactin, 175, 177, 219
Promazine, 177
Propranolol, 69
  Amnestic disorders and, 90
  Anxiety disorders and, 247, 250
  Impulse control disorders, 315
  Mental retardation and, 11
  Nicotine dependence and, 144
  Organic anxiety disorders and, 100
  Organic personality syndrome and, 108, 110
  Schizophrenia and, 172
  Sleep disorders and, 303
Protriptyline, 306
Pseudo-depressive, 107
Pseudodementia, 76
Pseudoparkinsonism, 176–177

Pseudopsychopathic, 107, 110
Psychogenic amnesia, 269-270
Psychogenic fugue, 269
Psychopharmacology. *See also* Specific names of drugs
  drug-drug interactions, 383-388
  in early hospitalization, 172-175
  fixed-dose combinations, 174
  generic and trade names of medications, 389-391
Psychosis
  Amphetamine intoxication and, 125
  Childhood, mental retardation and, 8-9
  Dementia and, 80-81
Psychosomatic disorders, 330-331
Psychotherapy
  Adjustment disorders and, 323, 326
  Anorexia nervosa and, 30-31
  Anxiety disorders and, 245, 251-254, 257-258
  anxiety states and, 28
  Attention-deficit hyperactivity disorder and, 21
  Avoidant disorder and, 27
  Delusional (paranoid) disorder and, 198-199
  Dissociative disorders and, 266-271
  Factitious disorders and, 312
  Identity disorder and, 43
  Impulse control disorders and, 315-316, 318
  Major depression and, 240-243
  opiate addicts and, 140-141
  Personality disorders and, 332, 334-336, 342-345, 347, 349-351
  psychosomatic disorders and, 330
  Schizophrenia and, 194-195
  Sexual disorders and, 274-276, 278-279, 282-283, 287-288, 293, 295
  Somatoform disorders and, 260, 262-263, 265
Psychotic disorders, not elsewhere classified, 200-203
Psychotropic medications, use with children, 4-6
Pyloric stenosis, 32
Pyromania, 318

Rabbit syndrome, 177
Reactive attachment disorder, 43
Relaxation therapy, 258, 263, 319, 322, 324, 331
Remoxipride, 172
Reserpine, 190

Resistance, 21
Restless leg syndrome, 304
Restraint, 268
Rumination disorder, 32

Schizoaffective disorder, 201-202
Schizoid personality disorder, 333-334
Schizophrenia, 163-196
  acute exacerbation, 163-167
  Alcohol halucinosis and, 92
  brief hospital treatment, 168-175
  in children, 6
  chronic, 187-194
    community resources for, 190-191
    hospital/residential settings for, 191-192
    prognosis, 192-194
    tardive dyskinesia and, 195-196
  outcome and prognosis, 185-186
  psychotherapy and, 194-195
  residual, 196
  treatment setting, 166-167
Schizophreniform disorder, 187, 201
Schizophreniform psychosis, conservative treatment of, 167-168
Schizotypal personality disorder, 334-335
School phobia, 25
Sedatives
  abuse/dependence, 141-142
  intoxication, 123-124
  withdrawal, 116-117
Seizures, 177-178
Self-destructive behavior, 11, 43, 127
Self-esteem, 14
  Attention-deficit hyperactivity disorder and, 16-17
  Oppositional defiant disorder and, 24
Self-mutilating behavior, 13, 312
Sensate focus exercises, 289-291
Separation anxiety disorder, 25-27
Sex therapy, 284-285, 287-291
Sexual disorders, 273-295
  arousal disorders, 289-291
  aversion disorder, 288-289
  desire disorders, 288-289
  dysfunctions, 284-288
  masochism, 281-282
  pain disorders, 293-294
  paraphilias, 273-284
  sadism, 282
Sleep
  Depression and, 238-239
  hygiene, 297
  variations of normal, 296
Sleep apnea, 305-306

Subject Index 413

Sleep disorders, 296-310
Sleep myoclonus, 304-305
Sleep restriction therapy, 298, 301
Sleep terror disorder, 308-309
Sleep-wake schedule disorder, 306-307
Sleepwalking disorder, 309
Social phobia, 249-250
Somatization disorder, 262-264
Somatoform disorders, 259-265
    Sexual pain disorders and, 293
Somatoform pain disorder, 264-265
Specific developmental disorders, 14-15
Speech disorders, not elsewhere classified, 41
Splitting, 43
Stereotypy/habit disorder, 43-44
    Mental retardation and, 8-9
Steroids, 105
Stress, 321
Stroke, 107
Strychnine, 93
Stuttering, 41
Suanzaorentang, 258
Substance abuse, 4, 133-145. *See also* Alcohol and Specific drug names
    Anxiety disorders and, 101
    Deliria and, 68-69
    Dementia and, 87
    Organic delusional syndrome and, 96-99
    Organic hallucinations and, 91-95
    Organic mood disorders and, 104
    Organic personality disorder and, 110
    patient management and, 57
    Personality disorders and, 343
    Post-traumatic stress disorder and, 255
    therapeutic principles, 134-136
Suicide, 22, 60, 66-68, 97, 104, 312
    Adjustment disorder and, 324
    Bipolar disorders and, 212
    intoxication and, 123, 125
    Major depression and, 214-215, 220
    pedophilic activity and, 278
    Schizoaffective disorder and, 202
    Schizophrenia and, 186-187
    withdrawal and, 113, 119
Surgery, 329
    sexual dysfunctioning and, 286
Sympathomimetic, *see* Amphetamines

Talk-down method, 94, 123, 126
Tardive dyskinesia, 11, 165, 180-182, 195-196
    Bipolar disorders and, 208, 211
Tardive dystonia, 179
Tardive-dyskinesia-like syndromes, 5
Temazepam, 305
Tetracyclics, 224-225
Tetrahydroaminoacridine, 84-85
Tetrahydrocannabinol, 93
Therapeutic communities, 139-140
Therapeutic plasma levels, 221-223
Therapeutic windows, 221
Thiamine, 73-74, 86, 88-89, 91, 115
Thioridazine, 177, 177-178
    Attention-deficit hyperactivity disorder and, 20
    Dementia and, 78
    Mental retardation and, 10-11
Thiothixene, 164, 334, 344
Thioxanthene, 172
Thyrotropin-releasing hormone, 190
Tic disorders, 36-37
Tourette's disorders, 36-37
Trade names, *see* Psychopharmacology
Transference, 342, 344, 346-347
Transient global amnesia, 90-91
Transient ischemic attacks, 71-73
Transsexualism, 34-35
Transvestic fetishism, 282-283
Trazodone, 225, 232-233, 243, 251-252, 286
TRH stimulation test, 217-219
Trichotillomania, 319
Tricyclic antidepressants, *see* Antidepressants
Tryptophan, 77, 227, 252
    Sleep disorders and, 299-301, 306
Tyramine, 223, 232
Tyrosine, 227

V codes, 44, 352-356
Vaginismus, 293-294
Valproic acid amide, 226
Vasodilators, 73
Vasopressin, 190
Verapamil, 172, 211
Violent behavior, 108-109, 126
Vitamin B-12, 198
Voyeurism, 283

Wernicke's Syndrome, 73-74, 88-90
Wilderness program, 338-339, 353
Withdrawal adjustment disorder, 326

Withdrawal and withdrawal deliria, 112–120
   alcohol, 114–115, 120
   amphetamines and, 119–120
   opioid, 118–119
   sedative, hypnotic, anxiolytic, 116–117

Work inhibition, 326

Zometapine, 226